Health Counseling
Application and Theory

Joseph Donnelly, Ph.D.
Program of Health Professions
Montclair State University

D1317029

Joan D. Atwood, Ph.D.
Director, Graduate Programs in Marriage
and Family Therapy
Hofstra University

Isabel Burk, M.S., C.P.P., C.H.E.S.
Director, The Health Network
New City, New York

Jon Carlson, Psy.D., Ed.D.
Division of Psychology and Counseling
Governors State University

Michele M. Fisher, D.P.E.
Graduate Program in Physical Education
Montclair State University

Eva S. Goldfarb, Ph.D.
Program of Health Professions
Montclair State University

Jerrold S. Greenberg, Ph.D.
Department of Public and Community Health
University of Maryland

Arden Greenspan-Goldberg,
M.S.W., A.C.S.W., B.C.D.
Clinician in private practice
New City, New York

Luis Montesinos, Ph.D.
Department of Psychology
Montclair State University

Gloria Pierce, Ph.D.
Department of Counseling, Human
Development and Educational Leadership
Montclair State University

Elizabeth Schroeder, M.S.W.
Independent Professional Trainer/Consultant

Len Sperry, M.D., Ph.D.
Professor and Coordinator of Doctoral Program in Counseling
Barry University
Clinical Professor of Psychiatry and Preventive Medicine
Medical College of Wisconsin

Shahla Wunderlich, Ph.D., R.D.
Department of Human Ecology
Montclair State University

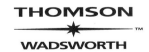

THOMSON
WADSWORTH

Australia • Canada • Mexico • Singapore • Spain
United Kingdom • United States

THOMSON
™
WADSWORTH

Publisher: Peter Marshall
Acquisitions Editor: April Lemons
Assistant Editor: Andrea Kesterke
Technology Project Manager: Star MacKenzie
Marketing Manager: Jennifer Somerville
Marketing Assistant: Mona Weltmer
Advertising Project Manager: Shemika Britt
Project Manager, Editorial Production: Sandra Craig
Print/Media Buyer: Judy Inouye
Permissions Editor: Elizabeth Zuber
Photo Research: Image Quest
Production, Design, Copy Edit, Illustration, Composition:
  Thompson Steele, Inc.
Cover Design: Roger Knox
Printer: Transcontinental Printing

Printed in Canada
1 2 3 4 5 6 7   06 05 04 03 02

For more information about our products, contact us at:
Thomson Learning Academic Resource Center
1-800-423-0563
For permission to use material from this text, contact us by:
Phone: 1-800-730-2214
Fax: 1-800-730-2215
Web: http://www.thomsonrights.com

Library of Congress Control Number: 2002113909
ISBN 0-534-60264-9

Wadsworth/Thomson Learning
10 Davis Drive
Belmont, CA 94002-3098
USA

Asia
Thomson Learning
5 Shenton Way #01-01
UIC Building
Singapore 068808

Australia/New Zealand
Thomson Learning
102 Dodds Street
Southbank, Victoria 3006
Australia

Canada
Nelson
1120 Birchmount Road
Toronto, Ontario M1K 5G4
Canada

Europe/Middle East/Africa
Thomson Learning
High Holborn House
50/51 Bedford Row
London WC1R 4LR
United Kingdom

Latin America
Thomson Learning
Seneca, 53
Colonia Polanco
11560 Mexico D.F.
Mexico

Spain/Portugal
Paraninfo
Calle/Magallanes, 25
28015 Madrid, Spain

Brief Contents

Contents

Foreword

Health Counseling: Application and Theory

It is not often one has the opportunity to review a text that has the potential to influence an entire profession, yet this is what *Health Counseling: Application and Theory* could do. Dr. Joseph Donnelly and the 12 contributing authors have developed a definitive work that should become a central part of the library not only of health educators, but of all those engaged in the health-related professions.

The approach and format of the text allows for ample coverage of the diversity of issues that constitute health counseling. It is a fresh and vibrant introduction to the current practice and scope of this relatively new profession. Students and professionals will benefit from the clear and comprehensive treatment of such challenging topics as sexuality, addiction, and relationships. Each chapter adds its own contribution to the richness of tools and knowledge that are essential for any health counselor or professional in today's complex health environments. Through the relative case studies in most chapters, this text goes above and beyond theory into pragmatic application in real-life situations a health counselor is likely to encounter.

Len Sperry and Jon Carlson set the tone for the text by explaining exactly what health counseling entails. They point out the difficulty of coming to a consensus as to a profession-wide definition of health, and how one defines health as a reflection of his or her philosophy in terms of practicing the health-education and health-counseling profession. They set forth, in clear fashion, the basic tenets of health counseling, and specify basic assumptions inherent within these tenets. In describing the various types of health counseling that may occur, Sperry and Carlson demonstrate the importance of knowing these types of counseling, and the settings in which health counseling is practiced. Regardless of the setting, they explain the importance of the counselor/client relationship, and return to the basic philosophy of Carl Rogers in developing a strong and trusting relationship between the counselor and client. They present and describe the stages of psychotherapy-based health counseling, and clearly explain each of the phases in language that is easily understood by those who are not in the psychotherapy profession. It is clear that maintenance of behavior change is the end goal of these processes. The chapter ends with a well-developed case study, in which the theoretic underpinnings discussed throughout the chapter are applied so the reader can see "theory in action."

Elizabeth Schroeder has done an excellent job in explaining the roots and history of the health-counseling movement. She expands on the basic information presented by Sperry and Carlson, and specifies not only what health counseling is, but also what it is not. She then explains how Hoffman and Driscoll's Concentric Biopsychosocial Model of Health Status can work in health counseling. This is a model that puts equal emphasis on the interaction of biological, psychological, and sociological factors that shape human behavior, and the importance of addressing all these issues in the counseling situation. She illustrates each part of the model with examples that clarify the points being made within the text. Schroeder describes several basic counseling skills, and the various defense mechanisms clients may use as each of these skills is manifest. She also explains how each of the defense mechanisms may be addressed and, in fact, turned into a therapeutic event. Schroeder clearly sets forth the concept of "boundaries" in terms of counselor–client disclosure, in both individual and group settings, and presents in a clear and forthright fashion a process for ensuring psychological ease for clients in individual and group settings.

The text then turns to the concept of ethics in health counseling where Jerrold Greenberg sets forth basic concepts of ethical processes for the health-counseling setting. Drawing upon the Code of Ethics for the Health-Education Profession, Greenberg describes the differences between ethics, morality, ethical principles, ethical dilemma, and values, and explains the difference between rule ethics and situational ethics. Using specific examples within each of these facets, Greenberg clearly demonstrates the importance of tempering absolutes with situations, when approaching a counseling situation. He describes four basic ethical theories, and how those theories mesh with the principles of proportionality and self-determination. The chapter concludes with seven ethical issues that health counselors may encounter. Rather than specify how to deal with each issue, Greenberg provides basic information so the reader can determine how he or she would respond to the situation.

Luis Montesinos further extends what has been presented in the first three chapters of the text and provides a compelling rationale for those in the health-related professions becoming involved in behavior change. He sets forth basic principles of behavior change, and applies basic techniques of behavioral analysis and therapy to that rationale. Montesinos explains how those involved in health counseling can help clients through a process of goal setting, and how behavioral strategies can be mutually developed by the counselor and client so the client's goals are reached. He provides a "painless" way of motivating clients, so the changes that are undertaken are internalized and have a greater chance of becoming the new "rule of behavior" for the client.

Building upon the work of Montesinos, Michele Fisher and Shahla Wunderlich provide a transition from the internal motivation to the physical benefits of changing behavior. Concentrating on the basic benefits of physical activity as a health-enhancing strategy, Fisher and Wunderlich describe the most recent recommendations for physical activity that have been developed by the U.S. Centers for Disease Control and Prevention, and the American College of Sports Medicine and point out some of the disparities that exist in terms of the amount of physical activity that should be undertaken in order for health benefits to accrue. They distinguish between the benefits that can be gained by moderate versus vigorous physical activity, and provide the reader with objective evidence upon which to base personal decisions in the physical-activity arena, and to develop a personal physical-activity plan designed to meet personal goals.

Arden Greenspan-Goldberg and Isabel Burk move the reader into the realm of addictive behaviors, and how to deal with those behaviors. Concentrating on substance abuse and eating disorders, she describes in detail the impact of these behaviors on the individual, family, and community. Using the Transtheoretical Model of Behavior Change, the authors explain how the counselor can identify what stage a client is in, and how that knowledge can be used as a basis for effecting behavior change. Rather than concentrating on health-damaging behaviors, Greenspan-Goldberg and Burk prefer to call these behaviors "health-compromising behaviors." This small terminology shift tends to put clients at ease, and become more receptive to the possibility that there are other behaviors that are less health compromising and that can become health enhancing behaviors. Several realistic case studies are presented, and the chapter concludes with one of the newest of the addictions, that of Internet addiction.

Joan D. Atwood expands the theory presented in the preceding chapter to the realm of healthy relationships. Although the focus is on the development of healthy one-to-one relationships, the principles presented can be applied to the development of healthy relationships across a wide spectrum of activities. She takes the reader through case studies wherein the basic principles of how to avoid relationship traps and pitfalls, are clearly evidenced, and processes to avoid these traps and pitfalls are explored. She explains how each of the traps and pitfalls can severely damage any relationship, and the reader can explore how avoidance of these issues can enhance relationships. Atwood concludes with a well-developed section wherein she presents the traits of health relationships. The reader is left with a basic set of traits that can enhance any relationship into which he or she may enter. Perhaps the key to all of this is that unless the individual feels comfortable with him or herself and his or her life, it will be most difficult to be involved in healthy relationships with others. Perhaps the adage of "cleaning one's own house first" is paramount.

In this chapter, Eva S. Goldfarb sets forth the concept that we are all sexual beings in one form or another. She distinguishes clearly between sexuality education and sexuality counseling, and explains the importance of understanding these distinctions. Goldfarb explains the characteristics of an effective sexuality counselor, and applies them to situations wherein individuals would seek sexuality counseling. She explains within the sexuality-counseling setting, the issues of sexual orientation, unintended pregnancy, encountering sexually transmissible infections, sexual dysfunction and sexual assault and abuse. Throughout each of these issues, case studies are presented and the theories of effective counseling are incorporated into the discussion of the case. The reader is challenged to consider what he or she would do, given similar circumstances. What is quite interesting about this chapter is that the information contained within it can be used as a personal reference point, so that the reader can make a determination related to identifying and resolving personal sexual issues he or she may face.

All people age, and as we age, we face numerous issues from decreased vitality and lessened income, to reliance upon others for meeting basic needs. Luis Montesinos again presents a cogent discussion of numerous issues that aging individuals must face, and how the health counselor can assist individuals deal with the process and effects of aging. He presents and describes basic theories of aging, and explores some of the myths and realities of aging. He clearly elaborates the basic theories of counseling as applied to these issues of aging, particularly in helping individuals "age successfully." Montesinos concludes by explaining, in easy-to-understand fashion, how the health counselor can best serve elderly clients, or even those clients who have issues they fear that are associated with aging.

In general, when one thinks of health counseling, issues associated with mental health arise. Joseph Donnelly approaches the concept of mental-health counseling from an historical perspective, and puts these concepts into an historical context so the reader understands the evolution of the profession of mental-health counseling. He sets forth a cogent definition of comprehensive health that includes five basic components of holistic health: physical, mental, social, spiritual and emotional. Donnelly explains the basic concept of psychoneuromunology, and why knowledge of this concept is important for the health counselor. He includes case studies that involve application of basic counseling concepts. The chapter moves toward an integrative nature of counseling that provides the reader with insight as to how and when to intervene, and the importance of understanding holistic mental health for the mental-health counselor.

Greenberg contributes yet another chapter to the text, only this time his focus is on stress and health counseling. Drawing upon basic tenets of stress-related theory, Greenberg clearly distinguishes between positive and negative stressors and how they both can affect one's health. He sets forth a model of stress and how intervention can affect that model, thus helping the client, or the reader, develop a realistic process for dealing with a wide range of stressors. Central to this chapter is the concept of cognitive restructuring, helping the individual control the way a stressor is perceived, thus making it less stressful. In case studies the reader is challenged to apply counseling processes to the cases being presented. Each of the skills being discussed can be applied to the individual's personal situation, thus allowing the individual to become his or her own health counselor. A series of stress-reduction techniques are presented, and the reader is advised to try these techniques not only as a means of counseling others, but also as a means of dealing with personal stressors.

Gloria Pierce draws a lot of the preceding chapter's theory together when presenting the concept of "Ecopsychology." This concept is defined as a holistic framework necessary to help people learn and develop positive, health-enhancing attitudes and behaviors. It is a process which, if understood, helps the individual see that all facets of life are interactive and can affect all other aspects of life. The theoretic basis for Ecopsychology is presented as an amalgamation of several prominent counseling theories. Central to this is the understanding of how individuals represent a microcosm that has to interact in a macrocosm of life. A discussion of the egocentric versus the ecocentric self underscores how people affect and are affected by the environment in which they live. A critical part of this understanding is to raise the consciousness of the individual so he or she sees this interaction and the effects of this interaction on oneself and on others. Once the effects of these interactions are understood, the individual becomes more aware of what he or she can do to help him or herself, as well as others, thus causing a positive result for everyone, including the environment in which individuals live, work, and play.

The text concludes with a compelling chapter written by Donnelly, who amalgamates all the theories presented within the text, and shows how modern technology can be used to enhance what we now know about individual and group behav-

ior. The Internet has provided many information-thirsty people with access to information heretofore not readily available, thus making it imperative for the health counselor to also be facile with the uses and ethics of technology. Donnelly discusses the ethics of conducting health counseling online and the legal issue of whether or not the individual's liability insurance covers "distance counseling." Clearly, the Internet makes counseling available to a broader range of clientele, but the ethics and legal requirements of client confidentiality must be safeguarded. It is important to understand that although the Internet is a wonderful tool, it does not replace the importance of in-person therapy. The counselor must make a decision as to whether or not the client would benefit from distance counseling, or if the more traditional methods are more likely to produce positive results.

Health Counseling: Application and Theory is a succinct text that contains a wealth of information provided by experts in a wide range of health and counseling techniques. The reader is challenged throughout the text to apply both health knowledge and counseling techniques to the many cogent case studies that are included in the various chapters. This is a textbook that can benefit anyone who reads it, from the novice to the experienced health worker. It is a book that provides theoretic underpinnings for the practical application of health-counseling techniques in a variety of practice settings.

Larry K. Olsen, Dr.P.H., C.H.E.S.
Associate Dean for Academics and Research
College of Health and Social Services
New Mexico State University
April 2002

Preface

Students preparing to enter the health education field increasingly need to know the ins and outs of counseling students who approach them with sensitive topics ranging from experimentation with alcohol and other drugs, to emotional difficulties, to a variety of sexual concerns and issues. It is also necessary for today's health educators to be able to connect with students in informal, sometimes impromptu, settings. The ways that health education and counseling are being practiced have been changing and evolving over the last 10 years. This text answers the need for an up-to-date source of information for students preparing to enter the fields of health education and/or counseling. Health counseling, as a distinct field, is necessarily bi-disciplinary in that it encompasses and infuses material from the fields of health education and counseling as they are practiced today. The approach of this text has been to consult the advice of experts who specialize in particular areas and to synthesize their contributions into a compendium of health-counseling concerns and applications.

The last textbook on health counseling was published by Judith Lewis, Jon Carlson, and Len Sperry in 1993 (*Health Counseling*. CA: Brooks/ Cole). It seemed appropriate and fortuitous, then, to have this text's first chapter, "What Is Health Counseling?", coauthored by two of the authors of that groundbreaking text (Sperry and Carlson). Subsequent chapters address specific subject areas such as addiction, exercise and weight management, relationships, sexuality, and stress manage-

ment. In these areas and others a health educator will often find him or herself in the counseling role. Very few health educators are given a broad overview of counseling skills they can use in responding to student issues both effectively and responsibly. Health educators need *specific examples* of applications of counseling for topics they are likely to encounter. This text's eclectic approach is its strength, since who better to guide health counselors in navigating specific areas than the professionals who have been immersed in those areas of practice for years?

While most colleges and universities require health counseling as a course for health educators, professors often find themselves at a loss for an adequate text. The need for a current text that infuses a whole decade of emerging trends and practices has been the driving force behind this project. Through conversations with several professors who instruct health counseling and countless students, the most popular and requested topics soon emerged and became the chapters of this text. As many aspects of health education and counseling overlap and encompass a wide range of concerns, it appeared unreasonable to have a health counseling textbook written by only one author. The contributing authors of the respective chapters of this text are professionals with a wealth of knowledge in the fields of counseling, health education, psychology, social work, and other related disciplines. Many chapters are extremely contemporary in scope, featuring cutting-edge topics that would not be found in a health counseling text of

10 years ago, such as counseling using new technologies, Ecotherapy, and Internet addiction.

This text aims to be highly accessible to students through its use of numerous case studies, vignettes, and examples of how health educators can connect with students in informal and nontraditional settings. Most importantly, the format provides students an opportunity to "apply" the material from this text to real-life situations. Five critical thinking/discussion questions are provided at the end of each chapter, along with related Web Sites for a student's further inquiry into Web resources and latest developments. Additionally, the text is accompanied by an instructor's manual of user-friendly lesson plans within each of the 12 chapters, and a test bank of proposed questions and answers by the author of each respective chapter.

It is my hope as author/editor of this text that it will help future health educators to connect with their students and mentor them through the sensitive areas and questions that will inevitably arise in the course of a career as health educator. And likewise, it is my hope that students of counseling will benefit from the health content and information offered in this text, as well as from the unification of the two disciplines as they are presented within these pages, as the diverse but unified whole that is health counseling.

This project would not have been possible were it not for my initial introduction to Wadsworth/Thomson Publishing through one of the sales representatives. In February 2001, this proposal idea for a health counseling textbook was received with great interest, and a meeting of myself and Wadsworth health publisher, Peter Marshall, was arranged. Peter saw the need for such a text and embraced the idea, providing me solid recommendations and great guidance throughout the entire project. My gratitude is heartily extended to Peter for his tremendous support in bringing about this text. April Lemons, health editor at Wadsworth, has continually kept the project on track and been enormously sup-

portive, with the outcome of making the text the very best it could be. I extend my gratitude to April Lemons, and to all at Wadsworth Publishing who accepted this project and made it possible.

Many thanks to Dr. Larry Olsen of New Mexico State University, who spent countless hours reviewing the text and writing the Foreword. Special thanks to Dr. Don Read who provided tremendous insight and support throughout the years in discussing the possibility and importance of this health counseling text.

I would like to express my personal thanks to each of the contributing authors who diligently prepared and revised these chapters. What has made this project so enjoyable and successful is the fact that I have worked these past 12 months with many associates and friends who truly supported this endeavor. This project has been a collective effort, made possible through the work of dedicated individuals. I thank the following contributing authors for their personal expertise and countless hours preparing their respective chapters: Len Sperry, M.D., Ph.D., Barry University; Jon Carlson, Psy.D, Ed.D., Governor's State University; Elizabeth Schroeder, M.S.W., Independent Professional Trainer/Consultant; Jerrold S. Greenberg, Ph.D., University of Maryland; Luis Montesinos, Ph.D., Montclair State University; Michele Fisher, D.P.E., Montclair State University; Shahla Wunderlich, Ph.D., R.D., Montclair State University; Arden Greenspan-Goldberg, M.S.W., A.C.S.W., B.C.D., Psychotherapy/Psychoanalyst/Private Practice; Isabel Burk, M.S., CPP, CHES, The Health Network; Joan Atwood, Ph.D., Hofstra University; Eva S. Goldfarb, Ph.D., Montclair State University; Gloria Pierce, Ph.D., Montclair State University. In addition, I would like to thank not only the contributing authors, but their respective institutions for providing necessary time to complete this project. It is with gratitude that I extend my appreciation to these authors and their families who have endured throughout this time-consumptive process. Also, I would like to thank my wife, Maryann, who has inspired and supported me throughout this process and has been willing to listen to countless ideas regarding the culmination of this health-counseling text. Many thanks.

It is with gratitude that I extend my deepest appreciation to Jennifer Ferraro who has provided tremendous editorial assistance, guidance, and support throughout this process. Jennifer has kept me on track and assisted in the transition process, which is essential in editing any text. Also, I would like to express my appreciation to Lisa Mathern who has provided tremendous assistance in the day-to-day tasks, which are essential to the success of any project.

Many thanks to the countless friends who have provided me insight and support throughout the writing of this text. The insights they have provided have been invaluable, along with their willingness to listen to the development of ideas at every step of the way.

Finally, I would like to thank the reviewers, who provided me with quality feedback and guidance:

Mary Jo Belenski
Montclair State University

Angela R. Burroughts
University of North Carolina at Chapel Hill

Jerry Carden
University of Illinois

Ellen Glascock
St. Francis College

Mark J. Kittleson
Southern Illinois University, at Carbondale

Simon Ogamdi
Florida Atlantic University

Kathleen Poole
Virginia Polytechnic Institute and
    State University

Patricia Richel
Montclair State University

Bill Roe
Phoenix College

John J. Zarski
University of Akron

Joseph Donnelly, Ph.D.

CHAPTER 1

What Is Health Counseling?

LEN SPERRY, M.D., PH.D. AND
JON CARLSON, PSY.D., ED.D.

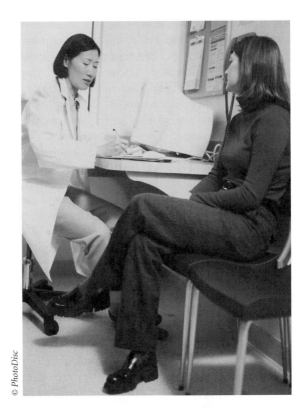

© PhotoDisc

OBJECTIVES

By the end of the chapter, the reader should be able to:

- Define health, health promotion, and health counseling

- Indicate two reasons why the need for health counseling has significantly increased

- Distinguish five types of health counseling

- Describe the curative elements of health counseling

- Describe the stages of health counseling

Case Study

Tina was a young woman who dreaded going to the women's clinic for any reason. She felt very uncomfortable and hated feeling like a number in the waiting room, and then having to be so vulnerable in front of a stranger during the exam. She put off going but this time she really needed to have something checked out for her own peace of mind. Something different happened this time when she got to the clinic. Another young woman, not much older than herself, came in to the small room where she was sent to wait for the nurse-practitioner. This woman was very friendly and asked Tina some questions about her health habits and history. The woman did not seem like a nurse and chatted amiably. She seemed very concerned that Tina feel comfortable. Tina was taken aback at first by the

1

sudden interest in her as a person. She felt a little mistrusting. Then she was called in for her checkup. Afterward, the woman came again and sat with her. She wanted to know if Tina had any questions and offered helpful information about birth control, exercise, and other topics, referring to Tina's health questionnaire. Tina found herself asking questions about things she never would have asked the doctor or nurse. They seemed too busy and besides, some things were too intimate to talk to a stranger about. She tried to politely ask the other woman what her role was, and felt silly even as she asked. "I'm a health counselor," the woman told her. If only this woman had been here at other times, when she could have really used some guidance and personal attention! Tina decided that this human touch made clinic visits much more pleasant. She would not dread coming next time.

The example above highlights some of the valuable functions that health counselors can have in the medical setting. This is just one context in which health counselors are used to great benefit. More and more often, people are asking for assistance in trying to achieve healthier lifestyles or adapt to changes in their physical, psychological, and emotional well-being. Health counseling is a process of helping people make these lifestyle changes. This chapter begins with a discussion of health, health promotion, and health counseling, and then describes some reasons why the field of health counseling has developed rapidly. It then describes four types of health counseling, followed by a discussion of some of the major theoretical and clinical contributions to health counseling from the fields of psychotherapy and counseling. Finally, the chapter integrates the preceding discussions of the scope and basis of health counseling by providing an extended case example that illustrates how one form of health counseling is actually practiced.

Defining Health and Health Counseling

Health

Since this text is about health, it may be useful to begin our discussion by defining health. There are a number of ways in which **health** is defined. Ask three individuals and you are likely to hear three different definitions. For example, one person might define health as "not feeling sick." However, that seems to be a rather limited definition since an individual can feel perfectly healthy and be harboring a serious or even potentially fatal condition such as cancer or HIV, the virus that causes AIDS. Another person may say health is the absence of symptoms and signs of disease. Again, a person can be asymptomatic (without symptoms) and have any number of serious diseases.

The World Health Organization (WHO) defined health over 50 years ago as "a state of complete physical, mental, and social well-being and not merely the absence of disease or infirmity" (World Health Organization, 1948, p. 1). This rather idealistic definition represents a vision that relatively few individuals, much less nations, have attained. However, it is a much more inclusive definition, made more so if it were to add the spiritual dimension. The spiritual dimension provides "important overlapping and interrelationship between spirituality and the other dimensions of human health" (Donnelly et. al., 2001, p. 178). It may be useful, therefore, to think of the definitions of health as spanning a continuum from "absence of symptoms" on one end to "complete, optimal well-being" on the other.

The way health is viewed and defined is more than a matter of semantics. Definitions are important because the way health is viewed has a direct bearing on the type and extent of health care that will be authorized and provided. For example, when health is viewed as the absence of the symptoms of disease, "disease management" will be provided. Disease management focuses on symptoms, not on the person exhibiting these symptoms. It is no surprise, therefore, that most health maintenance organizations (HMOs) define

Health. A state of complete physical, mental, and social well-being and not merely the absence of disease or infirmity.

health as the absence of symptoms and will authorize and pay for disease management–oriented treatment but typically will not pay for health promotion or preventative services. However, there are a few more enlightened HMOs that will authorize and pay for some types of prevention and health-promotion services because they recognize that such services are cost-effective because they have the potential to ward off more serious conditions.

Some counseling professions have found ways to compete in the health-care industry. For instance, mental health counseling has fared well in the managed-care era, with increasingly clinical training curricula including psychodiagnosis, psychopathology, psychopharmacology, and treatment planning (Hershenson & Berger, 2001). Health counseling too will establish its place in today's health-care industry.

Health Education and Health Promotion

The terms *health education* and *health promotion* are used with increasing frequency today. There are several ways of describing and defining health education (Glanz et al., 1997). Some definitions emphasize narrowing the gap between what is known about optimal health practice and what is actually practiced, while others focus on replacing detrimental health behaviors with behaviors that are more conducive to health. Still other definitions address the instructional processes and learning experiences necessary to facilitate the adoption of health-producing behaviors. Common to most definitions are instruction, informed behavior change, and the overall goal of health-status improvement. Beyond instructional activities to improve health status, health education can also include organizational, environmental, economic, and policy components. Recently there has been increased attention given to the importance of advocacy in health education. Health advocacy should include not only health-education professionals but also students and the individuals participating in community, medical care, and work-site programs (Tappe & Galer-

Unti, 2001). Health education is defined as "learning experiences that assist individuals in making informed decisions in order to increase their health status" (Sperry et. al., in press 2002). Health education, in a sense, is an umbrella term under which health promotion and other concepts fit.

Health promotion can be defined as "the science and art of helping people change their lifestyle to move toward a state of optimal health." Optimal health is defined by the *American Journal of Health Promotion* (O' Donnell, 1989, p. 3) as "a balance of physical, emotional, social, spiritual, and intellectual health." Physical health refers to such things as nutrition, medical self-care, and control of substance abuse. Emotional health refers to issues such as care for emotional crisis, and stress management. Social health refers to one's communities, families, and friends, while intellectual health refers to one's educational, achievement, and career development. Finally, spiritual health refers to a deep level of well-being that encompasses all these and includes positive feelings of love, hope, and charity.

Health promotion addresses the personal modifiable lifestyle habits and practices that lead to the disease process. According to the U.S. Department of Health and Human Services (U.S. Department of Health and Human Services: Healthy People 2000), nearly one-half of all premature deaths in the United States are caused by lifestyle-related problems. Many of these deaths could be prevented and the quality of life for millions could be enhanced through such lifestyle changes as regular exercise, eating nutritious foods (see Chapter 5), avoiding tobacco and excess alcohol, learning to manage stress, clarifying lifestyle values, achieving a sense of fulfillment in life, and more. Health counseling is a primary means of accomplishing this goal.

Lifestyle change can be facilitated through a combination of efforts to enhance awareness, change behavior, and create environments that support good health practices. Of the three, supportive environments seem to have a significant impact in producing lasting change. Effective health counseling involves all three strategies.

Health Counseling

So what exactly is **health counseling?** Health counseling is a broadly encompassing term that describes various approaches and methods for assisting individuals to reduce or prevent the progression of disease processes as well as to improve health status and functioning. Rather than being a new or separate health-care specialty, health counseling is more an attitude and orientation toward health and well-being. Service delivery professions such as health counseling are distinct for providing a synthesis of themes and emphases, rather than having one exclusive focus (Gelso & Fretz, 2001).

The goal of health counseling is to reduce symptoms and improve health status, to improve lifestyle and positive health behaviors, and to increase adherence to a health prescription. It is assumed that change occurs because the client is sufficiently engaged and collaborates with the tailored intervention process, and because barriers to change—that is, intrapersonal, interpersonal, social and/or cultural—are recognized and dealt with. Any type of health counseling requires that the client's motivation be sufficient before proceeding with the prescribed change effort. Accordingly, the counselor must be proficient in the use of motivational counseling strategies (see Chapter 4) to promote readiness (Miller & Rollnick, 1991). The assessment done in this approach to health counseling is more extensive than in the first two approaches to health education and health promotion and includes an evaluation of personality patterns, motivation, strengths, and barriers—psychological, relational, situational, and cultural—that have or could impede adherence to a change program. Health counseling emphasizes tailored interventions and relapse prevention. Several psychotherapeutic interventions such as reframing and cognitive restructuring, as well as

other systemic strategies, are utilized to reduce barriers to change.

Since health is impacted by social environment, health counseling tends to broaden the scope of the counseling process beyond the individual to include the social system. Interventions are designed to help the client build social support and, if possible, lessen environmental stressors. Furthermore, the aim of health counseling is to build up the individual's ability to engage in self-management. Self-management, in turn, requires a repertoire of health-oriented skills, a belief in one's own ability to address life's challenges, and an environment that encourages positive development.

Rather than imply or contend that health counseling represents a new theory or specialty, we simply suggest that health counseling is essentially an attitude. This "attitude" of health counseling reflects integrative, biopsychosocial, and proactive ways of viewing and working with patients and clients. This holistic and biopsychosocial orientation means that the focus is on the client's health status, interpersonal and social competence, as well as psychological and physical well-being. It is not simply on the psychological and emotional aspects that tend to be the focus of the majority of theories and systems of counseling. The biopsychosocial perspective has been articulated by Engel (1977) and is clearly based on systems thinking; it is called biopsychosocial therapy (Sperry, 1988) when related to treatment issues. In addition to having this holistic perspective, health counseling is proactive, meaning that it not only emphasizes restoration of previous levels of health and well-being or adjustment which is primarily a reactive function, but it also emphasizes prevention and increasing an individual's level of development and functioning.

Health counseling. A form of health education that describes various approaches and methods for assisting individuals to reduce or prevent the progression of disease as well as to improve health status and functioning.

Increasing Interest in Health Counseling

The fields of health education and health counseling have grown and developed dramatically in the past decade. There are several reasons for this phenomenon. This section will describe two of them.

Personal Expectations of Health and Longevity

Unlike previous generations, people today expect to live vibrant lives well into their eighties and nineties. This expectation is largely fueled by the prospects of increased life expectancy through the promise of age-defying supplements, prescribed medications, medical procedures, and particularly by the prospects of alternative medicine and health-promoting practices. This trend has also been impacted by a decrease in deaths from infectious disease and an increase in deaths from chronic conditions. It seems that at least some people have begun to understand, as we stated above, that many of the leading causes of death are lifestyle-related. Accordingly, many are attempting to make lasting lifestyle changes. Others need the help of health educators and counselors in order to do so.

For many people in today's society, health education and health counseling are the keys to living life to the fullest. These individuals do not welcome the later years of life as experienced by their parents. Their parents' generation, and others before them, accepted old age as synonymous with an inevitable array of chronic, degenerative diseases. Today's more health-conscious generation rejects the prospects of 20 or more years of progressively disabling illness and limited quality of life. Their hope is to live full, vibrant lives until shortly before they die. They understand the value of lifestyle change and have been sold on the prospects of defying the aging process. Not surprisingly, they constantly seek opportunities to learn more about increasing their health and well-being. Needless to say, they are prime candidates and consumers of health counseling.

Healthy People 2010

Today, an increasing number of highly educated adults in America are attempting to pursue the dream of life with little or no lifestyle-related disease. At the same time, many other Americans are experiencing unprecedented levels of acute and chronic diseases that *are* lifestyle-related. The fed-eral government has targeted certain acute and chronic illnesses as part of its agenda for promoting the nation's health. **Healthy People 2010** (U.S. Department of Health and Human Services, 2000) represents the third time that the Department of Health and Human Services (HHS) has developed 10-year health objectives for the nation. It reflects the scientific advances that have taken place over the past 20 years in preventive medicine, disease surveillance, vaccine and therapeutic development, and information technology. It specifies 467 objectives in 28 focus areas to achieve two goals: increasing the quality and years of healthy life, and eliminating health disparities among Americans.

Unlike its predecessors, Healthy People 2010 includes a set of Leading Health Indicators that will help researchers and practitioners target and track the success of these actions to improve health. Similar to leading economic indicators that are used to measure the health of the economy, these benchmarks provide a concise means for measuring the health of the nation. Five of the health indicators are lifestyle indicators: *physical activity, overweight and obesity, tobacco use, substance abuse, and responsible sexual behavior.* The other five are health-system indicators: *mental health, injury and violence, environmental quality, immunization,* and *access to health care.* Underlying each of these indicators are the significant influences of income, education, culture, and available support systems.

These indicators are intended to facilitate the development of strategies and action plans and health-promotion and disease-prevention efforts, and to encourage wide participation in improving health in the first decade of the new millennium. It is important to note that most of these indicators are behavioral, rather than medical in nature, and are lifestyle-related. Accordingly, such indicators lend themselves to modification by lifestyle change.

Healthy People 2010. Developed by the U.S. Department of Health and Human Services, a 10-year plan of health objectives for the nation based on two goals—to increase the quality and years of healthy life and to eliminate health disparities.

Healthy People 2010 is designed in such a way that its goals and health indicators can be carefully monitored. Furthermore, it is designed to impact not only health-care practice but also health-care research. Perhaps most significantly, unlike its predecessors, Healthy People 2010 emphasizes the importance of health counseling.

Types of Health Counseling

If it were only a matter of providing patients with health-related information about lifestyle change, the task of health counseling would be relatively simple. Unfortunately, studies of the effectiveness of lifestyle change programs indicate that there is no relationship between a client's knowledge about the need or means for change and a client's subsequent behavior change (Janis, 1983). For this reason, it is essential for health counselors to have sufficient knowledge and skills aimed at proper nutrition, exercise, management of stress, smoking cessation, and control of alcohol intake (Jordan-Marsh et al., 1984). Beyond Jordan-Marsh's recommendations, it is also vital for health counselors to have knowledge of and comfort with a range of sexuality issues throughout the human life span (see Chapter 8). They must also have an understanding of and sensitivity to the many different cultures that make up the United States' diverse population.

Four different approaches to the practice of health counseling will be described in the following sections (Sperry et al., in press 2002). The first approach to health counseling is provided by a physician and/or other clinician in a medical or clinical setting. This is called medical-care counseling. A second approach, offered by health-promotion specialists, provides health counseling information and services in private practice, corporate, or community settings. We refer to this as patient education. A third approach is called health-promotion counseling. A fourth approach is called health-focused psychotherapy.

Medical-Care Counseling

In the medical setting, clinicians typically broach the health matter, ask a few questions, give focused information, and prescribe some behavior change, all within a very short time frame. Usually, patients are given the prescription to change behaviors. For example, clients may be told that they need to lose weight, stop smoking, practice safer sex, or take up exercise. The goal of this type of **medical-care counseling** is to improve health status by implementing the health prescription or recommendation. This approach rests on a key assumption: that change or improvement will occur because the patient has confidence in and believes the providers' expertise and authority. Typically this type of counseling involves some limited advisement as to the need for the change and some general guidelines to follow. Usually there is a minimal degree of monitoring. If the patient is not able to follow this advice, for whatever reason, referral may be made to any of the other types of health counseling described in this chapter.

Patient Education

Patient education encompasses any health-education experience planned by both health-care provider and client to meet the client's specific learning needs, interests, and capabilities (Redman, 2001). It is a process of education and activity based on an intentional exchange and sharing of information that results in a positive change in the patient's behavior. It is best explained as a communication activity occurring within the context of a counselor/client encounter that influences client behavior toward improved health. It includes a variety of strategies designed not only

Medical-care counseling. A kind of health counseling that takes place in the medical setting, whose goal is to improve health status by implementing the health prescription or recommendation.

Patient education. Also called "psychoeducation." Is provided by physician extenders such as nurses, social workers, health educators, and so on, in a clinical setting. It is often directed at a specific health concern that the physician deems problematic. The goal is to improve patient understanding, skill, and compliance with health prescription.

to facilitate behavioral change, but also to help individuals to identify their social support and to maintain their achieved behavior over a long period of time. It is much more complex than the printed handouts or audiovisual aids so often associated with it. Personal interaction is a key dimension, although a variety of patient education can also be done in a group setting, such as a clinic waiting room.

Patient education is related to medical-care counseling in that it is typically provided by non-physician health professionals, such as nurses, nurse-practitioners, social workers, health educators, and/or medical assistants. Patient education, provided by other clinical staff, tends to focus on content first, rather than on skill-building or behavior-change strategies, which will come later. It may or may not be based on an assessment, but is usually directed at a specific health concern that the physician deems problematic. Less often the assessment involves a formal health-risk appraisal. It may or may not be tailored to the patient's needs and expectations.

The purpose of patient education is to improve patient understanding, skill, and compliance, along with a prescription for enhancing health. It provides patients with information that is designed to help them understand the factors that promote or threaten health. In doing so, the hope is that patients will then make informed choices in their lives (Levant, 1986). It is assumed that prescribed change occurs because the patient sufficiently understands and has adequately practiced or mastered the prescribed change regimen.

This type of health counseling can be illustrated by individuals who have been recently diagnosed with asthma. Usually the patient is given the diagnosis, medication, and brief instruction on using an inhaler. Because this often takes place in a clinical or emergency-room situation amid the distress associated with an asthma attack, medical-care counseling may not be enough to ensure effective compliance with the treatment regimen. Accordingly, ongoing patient education for this condition often involves one or more follow-up home visits by a health provider. By providing instruction and modeling for the patient in the correct use of the inhaler and then observing the patient's efforts to use it, the health professional monitors the patient's skills and provides corrective feedback. Since this is done in familiar and less stressful surroundings, the patient is more likely to effectively and successfully comply with the treatment.

Health-Promotion Counseling

Quite different from the physician and other clinicians who often work as physician extenders, the health-promotion specialist usually begins with a general screening assessment such as a formal health-risk appraisal instrument. The individual being assessed may not see himself or herself as a patient nor present the signs or symptoms of disease. At its best, this approach to health counseling is tailored to the individual's needs and expectations. It may also identify the individual's level of motivation and barriers to adherence to lifestyle change. More properly, health counseling provided by a health-promotion specialist could be called " health-promotion counseling."

The purpose of **health-promotion counseling,** as any other type of counseling, is to improve lifestyle and health behaviors. It is assumed that change occurs because of the client's collaboration in the process of establishing, practicing, and monitoring a tailored health-promotion intervention. Commonly, the interventions are tailored to the client's need and expectations. Relapse prevention is increasingly a component in successful health-promotion endeavors.

Lifestyle changes usually involve the development of health-oriented behaviors. Development of these behaviors depends as much on specific skills as it does on factual information. Although individuals need to know something about the health issues that they are addressing, they also need to believe that they know *how* to change their behaviors. Because personal skills are so crucial,

Health-promotion counseling. Provided by a health-promotion specialist to improve lifestyle and health behaviors. Uses assessment and educational methods aimed toward skill-building and often uses interventions designed to increase clients' perceptions of control and self-efficacy.

health-promotion counseling uses educational methods aimed toward skill building.

The literature on changing health behaviors suggests that a sense of personal control is vital to clients successfully optimizing their health (see Chapter 11). Because this sense of control seems basic to health enhancement, health-promotion counseling utilizes interventions designed to increase clients' perceptions of control and self-efficacy. Subsequent chapters in this book will describe other factors involved in successful health promotion.

Health-Focused Psychotherapy

There is much more to be said about the theoretical basis and actual practice of health counseling. This section briefly differentiates from **health-focused psychotherapy,** while subsequent sections of this chapter describe and illustrate the counseling relationship, interventions, and stages and the actual practice of this approach to health counseling. Since health education and health counseling share so many similarities, students may want to review the list of competencies established by the National Commission for Health Education (2000), which describes the skills needed by entry-level and graduate-level health educators.

Behavioral health professionals, such as social workers, professional counselors, psychologists, psychiatric nurses, and psychiatrists, have formal training and experience in counseling and psychotherapy. For this reason, they may tend to approach health counseling differently from health-promotion specialists or physicians and patient educators. This related approach to health counseling offered by some behavioral health providers, particularly psychotherapists, could be

Health-focused psychotherapy. Psychotherapeutic interventions for health issues that tend to focus more on core personality dynamics and psychotherapeutic assessment. Provided by a behavioral health provider or psychotherapist, it takes place in formal, ongoing scheduled sessions.

called "health-focused psychotherapy." Before proceeding further, it may be useful to make a basic distinction between counseling and psychotherapy. Generally speaking, counseling tends to focus more on improving everyday functioning, while psychotherapy tends to focus more on changing underlying dynamics that may be rooted in unconscious rather than tangible factors, such as low self-concept, irrational fears, depression, and more.

Individuals referred for health-focused psychotherapy may have challenges coping with the pain or disability associated with a severe or life-threatening illness, or difficulty accepting their health condition or status. Not surprisingly, the assessment process in health-focused psychotherapy is more consistent with traditional psychotherapeutic parameters than it is in general health counseling. Nevertheless, education on health matters is a part of both approaches.

There are a number of similarities as well as differences between health-focused psychotherapy and health counseling. In this section, we begin with the exploration of these similarities and differences as they relate to strategy, skill, and concepts. Briefly stated, strategies for individual psychotherapy center on formal, ongoing scheduled appointments, usually 50-minute sessions, in a private practice or mental-health office or consulting room. Conversely, strategies for health counseling are much more diverse, ranging from scheduled encounters in a physician's office to unscheduled, sporadic sessions at a client's bedside or in a hospital clinic. Although specific skills and interventions used in psychotherapy and health counseling are quite similar, the focus of each tends to be different. The need for clear distinction between professions has been recently emphasized. Browers (2001) has discussed the professional identity of mental-health counselors at length, and Gelso & Fretz (2001) have distinguished differences between counseling psychology and the general counseling profession. Pistole & Roberts (2002) have written about the importance of professional identity and why the shaping of a distinct identity has been difficult for mental-health counseling. While there is considerable overlap among professions, there are distinct differences in focus and approach. For instance, while such concepts as adherence, psychoeducation, relapse prevention, and systems influence are all common to both health counseling and psychotherapy, they are seldom discussed in the psychotherapy literature. Since these four concepts are so important to health counseling, they will be described in detail in this section and discussed further in subsequent chapters, in such topics as nutrition, exercise, and smoking cessation.

In psychotherapy, a confidential and more intensive relationship develops between a client with emotional and behavioral symptoms and/or dysfunctions and a trained therapist. The therapist uses verbal and nonverbal methods to help clients improve their ability to cope more effectively with internal and external stressors, both individually and within their relationships with others. Specific treatment methods are described as supportive, diagnostic, analytic, and reconstructive in nature. Although so-called "talking therapy" is the mainstay of treatment, it may be supplemented by such adjuncts as biofeedback, hypnosis, or in children, play. In addition, some medically trained and licensed psychotherapists (usually psychiatrists) may prescribe medications or other somatic treatments. Traditional approaches to psychotherapy usually involve regularly scheduled sessions with the same therapist for months and sometimes even years, depending on that client and the client's reason for seeing a therapist. There is also short-term therapy, usually focusing on a specific, isolated issue or crisis. This briefer type of therapy approach takes place over a shorter period of time—often 8 to 20 sessions.

Thus, there are four somewhat different forms of health-counseling practice. Each requires different skills, training and experience. Nevertheless, all four types share common elements.

The fields of general counseling and psychotherapy have much to offer the practice of health counseling. The following section briefly introduces the type of counselor-client relationship and intervention methods used in health-focused psychotherapy.

The Relationship Between Counselor and Client

The counseling relationship is the context in which the process of therapy is experienced and enacted. While there are notable differences in the way this relationship is described among the various psychotherapy approaches, most acknowledge the importance of this relationship. Across these various approaches, a correlation has been found between the therapeutic relationship and outcome of psychotherapy. It is estimated that about 30 percent of the variance in psychotherapy outcome is due to relationship factors as compared to 40 percent attributed to client resources or spontaneous remission factors (Lambert, 1992). Based on his analysis of psychotherapy research, Strupp (1995) concludes that the therapeutic relationship is "the sine qua non in all forms of psychotherapy" (p. 70). Furthermore, the research of Orlinsky, Grawe, and Parks (1994) suggests that the quality of the client's participation in the therapeutic relationship is the essential determinant of outcome. In short, clients who are motivated, engaged, and who participate actively in the work with their counselor benefit the most from the experience.

Important to the formation of a strong therapeutic alliance is what Carl Rogers (1951) called the "core conditions" of effective counseling and psychotherapy: empathy, respect, and genuineness. It appears that when clients feel understood, safe, and hopeful, they are more likely to take the risk of disclosing more, and to thinking, feeling, and acting in more adaptive and healthier ways. However, the client must actually *feel* these core conditions, which of course will be experienced differently by different clients. Duncan, Solovey, and Rusk (1992) contend that the most helpful alliances are likely to develop when the counselor establishes a therapeutic relationship that matches the *client's* definition of empathy, respect, and genuineness. This is a key component in client-focused health counseling, discussed in the following chapter.

Stages of Psychotherapy-Based Health Counseling

This section describes four stages or phases that evolve throughout the course of counseling and psychotherapy. The Phase Model has been adapted from the research of Beitman (1987) and consists of four stages of individual psychotherapy that reflect commonalities among both eastern and western therapy systems and approaches. The four **stages of counseling,** as described here by Sperry (1999), are useful in conceptualizing the health-counseling process. More information on Stages of Change can also be found in Chapter 6.

Phase 1: Engagement

Engagement is the first and most important stage of treatment. Effective treatment outcomes require that the client be sufficiently engaged—meaning the client is committed to and actively involved in the treatment process. In other words, client engagement is required for any therapeutic change to occur. Typically, therapists assume that a client who shows up for sessions and talks about their concerns is engaged in treatment. However, it only takes an instance or two of nonadherence with treatment activities, such as homework, for the therapist to begin to question the client's degree of engagement. A general rule is that until an optimal degree of engagement is achieved, formal treatment should not proceed. Engagement is also important because a high level of client motivation predicts collaboration, compliance, and positive changes—while a lower motivation predicts resistance, noncompliance, or no change. The goal of the Engagement phase, therefore, is to develop a working therapeutic relationship and maximize the client's motivation.

Phase 2: Assessment

We use the term *Assessment* here in a very focused fashion—meaning the assessment of the client's health and personality patterns. "Pattern" refers to the client's biological individuality as well as to his or her predictable and consistent health beliefs and behaviors. It also includes the manner in which the client thinks, feels, acts, copes, and defends him or herself both in stressful and nonstressful circumstances. Also assessed are the individual's motivation (see above), strengths, and previous successes in making health behavior or other personal changes. Finally, barriers and facilitators for successful adherence to a health prescription are assessed. Barriers include intrapersonal, interpersonal, and social and cultural factors that hinder client progress. In short, the focus of the Assessment phase of treatment is to determine a client's health and personality patterns, motivation for enhancing their health, barriers, and support systems or facilitators.

Phase 3: Intervention

The goal of the Intervention phase is to help the client to modify or transform her or his maladaptive patterns into more adaptive ones. Intervention methods potentially include all therapeutic intervention strategies and tactics. For example, these methods might include focused pattern-interruption strategies, cognitive restructuring, interpretation, and/or reframing methods (see Chapter 4).

In clinical settings, maladaptive patterns often manifest themselves with symptomatic distress and functional impairment. Thus, decreasing symptomatology and/or increasing life functioning are usually treatment goals related to Intervention. Individuals and couples who present for psychological treatment in symptomatic distress are seeking relief from symptoms they have not been able to reduce by their own efforts. Thus, symptom reduction or removal is one of the first goals of treatment. Usually, this goal is achieved with medication and/or behavioral interventions. Research indicates that as symptoms increase, one or more areas of life functioning decrease. Therapeutic efforts to increase functional capacity tend to be thwarted until symptomatology is decreased (Sperry et al., 1996).

Stages of counseling. Four stages or phases that evolve throughout the course of counseling and/or therapy. These are the 1) engagement, 2) assessment, 3) intervention and 4) maintenance stages.

Phase 4: Maintenance

The goals of the Maintenance phase of treatment are to maintain the newly acquired adaptive pattern, to prevent relapse, and to reduce/eliminate the client's reliance on the treatment relationship. Technically, relapse refers to a continuation of the "original" episode, while recurrence is the instigation of a "new" episode of what is a similar behavior or issue with different features. For example, a recovering alcoholic who begins to drink alcohol again has relapsed. A person who has suffered from depression, gone in for treatment, and recovered from the depression, only to become depressed again a few months later can be said to have recurrent depression. However, in this section, these terms will be used synonymously.

Relapse prevention is an intervention consisting of specific skills and cognitive strategies that prepares the client in advance to cope with the inevitable slips or relapses in compliance-to-change programs (Marlatt & Gordon, 1985; Sperry, 1986). In order to prevent relapse, the therapist must assess the client's risk factors and potential for relapse, and incorporate relapse-prevention strategies into the treatment process (see Chapter 6). Health counseling that does not recognize and emphasize the importance of relapse education and prevention is not likely to be effective. Relapse-prevention models grew out of both inpatient and outpatient treatment and recovery programs, often from those involving substance dependence. However, we believe the concepts embodied in these models have relevance to many other lifestyle-change and health-promotion programs.

Case Study

The Practice of Health Counseling

How is health counseling actually practiced? The following is one example of what health-focused counseling might look like.

Jack T. is a building contractor and has six construction workers and one estimator who report to him. He is also an avid part-time soccer coach at his children's private school. He is 41, has been married for 14 years and has a 12-year-old daughter and a 10-year-old son. For the past year, he has not had the energy and stamina that marked his earlier years. He admits his job is stressful, but no more so than it has been for the past several years. In addition to his declining energy levels, and occasional periods of moodiness and irritability, he logged 11 sick days for various maladies. This compared with previous years when he took no more than one or two sick days. Because he is the boss and coordinates the work of his employees, missed days mean lower productivity for his company. Being away from work only increased his stress level, to which he responds by eating, and subsequently gaining weight.

Jack was referred by his family physician for counseling for help with stress reduction and weight management. Over a period of four months, Jack had been given a diet plan and encouragement by the physician followed by weekly counseling sessions by the clinic's nurse practitioner on diet and stress management. Because the intervention did not match the client's needs, and his stress and weight levels remained the same, he was referred to a health counselor with training in psychotherapy.

The initial health evaluation assessed the client's energy pattern, stress-response pattern, body type, and weight-gain pattern, as well as personality and relational patterns. With some focused questioning (discussed more in Chapter 2), the counselor learned that Jack's diet consistently mostly of complex carbohydrates, no red meat, and only occasional fish and chicken. Jack said that he was embarrassed to admit that he craved snack foods including, chocolate-covered nuts, donuts, and chocolate-chip cookies. He added that he also snacked on apples, grapes, and bananas. Except for an occasional glass of wine, he used no other alcohol or recreational drugs and had never smoked. He took a number of vitamins, some minerals and herbs, but no prescription medicines.

Jack indicated that the nurse-practitioner he had met with previously started him on a high-carbohydrate, low-fat diet. He agreed to it since his wife had used such a diet to return to her ideal weight for the first time since the birth of their first son. Jack noted that it was ironic that while she had lost weight on this diet, he had actually gained an additional 15 pounds on it despite his four hours of exercise a week! He had been jogging for the past 20 years, even though his knee joints were becoming increasingly painful and arthritic. Jack made it clear that he was not interested in taking prescription medicine for either stress or weight loss. However, he was agreeable to a medical evaluation.

Before they met again, the counselor referred Jack for a comprehensive medical evaluation. It had been more than three years since his last physical examination. The evaluation included extensive lab testing and, given a family history of heart disease, a cardiac stress test. The report of that evaluation indicated that Jack was approximately 32 pounds above an optimal weight for someone his age and level of conditioning. His cardiac stress test was in the normal range and exhibited a level of exercise conditioning usually seen in amateur athletes. He was noted to have chronic sinusitis and mild to moderate levels of osteoarthritis in both knees and the right hip.

Two treatment recommendations were provided. To reduce sinus symptoms, it was recommended that he reduce sugar intake and eliminate dairy products from his diet. In addition, a trial glucosamine sulfate, an effective natural remedy, was suggested for 12 weeks and a referral to a joint specialist if the trial was not successful. The diagnosis of insulin-dependence, which the examining physician said was the first stage of adult-onset or Type-II diabetes, was also given along with the recommendation for an initial trial of either weight loss or medication. Overall, the physician assessed Jack's overall health status as being average to above average for individuals his age and gender.

Jack met with the counselor two weeks later to review the medical evaluation and continue the health assessment. An important focus of that session was on assessing client strengths and motivation for change as well as establishing an intervention plan. Jack reported that he stopped smoking when he was hospitalized for pneumonia four years previously. Although he had smoked two packs a day for 14 years, he responded well to nicotine gum and a short behavioral-counseling regimen. His current motivation level was high, and he appeared to be a good candidate for health counsel-

ing given that he had target symptoms, was reasonably motivated, and had been previously successful in making a major health-behavior change.

The counselor suggested a 10-session course of counseling over a six-month period. Sessions would be for 45 minutes, twice a week for five weeks, followed by biweekly and then monthly sessions. Two health-promotion target goals were proposed: first, stress reduction, and second, weight loss and maintenance within 10 percent of his ideal weight. Three intervention strategies would be involved: an individualized diet plan, an individualized stress management plan, and an individualized exercise program. A contract was made in which Jack agreed to the goals and to make the personal and time commitments to the intervention strategies.

Their next session focused on increasing motivation and identifying reasons why his recent efforts at weight loss and stress reduction with the nurse-practitioner had not worked. Not surprisingly, Jack noted his discouragement at gaining weight on the diet prescribed by the nurse-practitioner and the increase in his cravings for sweets. The counselor described Jack's unique health needs and the difference between one-size-fits-all health programs and individualized diet, exercise, and stress-management prescriptions.

A profile of the client's health concerns, health status, health behaviors, personality patterns, and body type was shared with Jack. The counselor noted that Jack's energy level was inconsistent throughout the day, that he craved sweet and starchy food, he was creative, impatient, irritable, and easily angered, and that he appeared to be carrying most of his weight around his waist and hips, that is, "love handles." Psychosocially, Jack had a variety of friends and colleagues and was most attracted to individuals who were original thinkers and stimulating conversationalists, and he seemed energized and exhilarated when initiating new projects but most stressed when finishing projects and engaging in work that was repetitive, detailed, and tedious. The process of describing and explaining Jack's unique dietary needs and his stress pattern, a key strategy in motivational counseling, fostered a shift from the decision to the action level of readiness.

They talked about the health patterns that Jack exhibited and they talked about ways to optimize his diet in order to both reduce his food cravings and lose weight. It appeared that the high carbohydrate diet that he had been on was a poor match for him. The nutritional strategy that better matched him was a higher protein diet, which emphasized eggs, poultry, fish, with some complex carbohydrates, but limited nonstarchy vegetables.

It appeared that Jack's exercise plan needed some fine-tuning. A more optimal exercise strategy would emphasize strength training with some aerobic conditioning. Jack expressed interest in working with a personal trainer who could design and monitor a strength-training program for him. It is interesting to note that given his joint pain and damage, the trainer urged Jack to replace jogging with lap swimming. Another key part of the recommended changes involved stress reduction and management. It was noted that Jack was overly stressed by job functions that required extensive involvement in detail-oriented oversight of ongoing construction sites. The counselor asked whether it was possible to shift much of this activity to one of his employees. Jack indicated that this was actually one of his foreman's duties. While it was not one of his stated job functions, Jack had believed he needed to roll up his sleeves and show his employees his personal commitment to these projects. It had become even clearer that he was a "big picture" person rather than a "detail" person. The delegations that were made about Jack's job fit considerably. It was mutually agreed to try these recommendations for four months and evaluate the outcome.

A major focus of the third, fourth, and fifth sessions was on Jack's operating belief that "if you want something done right, you have to do it yourself." His underlying schema of perfectionism came under therapeutic scrutiny. Through the use of cognitive restructuring and reframing, this operating belief was sufficiently modified so that Jack felt increasingly comfortable in reducing his micromanagement at each construction site. Reducing this level of involvement—in a job function that was actually not his but his foreman's—was a strategic part of his stress-reduction prescription.

During their eighth session, Jack indicated he was feeling considerably better. He felt less pressured and irritable since he had delegated many on-site management responsibilities to his foreman. Now he was simply monitoring progress at the various construction sites on a weekly basis. Using his creativity to conceptualize and plan new projects was not only immensely gratifying for him, but also more energizing and less stressful. Furthermore, being on the new diet plan seemed to be working. He was now within 5 pounds of his ideal weight, and his sinus and joint symptoms were considerably lessened. His physician indicated that his lab tests revealed no indication of diabetes or insulin resistance.

At six months Jack continued to do well. For the first time since college, he was at his ideal weight. He enjoyed lap swimming and strength training workouts with his trainer. He was able to exercise without joint pain, and the elimination of dairy products from his diet had nearly eliminated sinus congestion. He had taken only one sick day in 10 months.

The question can be asked: Why did this approach work rather than the interventions done by the physician and nurse-practitioner? At least two reasons can be noted. First, the diet plan suggested by the physician and nurse-practitioner was not a good fit with Jack's unique health needs. It was the standard diet prescribed at that clinic. Probably most of the health-education materials and handouts at that clinic endorsed that diet option. Although a high-carbohydrate, low-fat diet is appropriate and effective with certain individuals, it certainly was ineffective with Jack. Second, any health-education intervention that did not deal with Jack's psychological barriers to change would predictably be ineffective. Because health counseling assesses and addresses such barriers, this kind of intervention was more likely to succeed.

Summary

This chapter has defined and described health, health promotion, and several types of health counseling. It discussed three reasons why the need for health counseling has become increasingly evident in the past decade. Much of this chapter emphasized the contributions of theory and research in counseling and psychotherapy for effectively working with clients on health-related issues.

Two key points about the practice of health counseling were made. The first point is that health counseling is a broad, encompassing endeavor which spans the continuum from medical care to patient education to psychoeducation to health counseling and to health-focused psychotherapy. Although each of these types differs considerably, education is a central component of each type. Professional counselors and other psychotherapists have the formal training and experience to provide the type of assessment and intervention strategies needed for effective health counseling, and health professionals with other backgrounds can learn to utilize these intervention strategies and methods with individuals as well.

An extended case study was provided in order to illustrate the processes, stages and strategies of health counseling. Noteworthy is the fact that the counselor performed a comprehensive assessment that identified Jack's basic health and personality patterns, strengths, and motivation. This assessment permitted the development of an individualized health prescription for diet, exercise, and stress management. In addition, the counselor endeavored to engage Jack in a collaborative relationship and increase his level of motivation, rather than simply tell Jack what he needed to do. Furthermore, the counselor provided instruction, worked with Jack to develop an implementation and relapse plan, and utilized cognitive restructuring and reframing to reduce psychological barriers to adherence to the health-promotion plan. These counseling strategies and methods are examples of true health counseling and delineate it from other health-education efforts.

Those who practice health counseling, regardless of the settings in which they are employed, need to be able to help their clients make health-related behavior changes and cope with threats to their physical, psychological, and emotional health. Health counseling is an action-oriented process through which a helper enables a patient or client to make health changes that lead in the direction of improved health and well-being. This process depends less on the provider's job title or employment setting than it does on his or her point of view. Health counseling takes place in medical offices, human-services agencies, private practices, the workplace, and a variety of other settings. In short, it takes place wherever a provider with a biopsychosocial perspective can be found.

Key Terms

health, 2
health counseling, 4
health-focused
 psychotherapy, 8
health-promotion
 counseling, 7

Healthy People 2010, 5
medical-care
 counseling, 6
patient education, 6
stages of counseling, 10

Questions for Discussion

1. What aspects made the health-counseling intervention in the above case study work? What mistakes were made in the initial medical evaluation/intervention?

2. Why is assessment so important in a client evaluation? On what levels must a health counselor assess a client in order to have optimum success?

3. Discuss the reasons why the need for health counseling has become increasingly evident in the past 10 years. What are the advantages of health counseling as a distinct field and what are its limitations?

4. Describe the stages of psychotherapy-based health counseling. What kinds of presenting problems should a health counselor refer to a physician or therapist?

5. What are the four types of health counseling commonly practiced today? Which context appeals to you most? Why?

Related Web Sites

http:// www.samhsa.gov
The Substance Abuse and Mental Health Services Administration—Describes the programs of the Federal agency charged with improving the quality and availability of prevention and treatment of mental health and addiction disorders.

http://www.allaboutcounseling.com
All About Counseling—This site contains articles, FAQ, and self-help information and offers discussion opportunities, free listings in their professionals directory, and professional resouces for counselors.

http://www.psych.org
American Psychiatric Association—Features news, current information, jobs, and links to resources by the world's largest psychiatric organization

http://www.apa.org
American Psychological Association—A major clearinghouse for information of interest to students, professionals, and the public. Features current news, articles, programs information, a consumer help center, and more.

Health Counseling: Process and Skills

ELIZABETH SCHROEDER, M.S.W.

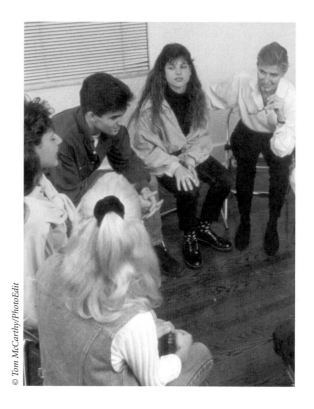

© Tom McCarthy/PhotoEdit

OBJECTIVES

By the end of the chapter, the reader should be able to:

- Identify the basic historical roots of health counseling

- Differentiate between what health counseling is and what it is not

- Explain the Concentric Biopsychosocial Model, and its applicability to health-counseling work

- Describe the basic components of climate setting with clients

- Explain several basic counseling skills, including attending, questioning techniques, and other nonquestioning techniques used in assessment and on an ongoing basis

- Describe at least three different kinds of psychological defenses and ways of responding effectively to these defenses

- Respond to questions relating to client–counselor boundaries, including confidentiality and self-disclosure

- Identify several different types of counseling groups, and the purposes they serve

Case Study

Jamal is a newly hired 24-year-old health teacher at a public high school. He graduated from his program with honors, and feels that he has mastered the content relating to health that he needs in order to be an effective health educator. He has also received rave reviews during his student teaching on his style, and feels ready for his first day at the school.

The first month goes well, and the students seem to both like and respect him. They are engaged in class, do their assignments, and seem to enjoy studying the material. One student, Mohan, is quieter than the others. He does not seem to be focused, has dozed in class a few times, and when he is called on to participate, jumps at the sound of his own name.

Mohan fails the first quiz, and his assignments are often incomplete if handed in at all. Jamal stops Mohan after class, and gives him a friendly punch on the shoulder, saying, "Hey, dude—you really need to get it together with this class, ok?" With a broad smile, Jamal dismisses Mohan, thinking he has related well to the student.

A few days later, Mohan asks if he can talk with Jamal after school. When Mohan returns at 3:15, Jamal suggests they walk down to the cafeteria to talk so he can get something to eat. Once in the cafeteria, Mohan looks around nervously and asks Jamal if he can talk with him about something completely confidentially. Jamal says, "Sure, you can talk to me about anything." Mohan tells Jamal that the reason he hasn't been doing as well in class is because his father has been beating him fairly regularly over the past two years. He tells Jamal that his grades are so low because he can't sleep at night— and this makes it hard for him to concentrate. He looks up at Jamal and asks, "What should I do?" Jamal stammers a bit, then feeling protective of Mohan, stands up and tells Mohan to follow him back to his office. Once there, Jamal picks up the phone and calls Mohan's father.

What happened here? What are some of the cues Jamal should have been tuned in to in order to have helped Mohan more effectively? What, if anything, do you think Jamal did well? What, if anything, do you think he did ineffectively—and what would you suggest he do instead?

As we read in Chapter 1, when people hear the word *counseling*, a number of different thoughts might come to mind. Some may think of it in terms of providing advice to someone, such as when a person seeks legal counsel or spiritual counsel. Some think of counseling in its most formal incarnation, psychotherapy. While millions of people in the United States avail themselves of some kind of psychotherapy each year, the concept of therapy remains an intimidating, uncomfortable topic for many. Even if therapy has proven helpful, many still regard it with suspicion or even shame. It is a stigma with which mental health professionals continue to struggle.

Health counseling, in its broadest definition, is neither of the above. But in some ways, it is more analogous to legal counsel, where an attorney provides an expert opinion and then lets a client decide for her or himself what kind of action to take. However, health counseling is not advice, nor is it therapy. It does, nevertheless, incorporate many of the concepts and skills that are used in the formal therapeutic process. These concepts and skills will be discussed and illustrated throughout this chapter.

A health professional who has the word *counselor* in her or his job title or description will have a clearer sense of the type and extent of counseling she or he is to provide. But what about other professionals?

Basically, any educational or health professional who is in a position to provide information or services to a client is a health counselor. This means that a health counselor could be a nutritionist, an educator, a social worker, a coach, an addictions specialist, a medical professional, or one of many other positions. As such, all of these professionals should be equipped with basic health-counseling skills. Since health-counseling encompasses such a broad spectrum of professionals, the generic term **counselor** will be used throughout the chapter to describe any and all of these individuals. In addition, the term **client** will be used to describe the individuals with whom the counselor interacts. This might be a student or team player, an individual seeking information, a patient, and so on. In doing so, we will emphasize the important point that any time a health or social-service professional interacts with someone who could come under our broad definition of *client*—including people who are affected by what goes on in the client's life, such as the client's family members—that health professional should have her or his counseling skills at the ready.

Counselor. Any educational or health professional who is in a position to provide information or services to a client.

Client. Any individual with whom the counselor interacts.

This chapter will provide an overview of some key counseling skills when working one-on-one with a client or in a group setting. The concepts and skills discussed in this chapter are basic but vital tools in providing effective, client-centered information and services regardless of who the client is and why she or he is seeking information or services. Since so much is based in the basic tenets of psychotherapy, it is important to first take a look at the sources of our society's concepts of counseling as we know them today.

Counseling 101: An Historical Perspective

Today, there are many different theories and types of counseling on which a range of professionals base their work with individuals and groups. While these different theories will sometimes build on and sometimes disagree with each other, the root of all counseling is generally traced back to the work of Sigmund Freud, the founder of psychoanalysis. Trying to summarize Freud's work in a few sentences would be like trying to provide the basic gist of Tolstoy's *War and Peace* in the same amount of space. However, there are a few basic facts we can share about Freud and a number of other theorists to put this chapter into context. The resource Web list at the end of the chapter can direct interested readers to supplemental information.

Freud (1856–1939) basically believed that human beings are constantly in conflict, conflict that has arisen from a mix of aggressive and sexual desires. Freud believed that if these conflicts, many of which are generated during childhood, are not resolved they serve as the bases for dysfunctions in adult personalities. People, Freud said, are governed by either the "pleasure principle" (which tells us to do what feels good) or the "reality principle" (the understanding that we must sublimate or suppress our desires in order to function on a daily basis) (Klages, 1997). Since this is a constant conflict, Freud believed that much of it goes on in our unconscious. As a result, it is necessary to reach into the unconscious to find out what a person truly thinks and feels. Freud did so by looking at people's dreams, as well as what he called parapraxes. Parapraxes are what later became known in our culture as "Freudian slips"—things people say, read, or write that reveal an unconscious, hidden desire. For example, say a person is working at an agency with a supervisor named Marnie. At the end of a meeting, the employee says, "Thanks. See you later, Mommy." While most people would laugh that off as a simple slip of the tongue, Freud would have said that this slip meant that the employee was having a mother transference with her boss. Freud would say that, unconsciously, there is something about Marnie that makes the employee see her as a mother figure and would explore the employee's feelings about her mother, authority, seeking approval, and more.

While much of Freud's work is still used and valued today, much of it is also dated, sexist, and even offensive to some. These are among the reasons why other theorists have challenged, supplemented, or built upon and gone far beyond Freud's premises on human psychological development. Some of them were students or contemporaries of Freud. Among the many theorists who came after Freud are Jean Piaget, Erik Erikson, Margaret Mahler, and Melanie Klein. Again, in the interest of space, only a few words can be said about each, none of which begin to pay tribute to the significant discoveries and contributions these professionals made to modern psychotherapy and counseling (see Chapter 10).

Jean Piaget (1896–1980) was interested in how human beings obtain knowledge and understanding as children. He created a sort of timetable by which children develop both physically and psychologically. Piaget observed, spoke with, and evaluated children (including his own) by spending time with them and then developing evaluation instruments that enabled him to assess the ways in which they viewed the world at different ages. In this way, his contributions went beyond child development into the area of education—specifically, age- and developmentally appropriate materials and learning (Savvides, 2001).

Both Margaret Mahler (1897–1985) and Erik Erikson (1902–1994) looked at human development in terms of stages. Mahler focused on infants, coining the term *separation/individuation* (Shane, 1989) to describe the significant experience a child faces again and again during infancy. Specifically, this refers to the relationship between the child and the child's love object(s)—most notably, her or his mother. Erikson was the first to look beyond childhood into a lifelong model. His stages of development start in infancy and go through advanced age, or "maturity." It is not a numerical age that enables a person to move from one stage to the next, he said, but rather the ability of the individual to face and complete a significant developmental task at each stage (Sharkey, 2001).

Melanie Klein (1882–1960) developed a theoretical approach called "Object Relations Theory." She is credited with establishing the foundations of play therapy with children, observing their interrelatedness with others and their drawings in order to understand their unconscious feelings (Martin, 2001). For example, a child may not be able to say to an adult, "My daddy hurts my mommy." However, while playing with dolls and other toys, the child may act out a scene between his parents that depicts an abusive argument.

There are volumes written on the works of each of these and other theorists. This brief summary is intended to provide a snapshot of the sources of the kinds of counseling we know today.

The Concentric Biopsychosocial Model

The transition from counseling to health counseling took some time, but it was a logical step. Among the many reasons why the term *health counseling* itself is so helpful is that it combines the concepts of physical and psychological health, recognizing the fact that each plays a key role in the other. Historically, medical professionals tended to look exclusively at the physical nature of symptoms without considering other potential causes. Yet according to Sobel (1995), nearly one-third of people who make appointments with their doctors or clinicians do so with symptoms that can be traced to psychological distress. One-third of the symptoms can be attributed to the behaviors of

the client, such as smoking, eating habits, and more. Thus the introduction of social factors became vitally important.

Looking at the physical (or biological) manifestations of health issues without looking at the psychological and social factors would be as useful as sitting on a stool that only has one or two legs. All three factors are equally important for effective health counseling. It does not mean, of course, that a health counselor must be well versed in all three areas. However, all three areas must be assessed so that appropriate information and referrals can be provided (see Figure 2.1).

Engel (1980) is credited as the first person to coin the term **biopsychosocial** to describe the role biological, psychological, and social factors play in a person's general health. Hoffman & Driscoll (2000) analyzed the biopsychosocial model and introduced a new way of looking at it. Their main criticism of the original model was that it looked exclusively at the way in which these three factors interact to cause disease. They believed that health professionals should focus less on disease prevention and more on health promotion. To do so, they created a Concentric Biopsychosocial Model of Health Status. They use the term *health status* because it does not look at disease or the absence thereof as the determining factor in whether a person is healthy.

Figure 2.1 shows the Concentric Biopsychosocial Model. The factors in the biomedical circle seem to speak for themselves. Here we will take a few moments to look at the biosocial and psychosocial contributors to a person's health status.

Hoffman & Driscoll (2000) explain that the psychosocial circle is positioned closest to the circle marked "health status" intentionally. This is because the factors listed in this circle can mitigate, aggravate, or have other direct or indirect effects on the biosocial and biomedical contributors. For example, a person with a strong coping style is going to be able to manage a cancer

Biopsychosocial. A term that describes the roles biological, psychological, and social factors play in a person's general health.

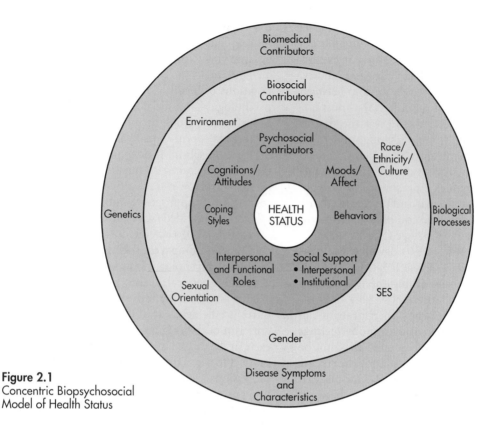

Figure 2.1
Concentric Biopsychosocial
Model of Health Status

diagnosis more effectively than someone with a weaker style. And a person with no family history or genetic predisposition toward cancer will still be at risk if she selects certain risky behaviors, such as cigarette smoking. In addition, a person with stronger social supports will be able to manage the stressful impact that many diseases and other deleterious health factors or diagnoses can have (Uchino, Cacioppo, & Kiecolt-Glaser, 1996).

The biosocial factors listed apply to the client's life outside the health or educational setting, as well as inside. Among the key factors listed, several pertain to race, ethnicity, and culture. A health counselor should be sure to keep these factors in mind along with the biomedical and psychosocial factors. Race, ethnicity, and culture play huge roles in the ways in which a person perceives health, the health system, seeking assistance, and much more. To discuss this issue, Fouad & Brown (2000) developed the term differential status identity. This de-

scribes the ways in which a person's differences in social standing—whether real or perceived—affects that person's psychological well-being. In turn, a person's psychological well-being has a significant effect on a person's physical health.

For example, the poverty rate of African American people in the United States is three to four times that of European Americans (Rossides, 1997). Unemployment is higher among African American people, and the rate of higher prestige, higher-paying jobs is lower. This factor is not something a person can acknowledge and then move on—it is one of the many realities many people have to face each day. Just as a lesbian or gay person must live with the daily pressure of deciding whether or not to disclose her or his sexual orientation to any number of individuals, people with a low differential status identity will carry that with them. And it will always be in the room with a health counselor, whether that room is a medical exam room, a classroom, or a clinic waiting room.

This does not mean that a health counselor has to be self-conscious or apologetic about who he or she is. Nor should she or he make the assumption that just because a client is of a different race, ethnicity, gender, and so on that she or he lives with all or any of the stressors that others with low differential status identity do. However, when screening for stressors—when making an assessment of factors that affect a person's overall health and well-being—the social factors must be taken on an equal level with the biological and the psychological.

The Purviews of Health Counseling

Counseling itself is a very broad term that can apply to many different methods of providing individuals and/or groups with some kind of support. Health counseling *may* include:

- **Providing information,** either one-on-one or in a group setting. This might include, for example:

  - a workshop on smoking cessation, birth control, healthful eating habits, and more

  - instructing someone who has been diagnosed with diabetes how to administer injections

  - supplying someone with printed information and Web-site addresses

  - making referrals to support groups, medical specialists, mental-health professionals, and others.

- **Options counseling** applies to situations in which a client has a challenging decision to make. A counselor can lay out the options for her or him so that the client has all the information he needs before making a decision. For example, a 14-year-old girl who is faced with an unplanned pregnancy comes to a counselor and asks for advice on what she should do. The counselor may feel very strongly that the girl should terminate the pregnancy by having an abortion. Another counselor may be strongly against abortion and feel that the girl

should give birth, regardless of whether the girl intends to place the baby with an adoption agency or chooses to parent. In this situation, it is the counselor's responsibility to lay out the choices and explore the pros and cons of each. A counselor should *not* try to influence the client's decisions in any way. This can be difficult, particularly if the client makes a decision with which the counselor disagrees. However, any kind of information, care, or support should be client-determined so that it is client-focused, a concept discussed in more detail later.

When looking at what counseling *is,* it is equally important to consider what counseling is *not.* Counseling is *not* :

- **Therapy.** Certain techniques that are part of the therapeutic process can and should be used during other types of interactions with clients. However, once a particular issue has been resolved or a referral made, a health counselor should not try to fall into the role of therapist. A therapist has very specific training, and the therapeutic process requires knowledge of and experience with this process. Some clients will feel comfortable with a particular health counselor and want to talk with her or him about issues that may not be within the health counselor's role or responsibilities. If this were to happen, the counselor would need to make an appropriate referral rather than try to handle the issue himself.

  Let's think about Jamal (in the Case Study) for a moment. Although prepared to teach health education, he was clearly unprepared for any other issues that might come up with a student. Even though his motivation may have been noble, Jamal should have recognized his limitations and referred Mohan to the school counselor rather than jumping in to help.

- **Advice.** Often, a client will ask, "What should I do?" or "What would you do if you were in my situation?" A counselor must resist the temptation to direct the client toward a particular outcome. This is true even if the client seems to be leaning toward a decision with which the counselor disagrees. Using the previous example of the 14-year-old girl who discloses that she is pregnant, a counselor may be tempted to encourage the girl to do one thing or another. She may feel very strongly that the girl would be ruining her life if she were to keep the pregnancy and become a pregnant teen. However, if the girl has made it clear that abortion is out of the question, the temptation for this counselor may be to try to convince her otherwise. Instead, the counselor needs to be **client-centered.** Client-centered means helping a client to make a well-informed decision. It does not mean doing what a counselor thinks is in the best interest of the client. Appropriate steps would include helping the client to evaluate her support system—can she continue to live with her family after the baby is born? Does the baby's father intend to play a role? Can he help financially and/or by baby-sitting so that they can both finish school? Also, the client would need to get prenatal care as soon as possible. The health counselor can help by referring the girl to health centers where prenatal care is available.

A counselor should not tell a client what to do. There are a few reasons for this. From a humanistic standpoint, each person must be able to make decisions for her or himself, as long as that person is competent to do so. From a practical standpoint, giving advice can come back around to haunt a health counselor, both personally and professionally. For example, a counselor who tells a woman in an abusive relationship to move out immediately will have to live with the consequences if the woman were to do so, only to be caught by her husband and then beaten or killed. In addition, it is exceedingly self-centered to think that one's status as teacher, nutritionist, social worker, or even adult, gives one the right to be able to dictate how another person should live. Starting a sentence with, "When I was your age, I . . ." or "When I had my surgery, I opted for . . . " makes the erroneous assumption that the counselor knows what the client is going through or feeling. Again, while the counselor's motivation here may be good—an attempt to show the client that he and the coun-

selor have something in common—it can, instead, belittle the client's experience by not allowing him to react to it in his own way. He might think, "Wow, my counselor has diabetes, and says it's no big deal. But it's really hard for me. What's wrong with me that I'm feeling this way?"

Counseling Skills Overview

When a client first comes to a counselor, the counselor will have little or no information about the client's needs. The counselor must assess these needs to determine the presenting problem. She must focus on setting the climate in an effort to build rapport with the client. In this section, we will discuss what these interventions involve.

Assessment

To "assess" a situation means to evaluate it—to look the entire situation over and determine which aspects are significant or relevant, and which are not. An **assessment** in a counseling situation refers to when a counselor collects information about a client in order to work with that client to determine what, together, they can do to deal with the client's presenting problem (defined below) (Gladding, 2001). It involves asking questions, reading information that may have already been gathered from other sources, and based on that, working with the client and other appropriate individuals to plan a course of action. This can be done by using a standardized intake form, as one might do in a health clinic. In a sense, part of the initial and ongoing work of a counselor is similar to that of a detective. At the beginning, the counselor must gather as much information as possible. If the counseling relationship continues, the counselor will continue to gather this information, which can result in changes in a client's action or treatment plan.

Client-centered. Helping a client make a well-informed decision, rather than doing what a counselor thinks is in the best interest of the client.

Assessment. An initial estimation of the patient's understanding of the need for treatment, the treatment regimen, and the degree of mastery of any requisite skills necessary for compliance.

The Presenting Problem

The very first thing a counselor needs to find out about the client is why she or he has come to the counselor. Even if a counselor knows why a client has been sent to her or him—if, for example, a coach has heard rumors from team members that a teenage girl may be suffering from an eating disorder—it is important to determine what the client perceives to be the reason for her or his visit. In assessing this, the counselor will learn valuable information, such as:

■ **Is the client there of her or his own free will?** A client who seeks help on his own will have a much different attitude towards the situation than one who has been brought in by his parents or mandated to come in. This is seen clearly when individuals who break the law are mandated for some kind of counseling as part of their sentence.

■ **How does the client feel about being there?** Again, this will help the counselor to get a sense of both the client's motivation and how the counselor may or may not wish to proceed. For example, a client who says, "I came in because one of the other girls on the team said you were really easy to talk to about stuff" is different from someone who says, "My girlfriend told me I should talk to you, but I don't know why I'm here—there's nothing wrong with me."

Climate Setting

Climate setting basically refers to the environment in which the counselor provides information and support. This includes:

Environment. The environment in which counseling or an intervention takes place is key to setting a climate of safety, reliability, and respect. It has to do with the physical environment, as well as with how the environment is managed by the counselor. As people often do when they enter another person's home for the first time, a client looks around a counselor's office to try to learn something about the counselor. Therefore, a counselor can set a comfortable environment by having posters up on the wall featuring positive, encouraging, and/or healthful messages. A counselor can also reinforce her or his comfort with diversity by ensuring that posters include people of different racial and ethnic groups, ages, and physical abilities. Brochures and books on the bookshelf might include a resource for working with lesbian, gay, bisexual, and/or transgender individuals. In this way, a counselor is saying to her clients, "Whoever you are, I am here to provide you with information and services."

A client will feel much less comfortable discussing a personal issue in an open cubicle than in a room or office with a door that shuts. For this reason, a counselor should always aim to find a private place for talking with a client, even if the counselor does not have a private office. Jamal's choice of the cafeteria for speaking with Mohan was clearly unwise. If Jamal had not had lunch all day, he could have suggested a trip down to the cafeteria that included conversation about a general topic and waited to discuss the issue when they returned to his office.

In addition, a counselor should make the decision not to answer the phone unless completely necessary. If a counselor knows in advance that she or he will need to answer the phone if it rings, it is a good idea to let the client know that. If counselors are in settings where colleagues may occasionally knock on the door and ask to interrupt, they should let colleagues know when a meeting with a client cannot be interrupted. This will let the client know that his meeting with the counselor is being taken seriously.

Thinking about environment: What does your school or clinic look like? Is it well lit and inviting, or is there paint peeling everywhere? Do you have your own office? If so, what does it look like? Are there papers strewn about, or are you able to make some order amid the chaos? Do you have posters on the wall with positive, healthy messages? Do your materials represent diversity in race, age, gender, sexual orientation, and physical abilities? These are all a part of climate setting. It's important to make a good first impression!

Language. Health professionals are always encouraged to avoid making assumptions. However, the language we use can often make assumptions for us. Doing so can shut a client down almost immediately. We must also listen carefully to the language a client uses, use the same or similar language, and determine whether the client is providing us with important information through the language used.

A specific example of this pertains to working with lesbian, gay, bisexual, and/or transgender clients. For example, say a young girl goes to her coach and tells the coach that she's really upset because she's in love with someone at school and doesn't know what to do. If the coach asks "What's his name?", he has made an assumption that this girl was talking about a boy. The girl has said that she likes "someone"—she has not identified the gender of that person. The coach should instead use a gender-neutral term until the girl is specific. She may very well be telling the coach that the person she's in love with is another girl, and is seeking advice about how to deal with that. Then again, she may have used the word *someone* and is talking about a boy. Regardless, the counselor who makes a heterosexist assumption—the assumption that everyone is heterosexual—will give the message to any client who is or thinks she or he might be lesbian, gay, or bisexual that the counselor is not a safe person to go to with her or his issues.

People who are transgender do not necessarily identify as male or female. Or, they may identify as one gender even though their biological makeup would suggest otherwise. Transgender individuals face a unique kind of bias—they are forced daily to choose whether they are more *like* someone who is female or male in order to navigate in society. A clinic can be more sensitive to this by making their intake forms more inclusive—for example, instead of asking clients to check off "male" or "female," they can have a space for "gender" with a blank line so a person can fill it in for her or himself. In addition, more and more health centers have single-occupancy rest rooms that can be used by anyone regardless of gender. The simple removal of gender specification from a rest room can make a health center more welcoming to transgender individuals.

Paying attention to language also refers to the language in the materials health counselors supply to their clients. If a health center sees clients for whom English is not their first language, it should offer health information in different languages. In addition, people have different levels of education. Health brochures and information should therefore be written at a reading level that is appropriate to a client population, including large, descriptive drawings in areas where literacy may be lower.

Active listening. Activing listening refers to when a counselor is cognizant of the client's verbal and nonverbal communication without judging the client, either positively or negatively (Gladding, 2001). Among the nonverbal communications a counselor is assessing is the client's **affect.** A person's affect is basically how they express their emotional state. For example, a person who does not seem to display any emotions, either positive or negative, is considered to be displaying a blunted affect. Taking note of a client's affect can aid in assessment and treatment in a number of ways. A person's affect will usually reflect the circumstances in a client's life. If it does not—if a client were not to react at all to a diagnosis or show no emotion during a session or meeting—the counselor would be able to explore whether the client had heard the information correctly. Or, if the client appears to be in **denial,** the counselor will know to deal with this defense (discussed later). This would be important information for the counselor to record, particularly if the counselor will need to make a referral to another professional within their own setting or elsewhere.

Affect. How a person expresses their emotional state, usually reflecting the circumstances of a person's life.

Denial. A defense in which a person acts as if something is not real, or ignores a situation or circumstance.

The Counselor's Presentation. Just as counselors need to be aware of a client's body language during assessment, they need to know that the client will be aware of theirs. Counselors need to think about what their appearance presents to the client. In addition to things like clothing, this includes the counselor's tone. In fact, *how* a counselor conveys information is often just as, if not more important than, *what* is actually said. Sexuality educator and author Pamela M. Wilson (1991) talks about communication in terms of "the words and the music." She makes the important point that, just as when we listen to a song on the radio, the content (or words) are often less memorable at first than the way in which the content is delivered (the music). A client will look to the counselor for cues when hearing difficult information. A client will respond more calmly to a counselor whose voice is soothing and quiet, rather than to someone who bursts into the office with great energy and fanfare. It is all a part of being client-centered.

How a counselor carries her or himself is also important. Counselors should attempt to keep their body language open. This includes sitting without a barrier between the counselor and client, such as a desk. It also includes making eye contact*, and smiling when first greeting the client. Examples of closed body language include folding one's arms in front of one's chest, hugging a file or folder against the body, and sitting turned away from the client. These types of gestures imply, respectively, that the counselor is feeling defensive, that she or he has something to hide, and that she or he is either angry with or unconcerned about the client.

Clients respond to nonverbal cues as well as to verbal statements. In an age where casual dress in the workplace has become the norm, professionals need to be even more careful about the messages they give to their clients by their appearance. This is not about whether a counselor is perceived to be attractive, it is about the counselor making a thoughtful decision about what she or he wishes to convey nonverbally to the client. A counselor who wears a business suit when everyone else working at the clinic is wearing jeans will stand out and may be off-putting. On the other hand, a counselor who is dressed more casually than a client may be perceived as inexperienced.

Attending to the Client. Whether a counselor has just met a client, or has been working with or known the client for some time, she must always "attend" to the client. Attending refers to the ways in which a counselor lets the client know that she or he is completely focused on the client, and is not judging her or him in any way (Gladding, 2001). Attending can be done physically or verbally. Physically attending to a client might include making eye contact with the client, leaning forward, or even touching* a person's hand or arm to convey understanding.

A note about touch: While some counselors choose to take a person's hand to convey serious news or to comfort someone who may be crying or otherwise upset, it must be done with caution. People have very individual boundaries, which include physical touch. What a counselor might consider to be an empathetic gesture could alienate him from the client. In addition, when there is a significant difference in age, such as an adult counselor and a teen or child client, there is also a potential for the client to misconstrue the touch as a more intimate gesture than it had been intended. Many clinics and schools have developed policies that outline the types of interactions that are permissible between staff and clients. Some very explicitly forbid any physical touch between clients to avoid misunderstanding and accusations of inappropriate conduct or abuse. All health counselors, regardless of the setting in which they work, should become familiar with policies relating to counselor–client boundaries.

Verbally attending behavior can include minimal encouragers. These are sounds or brief statements that show the client that you are listening, but that don't interrupt the client's train of thought (Gladding, 2001). This might include saying, "unh-huh" or "I see." Caution should be taken when using minimal encouragers, however. They can easily be overused, becoming more like a verbal tic than a counseling technique. For example, saying, "unh-huh, unh-huh" or "right, right, right," after every statement the client makes can sound dismissive, as if the counselor is trying to rush the client through a story or session. This, of course, defeats the purpose of using minimal encouragers in the first place.

A nonverbal tic might include tapping a pen against a desk or file folder, or bouncing one's knee up and down quickly. Nonverbal tics can send particular messages to the client—again, that the counselor is uncomfortable, trying to rush the client, and so on.

Another element of body language a counselor must be aware of is his or her facial expressions. Even if a counselor does not say, "I disagree with the decision you've made," this information can be conveyed loud and clear through a frown, shrug, or other types of nonverbal communication. While a counselor does not necessarily need to remain expressionless throughout the entire meeting with the client, she or he must remain aware of what is conveyed through nonverbal body language as raised eyebrows, smiles or frowns, shrugs, sighs, and more.

A note about eye contact and body language: In some cultures, it is inappropriate to make eye contact with other people. If you notice that a client is not making eye contact with you, you may wish to note it. In some cases, this will indicate that he or she is uncomfortable in the setting. In other cases, they may be indicating respect by not making eye contact—or feeling uncomfortable that you are making eye contact with them.

Paying attention to the climate is an important part of building something called **rapport**. Rapport is a process by which a counselor creates a comfortable, warm, trusting relationship with a

---

Rapport. A process by which the counselor creates a comfortable, warm trusting relationship with a client.

---

client (Gladding, 2001). Most of us have experienced working with a health-care professional or health counselor who has not seemed concerned about building rapport. The counselor enters the room, does not address us by name, does not introduce her or himself, then begins firing question after question at us. The result is that we end up feeling uncomfortable, mistrustful, and perhaps even belligerent in return. There is no incentive for us to provide information because we do not have faith in this professional and what she or he may do with the information.

Conversely, a health counselor who cares about building rapport with her client will:

1. Walk into the room, make eye contact with and then smile at the client.

2. Introduce herself and ask the client what she or he would like to be called. (Some clients, particularly older clients, may prefer a more formal address of "Mr." or "Mrs." Others might prefer a nickname that does not appear in their formal records.)

3. Explain up front what her role is, how long they will be meeting together, and what, if anything, the client needs to do next. For example, a health counselor might say, "Hi, my name is Jessica Rodriguez. I'm going to be asking you some questions from this form to see how we can best help you today. This should take about twenty minutes, and then I'll take you in to see the doctor."

A client usually needs to deal with a number of people in the same setting. For example, a woman who has an appointment at a reproductive health clinic may see a receptionist, an intake counselor, a gynecologist, a social worker, and any number of other professionals, depending on why she has made her appointment there. If everyone, from the receptionist to the social worker makes the effort to build rapport with the client, the client will see the entire clinic as a safe, warm, inviting atmosphere. If only a few out of however many professionals she sees incorporates rapport-building skills, she will leave with a mixed experience. And if only one person or none of the professionals she sees seems invested in building rapport with her, she will leave feeling vulnerable, angry, and hesitant to return. Building rapport is very strongly valued within the formal therapy environment. However, a health-care setting, school, or any other environment in which a health counselor may work should consider rapport equally as vital to being client-centered.

All of the techniques we just discussed are part of the counselor's attempt to convey something called empathy. Empathy is very different from sympathy. When a person feels sympathy for another person, it involves feeling sad for that person. Sympathy involves an emotional response, where the person feeling sympathy experiences actual sadness, anger, or any other negative emotion the other person is experiencing. For example, if a client came in and said her mother had just died and was clearly distraught, the counselor might begin to feel sympathy for the client, even feeling sad herself. A person does not have to experience the same event or circumstance in order to feel sympathy. It is clear that death of an intimate would be a hurtful experience. Therefore, the counselor may feel sympathetic, regardless of whether he had lost a parent himself or not.

Empathy, however, refers to the ways in which a counselor can understand and effectively communicate back to a client what the client is or has been experiencing. (Gladding, 2001). For example, if a client were a trader at the stock exchange and were to talk about his 70-hour work week and the pressures of working in such a high-stress environment, the counselor could respond to this in one of two ways. An ineffective response would be to minimize the client's experience, or try to make it seem less stressful than it is. He might say, "Oh, it really can't be *that* bad. It's all in how you deal with stress." Another ineffective, although unfortunately overused response is, "I know how you feel! Last week, I had 15 clients in one week." A counselor who gives either of these responses is not demonstrating an understanding of the client's experience. The counselor is not a stock trader, so he cannot know what the client's experience truly is. In addition, the client's experience of his workday is irrelevant. A comparison is, therefore, inappro-

priate. Even if the counselor had experienced something similar to the client—as in the previous example of losing a parent—no one knows exactly how another person experiences loss, pain, excitement, or any other emotion, positive or negative. Saying "I know how you feel" is not only disrespectful to the client, but it is also false.

A more appropriate response might be, "Wow, it sounds like you have a lot going on right now." This statement acknowledges that the counselor understands that the client's work is stressful to the client without trying to offer a solution just yet. This is similar to paraphrasing, discussed later.

Setting Boundaries with a Client

Generally speaking, the concept of boundaries often gets a bad rap. Parents sometimes fear that putting up boundaries with their children will stifle creativity and growth. Partners and spouses often fear that putting a boundary up in a romantic relationship will be perceived as an ultimatum and imminent end of the relationship. Professionals, particularly those in the so-called "helping professions," feel like they are not fulfilling clients' expectations if they put up a boundary, or acknowledge that there is something that they cannot do for their clients. However, quite the opposite is true. Boundaries serve very important purposes, for clients and counselors alike.

A **boundary** is a physical or psychological parameter within which a counselor works with a client (Gladding, 2001). There are environmental boundaries, such as restricted areas of a hospital with entrances marked "Staff Only." There are physical boundaries, such as whether a counselor and client have any kind of physical contact like a handshake or comforting touch (mentioned earlier). There are service boundaries, such as if a client were to go to a health center and ask a phlebotomist to help her apply for social security benefits, which is not the phlebotomist's job. There are

Boundaries. Physical or psychological parameters within which a counselor works with a client.

process boundaries, which include starting and ending a session or meeting on time, even if a client comes late to an appointment. Finally, there are personal boundaries, which include how much a client or counselor shares of their personal lives. The most common personal boundaries deal with confidentiality and self-disclosure.

Confidentiality

Medical professionals, counselors, therapists, social workers, and any others employed by a health center are bound by confidentiality. This refers to the professional's obligation not to disclose anything about the client without the client's written consent (Gladding, 2001). A standard line many counselors use is, "What is said in this room, stays in this room." However, this is not necessarily accurate for two reasons: first, confidentiality often binds an entire health setting, not just an individual. In a multiservice setting, it is imperative that the counselor share information with the other professionals involved in the client's case. If a nutritionist were working with a client who was recovering from a heart attack and the client's doctor asked what the client's progress was, the nutritionist certainly would not say, "I can't tell you that, it's confidential." However, if the client were working with a doctor who was not a part of the same hospital, clinic, or health setting as the nutritionist, the nutritionist would need to obtain a signed consent form allowing her to share any information about the client with that doctor. Most health centers have standard forms that will be signed by the client during the intake process.

Another reason why a health counselor cannot guarantee confidentiality is that there are times when a counselor must, legally, break confidentiality. The general guideline for this is if the client says that he intends to seriously harm himself or someone else. With a minor (someone under the age of 18), confidentiality must also be broken if the young person is being hurt by someone else, including a family member. Teachers and health professionals are what are called mandated reporters. This means that if a child were to reveal that she was being sexually abused, or if a client of any age

were to say that he intended to go home and kill himself or his partner, the counselor would be required by law to intervene. The intervention is usually made with the support of the counselor's supervisor—although sometimes the counselor must act more quickly than that, especially if the client prepares to leave before the intervention can be made. Doing so always involves breaking confidentiality, which is why the purviews of confidentiality *must* be stated at the beginning of a meeting or formal session. A counselor can do this by saying to a client, "Whatever you share with me will be confidential within our health center. We will not share any information with another person unless you give us written permission. The only situation under which we would not need your written consent is if you were to tell us that you were going to seriously hurt yourself or someone else." Again, with a minor client (someone under 18), it is important to also explain that the counselor would need to break confidentiality if she learned that the child was being hurt in any way. Guaranteeing confidentiality and then breaking it can be quite traumatic to a client. Imagine how Mohan was feeling when Jamal, who had promised to keep their conversation confidential, picked up the phone and began calling Mohan's father!

Counselors are sometimes concerned that making a disclaimer up front about breaking confidentiality will dissuade a client from speaking openly. However, the contrary is often true, particularly in cases where a child is being sexually abused and does not know what to do about it. The client may actually be *more* likely to disclose the abuse knowing that the counselor is the one who would report it, not her or him.

Client and Counselor Self-Disclosure

Self-disclosure refers to when a person shares personal information about her or himself. People disclose personal information about themselves

---

Self-disclosure. Refers to when a person shares personal information about him or her self with another person.

every day without even thinking about it. In a counseling relationship, the client is often asked to provide and discuss very personal information. Client self-disclosure is to be encouraged, since it provides the information the counselor needs for assessment, treatment plan, and referrals.

When it comes to counselor self-disclosure, however, the counselor has some careful thinking to do. Sometimes, the client will ask the counselor personal questions. This is usually done for any number of reasons. A client may feel self-conscious that she or he has been talking for so long and need a break. A client may be feeling curious about the counselor and want to know more about her or him. A client may want to know more about the counselor's background in order to assess for her or himself whether the counselor is qualified to be discussing a particular topic. Some questions a client might ask could include, "Have you ever had a heart attack?" or "When you were my age, did you ever have an eating disorder?" A client may also want to know that she or he is not alone in the health concern. This tends to arise most frequently when the counselor and client have certain characteristics in common—such as age, race, gender, and so on.

Regardless of the reason for asking the question, counselor self-disclosure is often a slippery slope. Health professionals have quite a range of thoughts and feelings on the issue. Traditional therapists from the Freudian school will say that the counselor should disclose absolutely no personal information whatsoever. Some types of counseling, such as drug and alcohol counseling, often use a counselor's past as a significant part of the client's treatment. Therefore, the expectations are that a drug and alcohol rehabilitation counselor would disclose more personal information than another type of counselor. There is also a range of thoughts and beliefs in between the two extremes.

One way of thinking about self-disclosure is in terms of a five-point scale (see Figure 2.2). A counselor who is at 0 would disclose little more than her name, title, and function at the agency or school. The advantages of doing this is that the focus of the treatment remains completely on the client. No personal information about the counselor is discussed; therefore there can be no distraction from the needs of the client. The potential disadvantages are that the counseling relationship is one-sided, and some clients may misinterpret the counselor's lack of disclosure as discomfort, distance, or indifference. In ongoing relationships, such as a school environment, it is virtually impossible to remain at 0 with students or team members.

A counselor at 3 or above puts absolutely no limits on what she shares with the client. Personal information is disclosed without forethought or care. Doing so serves only the counselor, not the client. A counselor who uses her own personal experiences so openly and frequently in the counseling process is more interested in talking about herself. She assumes that, as a counselor, her decisions were the best decisions. This puts the focus on her, not on the client.

Most counselors fluctuate somewhere between 1 and 2—they use personal stories in their work with clients, particularly young people, to make an important point. For example, a counselor who grew up in a low-income neighborhood and returns to work with young people in that neighborhood can serve an important purpose by demonstrating that someone similar to them was able to become a successful professional. At the same time, however, this technique could backfire on the counselor. The implication that "If I could make it, you can" may set the clients up for added disappointment if they are, for any reason, unable to break from poverty and

Figure 2.2
A Five-Point Scale of Self-Disclosure

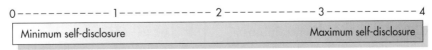

succeed as she did. Basically, a counselor who thinks that by telling her story she will make a difference in the client's life puts much too much stock in her own power. Behavior change does not happen just because a person says, "If I was able to quit smoking, anyone can!"

Although every counselor must make her or his own decisions, it is generally recommended that a health counselor find a comfortable place between 0 and 1, especially at the beginning of the counseling relationship. How close to or beyond 1 a counselor goes will be based on the length and context of the counseling relationship, on the role of the counselor, and on the information shared. For example, a teacher who has been tutoring a student after school for several months may feel more comfortable answering questions in the realm of relationship status, whether she or he has any children, what she or he was like as a teenager, and so on. However, care should always be taken whenever a counselor begins to disclose personal information about her or himself. Always remember that *once information is shared, the counselor has absolutely no control over how the listener interprets or may use it.* Also, sharing one piece of personal information sets a precedent that additional questions relating to the counselor's personal life are also appropriate. If boundaries have not been established up front, it may be difficult for the counselor to establish them at a later date.

Finally, a counselor who puts himself at 3 or higher is someone who may have serious boundary issues himself and needs to work with a supervisor to look at this. Someone at 4 might be among those misguided professionals who would unwisely pursue a social or romantic relationship with a client. This is *never* appropriate. Most clinics, schools, and social-service agencies have clear policies prohibiting these types of relationships. A counselor who ignores these policies puts his job in jeopardy, and betrays the sanctity of the counselor–client relationship. In addition, having a sexual or romantic relationship with a client in some cases may be illegal, depending on the age of the client. Any counselor considering an intimate relationship with a client must seek guidance and

support immediately before doing himself and the client any harm.

The bottom line is, any self-disclosure, whether a part of casual conversation or a part of the intervention or treatment process, should be well thought-out, and done with great care. Hedgepeth & Helmich (1996) offer the following questions a health counselor can ask her or himself as guidelines for determining whether and when self-disclosure by the health counselor is appropriate:

- Is this disclosure really necessary in order for me to make my point effectively?

- Is what I am thinking about disclosing developmentally appropriate for the age and experience level of the individual or group in front of me?

- Will disclosing this information have a potentially positive or deleterious affect on my relationship with this individual or group? How might it affect issues of trust between the client or group and myself? How might it affect the client's or group's level of comfort?

- Is my timing for disclosing this information appropriate, keeping in mind that if it is shared too early in the relationship it could limit further discussion or turn the focus on me, or too late in the relationship it could make it appear as if I am trying to bring the discussion to a close?

Depending on the answers to any or all of these questions, the counselor may choose to share the information as originally intended, less information, or nothing.

Hedgepeth & Helmich (1996) urge health counselors and educators to "separate the message from the messenger." This means that personal experience is not necessarily a prerequisite for being able to provide information and a caring, nurturing environment.

Thinking about self-disclosure: If you went in to be tested for a sexually transmitted disease (STD), and the clinician told you that he had had gonorrhea before and it was no big deal, how do you think you'd feel? How might he be able to make you feel more comfortable about the testing process rather than to disclose his previous experience with an STD?

Asking the Right Question

Over time, counselors must learn to become proficient in the art of questioning. There are different kinds of questions, each of which serves its own purpose within the counseling process:

■ The **open-ended question** is used primarily at the beginning of a counseling relationship, or when a new issue is brought up within the context of an ongoing relationship. An open-ended question is one that cannot be answered definitively with a "yes," "no," or other one-word answer.

For example, a client thinks she has been exposed to HIV, and goes to a local health department for testing. After the counselor introduces himself, he should ask open-ended questions to assess the client's knowledge and risk for HIV. The following are examples of open-ended questions the counselor might use:

"Can you tell me why you came here today?"

"What do you know about how HIV is transmitted?"

The first question assesses what the client is expecting from the clinic. This will help the counselor know up front if the client is expecting anything that is not available (service boundaries). The second question provides the counselor with vital information about what the client knows about HIV and whether she was truly at risk. For example, if she says, "Well, I shared a soda with a friend and later found out that he was HIV positive," the counselor will be able to both correct the client's misinformation and determine whether there was any other way in which the woman may have been exposed to HIV. Open-ended questions are used during assessment because the counselor is trying to obtain as much information about the situation as possible.

■ A **close-ended** or **closed** question is one that has a specific answer to it. This could be a "yes," "no," or a particular piece of information. Closed questions might include, "Have you ever had trouble breathing before?" or "How old are you?" Because closed questions tend to feel more direct, they are usually used later in the counseling relationship. If they must be used earlier on, they should be prefaced by an explanation of why the questions are necessary. For example, "I need to ask you some direct questions about your relationship. These are standard questions that we ask all our clients."

Waiting for the Answer

When asking questions, the counselor must learn two important techniques: to tolerate the silence that clients often need while formulating their answers, and to wait for the answer to a question before asking another.

Silence can be difficult to tolerate. Counselors are often uncomfortable with silence because they feel they should be doing something. And if the counselor has limited time with her client, she may feel pressured to move the appointment or meeting forward. Even in this situation, it is important to tolerate silence whenever possible. It can take a client a few moments to formulate an answer. He may need some time to recall information, or to figure out how to answer in a way that feels comfortable to him. A client who is asked a barrage of questions, one right after the other, will feel like he is being interrogated. Timing questions is something a counselor learns with time and experience.

Alternatives to Asking

Sometimes, asking a particular question can lead a client down one road, when she or he may have gone down another if left to her or his own devices. For this reason, a counselor can try two different techniques that are used to obtain information without asking a question. One is noticing, and the other is paraphrasing.

Noticing involves sharing with the client something the counselor has observed. For example, "You seem to get angry every time we talk about your parents," or, "You're really quiet today." Noticing is different from questioning because there is no question involved. It puts the onus on the client to talk about what she or he wants to talk about.

Another technique a counselor can use when working with a client is called **paraphrasing.** When a counselor paraphrases what a client has just said, he takes a statement or concept and puts it into simpler, more concise, yet still nonjudgmental terms (Gladding, 2001). This serves several purposes. First, it reinforces for the client that the counselor is listening to and understands what the client is saying and has been experiencing. Second, if the counselor paraphrases a concept incorrectly, the client can clarify what she has said. That way, the counselor will be sure to understand the issue from the client's viewpoint. Third, it can help a client, particularly one who may be feeling particularly emotional or unfocused in the moment, break through the many different emotions they may be feeling and focus on the issue at hand. Finally, if the client is expressing negative feelings about her or himself, the counselor's paraphrasing in a nonjudgmental way will serve to mitigate the negativity rather than reinforce it for the client. Paraphrasing statements might start with, "It sounds like . . . " or "So what you're saying is . . ." or "Let me see if I understand what you mean. You seem to feel like . . . ", and so on.

For example, a teen gymnast who is speaking with her coach after what she considers to be a bad practice might go off, saying "I told my mom I couldn't stay up so late baby-sitting my little brother last night! I was awful today, and it's all her fault. She doesn't understand how important this is to me. She never supports me in anything." The counselor (who in the case is her coach) might paraphrase what she just said by saying, "It sounds like you're really frustrated with your mom," or "So what you're saying is, you had an off practice and you feel your mom's responsible for that."

In the first sample response, the gymnast will very likely respond in the positive, saying, "I am frustrated. She makes me really mad sometimes." In this way, the client has confirmed for the counselor that the paraphrasing was accurate. Once this is done, the counselor can make an intervention. She might say, "Have you considered talking with your mom and telling her how much this means to you?" Note that this is different from saying, "Well, if you're so frustrated with your mom, then you need to tell her so." By putting this in the form of a question, the counselor is giving the client something to consider—and letting the client decide for herself whether the suggestion has any merit.

In the second sample response, the counselor is paraphrasing in a way that gently points out a disparity in the client's thought process. While she may very well have had an off practice, she seems to be displacing her frustration onto her mother rather than owning the fact that she simply had an off day. The client might respond to the counselor by saying, "No, it's not her fault I had a bad practice. But I do wish she would ask me about practice more and come to a meet once in a while." If this were to happen, the counselor will have helped the client understand and accept her responsibility for performing inadequately during practice. She will also have helped the client reveal the true source of her frustration: that gymnastics means a great deal to her, and she wants her mother to support her in her enthusiasm by watching her from time to time.

Defense Mechanisms

Counseling is never as easy as simply asking questions and getting clear answers. Many elements can serve as barriers within the counseling process. Among these are **defenses.**

Noticing. When a counselor shares with the client something the counselor has observed.

Paraphrasing. When a counselor takes a client's statement or concept and puts it into simpler, more concise, yet still nonjudgmental terms.

Defenses. Ways in which a person attempts to protect her or himself against anxiety. These can include denial, rationalization, regression, and so on.

A defense is a way in which a person attempts to protect her or himself against anxiety (Gladding, 2001, p. 35). Defense mechanisms are psychological guards that keep people from facing very stressful situations. Some of the more common defenses that a health counselor will come across are denial, rationalization, regression, and intellectualization.

- **Denial** is a defense that has made its way into society's lay language to the extent that most people have a sense of what it means. A person who acts as if something is not real, or ignores the situation or circumstance, can be said to be "in denial." (Gladding, 2001, p. 36). For example, a person who is diagnosed with HIV but takes no steps in her treatment or to practice safer sex may be in denial. The concept of having HIV is so overwhelming that her mind cannot acknowledge it as real.

- **Rationalization** is when a person tries to explain a situation or behavior in a way that will make what is clearly unacceptable (or, in the context of this textbook, unhealthy) acceptable. For example, a man who smokes a pack of cigarettes a day and says, "Hey, I'm not at risk—no one in my family ever had lung cancer" is rationalizing his unhealthy behavior. His mind does not want to accept the risks smoking carries with it, and therefore must come up with a valid reason, one that he can accept, to continue smoking.

- **Regression** is when a person responds to a stressful for anxiety-inducing situation by returning to a previous developmental stage (Gladding, 2001, p. 103). For example, an adolescent whose parent dies may deal with this stressor by wanting to sleep in his other parent's bed, by wetting himself in his sleep, by sucking his thumb, or by performing any other behaviors that are characteristic of early childhood, rather than adolescence.

- **Intellectualization** is a defense mechanism that is seen when a client deals with a stressor or issue by talking about it abstractly, focusing on the process of discussing a topic to avoid the feelings the stressor induces. (Gladding, 2001, p. 64). For example, a client who is diagnosed with inoperable cancer may respond to the news by talking about how much he knows about cancer. He will not respond to the news directly, or show any emotion. Instead, he will launch into a soliloquy of complicated medical terms, statistical facts, or anything else relating to the topic, but not to him. By keeping the focus on the information itself, the client's mind does not allow itself to deal with the reality of the devastating news.

A health counselor who suspects that a client is using a defense in order to cope with a given situation should never confront the defense. A defense serves an important purpose. Most health counselors have neither the training nor the time to work through a defense in the way it should be done to best serve the client. A health counselor can certainly note in a client's file or for her own edification that the client seems to be in denial or regresses under circumstances. However, a therapist, psychologist, or psychiatrist should determine whether it is necessary to confront a defense, and if so, when and how.

This is an important concept, particularly for the health counselors who end up in the role of counselor without much formal training. Recall the example given earlier of the gymnast who voices frustration about how she perceived her mother to have affected her practice. An adult may feel tempted to say, "Come on, your mother wasn't even here. You had a bad practice, and that's it. Move on." A response like this minimizes the young person's experience, embarrasses her, and will pretty much guarantee that she will never seek this adult out again for help or support.

Working with Groups

Health counseling is not restricted to one-on-one interactions between counselor and client. Health counseling can be provided in a group setting, within a number of contexts. However, as mentioned at the beginning of the chapter, group counseling skills can be applied to any group environment, whether it is a classroom environment, professional meeting, team discussions, or other situation. Just as there are tomes written about the history of counseling, there are myriad resources available about group work in a range of settings. We will touch on only a few elements of group work here.

Some agencies offer groups on a variety of topics. More formal support groups include:

- bereavement groups for people who have lost a loved one

- sexual abuse, rape, or incest survivor groups to help the members heal from their trauma

- family therapeutic groups, where an issue comes up for one family member that affects and/or requires the support of the rest of the family

- "anonymous" groups, which provide much-needed support to people recovering from addictions. These include Narcotics Anonymous, Alcoholics Anonymous, Overeaters Anonymous, and more

Formal group work, which is done by a therapist or counselor trained in this area, has a number of benefits that are different from, although in some cases supplemental to, the benefits gained from individual treatment. Among the benefits Ormont (1992) describes are the following:

■ **Group work encourages people to exhibit their negative behaviors in a safe environment.** Because there are a number of people in the room to which an individual can respond, that person is more likely to demonstrate some of the behaviors that she has come to identify in her own life as problematic. Quite simply, in individual work a person is quite often recounting an experience or aspect of who she or he is. In group work, a person cannot help but behave in this way. It enables the counselor as well as the rest of the group to observe the person as she truly is.

■ **Group work provides an atmosphere in which people can not only be themselves and demonstrate the self-destructive behavior, but also see how others respond to this type of behavior.** In this way, group work provides an excel-lent learning environment for a client. For example, a person in a group may consistently snort impatiently whenever another person expresses how he or she feels. The counselor can intervene by pointing out to the person that he does that, and by asking the group how it makes them feel when that person reacts in this way. In some cases, the person might not be aware that they even have this habit. Pointing it out in a safe environment can help a person take greater responsibility for who they are and how the manner in which they act can affect other people.

■ **Groups provide an opportunity for people to practice different kinds of behaviors before trying them out in the real world.** Once a person has become aware of his challenging behavior, he will hopefully work within the group to find ways of managing his feelings and behaving in ways that are less self-destructive and more respectful to others. As we all know, we have people in our lives who are perhaps kinder than we would like them to be. A therapeutic or support group contains members who do not hold back. While not intentionally hard on a particular individual, the group will be honest in its feedback. This is among the most valuable aspects of a group experience.

The level of intensity of a particular group should dictate the level of training the facilitator should have. For example, the coach's informal groups might result in disclosures of sexual abuse, eating disorders, and more. This coach should immediately take steps to provide referrals to the affected team members. She should not, however, turn her group into a support group for sexual-abuse survivors. Without the training in this specific topic, she could end up opening discussions that neither she nor the team is prepared to handle. In the end, this could do much more harm than good.

Health counselors frequently offer groups that are informational in scope. For example, health educators working in a school setting often are charged with providing classes on health education. Health educators in a social-service agency or clinic setting will provide group workshops on a range of health-related topics, either in-house, at schools, or in other social-service settings. For the purposes of this chapter, we will focus more on informational sessions, although the skills discussed can apply to just about any group environment.

A vital concept in group work is to always keep the best interest of the entire group in mind. One way in which a health counselor can do this is by establishing ground rules. Ground rules are used most effectively in educational settings—for example, an informational workshop on nutrition, health education, and so on. Ground rules are particularly important in settings where the topic to be discussed is particularly sensitive. For example, some health educators provide workshops on sexuality, reproductive health, and other intimate topics. Ground rules set an equal stage for everyone present, laying down expectations for how everyone, including the counselor (or in this setting, facilitator), will act.

It is important for ground rules to be established by the group, not by the group facilitator or health counselor. The health counselor can provide suggestions if the group is unable to come up with any, or if the group leaves out a ground rule that is particularly important. However, groups must feel that they, not the health counselor, have established their own guidelines for conduct. That way, they will be more likely to adhere to the rules and refer back to them if they feel that someone in the group is not abiding by them.

Some examples of standard ground rules are:

- **Respect.** This means that people will allow differences of opinion, agreeing to disagree as necessary.

- **No put-downs.** In line with respect, this ground rule reinforces the concept that there is no such thing as a stupid question. People in the group should feel that they can say or ask anything, and not be ridiculed by other members for what they say, how they say it, or the fact that they do not know the particular information.

- **The right to pass.** In any group, the health counselor should encourage people to participate as much as possible. However, particularly when dealing with a sensitive topic like sexuality, participants should also be allowed the right to *not* participate in a given activity without repercussion from the health counselor or the group.

- **Confidentiality.** We frequently hear people say, "What's said in the room stays in the room." This is not exactly accurate. We do want people to leave the group and discuss concepts and information with others and in their own lives. What this rule refers to is really not using a piece of information against a person at a later date. For example, if during a workshop on birth control a 14-year-old boy discloses that he is still a virgin, he should not have to fear being ridiculed about that by his friends during the group or later in school. Counselors must remember, however, that the disclaimer relating to confidentiality between a counselor and individual client still applies to a group setting. If anyone were to share that someone was hurting them, or they were thinking of hurting themselves or someone else, the counselor would need to break confidentiality in order to protect that person.

- **Use "I" messages.** This means that a person will speak for her or himself, rather than make generalizations about an entire group of people. Let us use the example of the workshop about birth control given above. If a girl were to say, "All guys want from a girl is sex," the counselor should point to the ground rules and ask her to speak for herself and her own experience. This might sound more like, "The guys I've met have always been more interested in sex than in a relationship." In that way, she is not generalizing about boys and men in general. This demonstrates respect for the safety and dignity of everyone in the room.

There are other ground rules that the counselor may wish to introduce, such as "no cell phones," "avoid side conversations," and "start and end on time." These serve to ensure that everyone in the group has as productive an experience as possible, while continuing the process of setting boundaries.

Once ground rules are established, the group will evolve on its own. The leader or facilitator must be clear on his relationship to the group. He plays an important role, but he is not an equal member of the group. Therefore, the issues discussed earlier in this chapter in relation to boundaries, climate setting, and building rapport still apply in a group setting.

Summary

Health counseling is rooted in the teachings of psychoanalysis, founded by Sigmund Freud. Other theorists, including Margaret Mahler, Erik Erikson, Jean Piaget, and Melanie Klein, also made significant contributions to understanding counseling techniques. Health counseling is currently considered from a biopsychosocial standpoint, regarding each of the three as equally important parts of the whole.

Health counseling may include information provision and options counseling, but it is neither therapy nor advice. It should, however, always be client-centered in its approach.

Health counselors must pay close attention to climate setting when first meeting a client. This includes how the physical environment looks and is managed by the counselor. It also includes ensuring that materials and posters reflect our society's broad diversity, including different races, ethnicities, and cultures, genders and sexual orientations, ages, and physical abilities. It has to do with the language used, how a counselor lets the client know she or he is being heard, and how the counselor presents her or himself to a client. A counselor can give positive messages by attending to a client, although care must be taken in order to do so effectively.

After making an initial assessment and determining the client's presenting problem, counselors must seek to build rapport. They can do this by displaying empathy toward the client, setting appropriate boundaries, and maintaining confidentiality—unless a circumstance requires that confidentiality be broken. A counselor must think before disclosing personal information about her or himself, doing so only when the information could benefit the client's situation.

Health counselors can learn a great deal about their clients by asking the right questions. These include open-ended questions at the beginning of a counseling relationship, and closed questions for specific information-gathering purposes. As an alternative to asking questions, counselors can notice things about their client's affect, or paraphrase something the client has just said to incite further comments or discussion.

When a person is faced with a particularly stressful situation, she or he may cope by setting up defenses. Among these are denial, rationalization, regression, and intellectualization. A health counselor should always respect these defenses, referring the client to a mental health professional who is trained in negotiating whether and how to confront and deal with a particular defense.

Health counseling can also include group work, such as support groups for abuse survivors, bereavement groups, family-therapy groups, and so-called "anonymous" groups. Group work can be very beneficial to certain individuals, although in setting a safe environment it is important to establish ground rules with the group.

Health counseling is a vastly growing field. Many health students find themselves faced with situations where their knowledge of the content is more than sufficient, but their facility with handling the social and psychological aspects of a relationship with a client is lacking. For this reason, it is imperative that future health counselors focus as much on the "counseling" aspect as they do on the "health."

> Thinking about health counseling: Having read this chapter, go back to the case study at the beginning of the chapter. Certainly, Jamal had many options open to him, but because he did not have much experience and was not trained in basic counseling skills, he made some unwise choices. What would you do differently if you were the health counselor working with Mohan?

Key Terms

affect, 24

assessment, 22

biopsychosocial, 19

boundary, 27

client, 17

client-centered, 22

counselor, 17

defenses, 32

denial, 24

noticing, 32

paraphrasing, 32

rapport, 26

self-disclosure, 28

Questions for Discussion

1. How much information do you think you would feel comfortable sharing about yourself with a client? On what do you base your reasons for sharing this information, but not something else? Where do you draw the line, and how do you justify doing so?

2. What is the most challenging prospect about being a health counselor for you? What makes this aspect of health counseling more or less challenging? How do you think you will deal with overcoming this challenging if you are faced with it in the future?

3. Should parents be able to know everything their teen or adolescent children discuss with a health counselor? Why or why not? Is it different if the health counselor is in a medical field vs. an educational setting? Why or why not?

4. What would be an issue that you do not think you would be able to remain neutral about? For some counselors, this is abortion, for others it might be sexual or relationship abuse. Figure out what it might be for you, and then think about how you might respond if a client were to come to you with that as the presenting problem.

5. If a client is no longer under the care of a counselor, and they are both consenting adults, would it be all right for them to have a romantic relationship? Why or why not? Would your answer change if the person had not been a client for more than a year? More than five years? On what do you base your thoughts?

Related Web Sites

http://www.allaboutcounseling.com
All About Counseling—This site contains articles, FAQ, and self-help information and offers discussion opportunities, free listings in their professionals directory, and professional resources for counselors.

http://www.psych.org
American Psychiatric Association—Features new, current information, jobs, and links to resources by the world's largest psychiatric organization

http://www.apa.org
American Psychological Association—A major clearinghouse for information of interest to students, professionals, and the public. Features current news, articles, programs information, a consumer help center, and more.

http://www.naswdc.org
National Association of Social Workers—This site features links related to ethics, publications, continuing education, career opportunities, certifications, advocacy, practice and diversity issues, among others.

http://www.psychlinks.cjb.net
Psychology Information and Research—Features many useful psychology-related links.

CHAPTER 3

Ethical Issues in Health Counseling

JERROLD S. GREENBERG, PH.D.

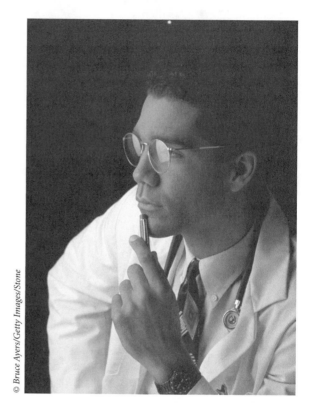

© *Bruce Ayers/Getty Images/Stone*

OBJECTIVES

By the end of the chapter, the reader should be able to:

- Define and differentiate between ethics, morality, ethical principles, ethical dilemmas, and values

- List and describe at least five ethical principles

- Differentiate between rule ethics and situation ethics

- Describe the four ethical theories of natural law, utilitarianism, paternalism, and distributive justice

- Justify the use of coercion using the Principle of Proportionality and the Principle of Self-Determination

- Cite the purposes of codes of ethics and differentiate between standards, principles, and rules

- List four sections of the Code of Ethics for the Health Education Profession that is applicable to health counseling

- Describe three ethical issues that might be encountered by health counselors

Case Study

Linda is a 23-year-old woman who has been trying to get pregnant with no success over the past few months. It is difficult to get a coherent medical history from her. She has a hard time focusing on your questions and doesn't understand about the different ways to determine if she is ovulating.

Linda has a 3½-year-old son who is developmentally delayed with mild cerebral palsy. He does not speak yet. However, Linda does not acknowledge this unless asked about it directly. She is married to a man who she describes as physically abusive. This man is not the father of her child. She tells you that they are in family therapy to work on the problem of his physical abuse.

She asks questions about using inhaled propellants, easily purchased at "head" shops, and wonders whether that could keep a person from becoming pregnant. When asked directly, she does not admit to any drug use. She is having trouble taking care of herself and her child at the present time. Although her relationship is problematic, she is in therapy to work on these concerns.

She wants to have a child with her husband and seeks your help in getting pregnant (Razak & Schoenwald, 1989).

Facing A Difficult Choice

How is a health educator/counselor who is assigned to Linda to respond? The temptation might be to involve Linda in a lengthy discussion regarding her lifestyle and the additional stressors that would accompany another child. Given her abusive relationship, the possibility she is involved with drugs, and the responsibilities associated with raising a developmentally delayed child, which she already finds overwhelming, the health educator may believe it is unwise—maybe even unhealthy—for Linda to get pregnant. On the other hand, Linda has determined she wants another child. Is it appropriate, then, for the health educator/counselor to withhold information from Linda that would help her achieve that goal? A dilemma arises for the health educator/counselor when clients, students, and others they counsel make decisions the health educator/counselor believes are not in the best interest of the person being counseled. Is it appropriate—ethical—for the health educator/counselor to determine what is best for those they counsel and then attempt to influence the person to behave as the health educator/counselor has predetermined to be healthy? Is it appropriate for the health educator/counselor to facilitate an action desired by the person being counseled that the health educator/counselor believes is unhealthy?

These dilemmas are not uncommon to the experience of health education/counselors. Yet, it is beyond the scope of this chapter to propose solutions to each and every ethical issue encountered by health education/counselors. In fact, even if this were possible, it would probably be unwise. Health education/counselors need to employ their *own* values and perspectives to resolve ethical dilemmas to their satisfaction, rather than seek the Holy Grail that will instruct them what to do in all situations. That is not to say that a consideration of ethical issues in health counseling is not useful. We believe that a method—a system—can be learned and employed by health education/counselors to better resolve ethical issues. Consequently, we present this system in this chapter. We also believe that when health education/counselors can anticipate the ethical issues they might be likely to encounter, they will be better prepared to respond to them. Consequently, we discuss some of the more common ethical issues as well in this chapter.

A System for Resolving Ethical Issues

Before we discuss how to systematically resolve ethical issues, several terms need to be defined.

Ethics. Ethics is "a branch of philosophy that deals with systematic approaches to understanding morality" (Hiller, 1987). The key to remember is that **ethics** is a system by which one determines whether an action is moral or immoral.

Morality. Morality is a judgment about whether an action is "good" or "right," or "bad" or "wrong." **Morality,** therefore, refers to a specific situation or event that requires a decision regarding its "rightness" or "wrongness" (Greenberg, 2001; Thiroux, 1995). Consequently, the system of ethics is employed to determine whether an action, situation, or event is good or bad, right or wrong. To make this determination, ethical principles are employed.

Ethics. A system by which one determines whether an action is moral or immoral.

Morality. A judgment about whether an action is "good" or "right," "bad" or "wrong." Refers to specific situations or events.

Ethical Principles. **Ethical principles** are guidelines used to determine whether a situation or decision is moral or immoral. Examples of ethical principles include:

- Nonmaleficence—Whatever else is done, do no harm. For example, **nonmaleficence** has been applied "to several major issues in biomedical ethics, including the distinction between killing and letting die, the difference between withholding and withdrawing life-sustaining treatments, the judgments of quality of life, the treatment of seriously ill newborns, and the duties of proxy decision makers for incompetent patients" (Beauchamp and Childress, 1989). Nonmaleficence can be broken down into several components such as not inflicting harm, preventing harm, and removing harm when it is present.

- Beneficence—Beneficience is an obligation to do good; not doing harm is not good enough (Jecker, 1997). **Beneficence** has two components: providing benefits, and balancing benefits and harms. Since benefits are often accompanied by potential risks, this distinction is an important one. Consequently, it is imperative that health counselors make sure that benefits derived from an action exceed the risks associated with that action.

- Autonomy—Autonomy means people should be free to decide their own course of action as long as they do no harm to others. **Autonomy** is synonymous with individual choice, liberty, and being one's own person. Recognize, though, that no one is absolutely autonomous. There are numerous restraints that limit a person's autonomy such as social constraints and laws (Butler, 2001). The concept of informed consent is a reflection of the value of autonomy (Last, 1998). Without informed consent, one is not knowledgeable to decide for one's self. To withhold information from a client or student during counseling is to deprive that person of the ability to be autonomous. Similarly, if a person is coerced into an action, that person has not made an autonomous decision. Consider the implications of this last statement for persons referred to counseling and required to participate by the courts or the motor vehicle administration.

- Justice—Each person should be treated fairly and similarly given the circumstances. This does not mean that each person ought to be treated the same, just fairly. For example, someone who uses tobacco products might be expected to have his or her health-insurance premium be higher than someone who does not. In that instance, one might argue that the smoker is treated fairly since he or she is expected to access the health-care system more frequently and, thereby, use more of the health resources provided. Ethicists, therefore, interpret the ethical principle of **justice** to be more related to what people deserve than to treating them the same. They argue that people ought to be given their due. As Aristotle advised, equals must be treated equally, and unequals must be treated unequally. Some have referred to this interpretation as distributive justice. The conundrum raised by the ethical principle of justice—that is, distributive justice—relates to issues such as whether wealthy people ought to have access to the same health resources (for example counseling) as poorer people, or

---

Ethical principles. Guidelines used to determine whether a situation or decision is moral or immoral; for example, nonmaleficence, beneficence, autonomy, and so on.

Nonmaleficence. The ethical principle that describes the position "whatever else is done, do no harm."

Beneficence. The ethical principle to do good—not doing harm is not good enough. Includes benefits and balancing benefits and harms.

Autonomy. The ethical principle that people should be free to decide their own course of action as long as they do no harm to others.

Justice. The ethical principle that each person should be treated fairly and similarly given the circumstances, not treated the same.

whether their income ought to allow them access to a great array of health resources.

- Other Ethical Principles—There are other ethical principles as well. Among these are promise keeping, truthfulness, privacy, and confidentiality.

When we decide about the morality of a situation or action, we use these ethical principles to guide that decision. For example, to decide whether abortion is moral one might use the ethical principle of autonomy and state that a woman should be free to choose to do whatever she decides with her body and, therefore, abortion is moral. On the other hand, if we use the ethical principle of nonmaleficence and believe that life begins at conception we might decide that abortion is immoral since it does harm to the fetus, a living being.

Ethical Dilemmas. In many instances, however, two or more ethical principles compete with each other. That is, they lead to different determinations of the morality. These situations are called **ethical dilemmas.** Consider the health counselor who is counseling a client with a sexually transmitted disease. The health counselor might believe in autonomy and conclude, therefore, that the person being counseled ought to be free to decide whether to disclose his or her STD status with sexual partners. Yet, the health counselor might also believe in beneficence and, therefore, conclude that he or she has an obligation to inform a sexual partner of the client's STD status in order to benefit that person's health. Making decisions about morality is multifaceted.

Values. Ethical dilemmas are resolved by weighting the operative ethical principles and deciding which one(s) is more applicable in the particular situation. We call these weights values. A **value** is

Ethical dilemmas. Instances when two or more ethical principles compete with each other, leading to different determinations of morality.

Value. Estimation of worth developed over many years through numerous experiences and encounters that determine the weighting of ethical principles.

an estimation of worth. The greater the value, the more worth. As regards ethical dilemmas, when two or more ethical principles are in conflict with one another, we determine which one is more valuable and use that to guide our decision about the moral nature of the situation or action.

The interesting thing about values is that no two people have the exact same values. Values are developed over many years through numerous experiences and encounters. Values are affected by parents and upbringing, by teachers and education, by clergy and religious beliefs, by cultural influences, and by interactions with friends and coworkers. Given that no two people have all of these experiences in common, it is understandable that people differ in their values, and some differ more than others. So, since people differ in their values, and values are the determinants of the weighting of ethical principles decided on to guide decisions about morality, it is no small wonder that people will differ on judgments about the morality of a particular situation or action. Understood in this way, it becomes clear that most of the time when people argue about the morality of a situation or action (for example, abortion) it is not a group of bad or uninformed people arguing with a group of good or educated people but, rather, people who differ in their valuing of ethical principles because of their different backgrounds. Perhaps with this perspective, people will be more tolerant and open to different points of view regarding morality. This is an important understanding for health counselors to come to.

Using the case study presented at the beginning of this chapter, the health education-counselor would use the system of ethics to determine whether to provide Linda with the information she seeks that would help her get pregnant. In doing so, the health education/counselor would identify the ethical principles operative and value these before coming to a decision. For example, counselors who value autonomy most highly might conclude that Linda has a right to decide whether to have another child and, therefore, she is entitled to the information she requests. On the other hand, a health educator/counselor who most values maleficence might conclude that to provide information to Linda that would help her get pregnant would be doing harm to her family, to her young son, and to the child who would be borne if the information were provided.

Rule Ethicists and Situation Ethicists. Another distinction necessary for the discussion of ethical issues in health counseling is the difference between rule ethics and situation ethics. Rule ethicists believe there is a rule that governs all situations. For example, a rule ethicist might argue that all killing is immoral. Such a person might become a conscientious objector and refuse to serve in the military. On the other hand, situation ethicists believe that no one rule can be applied in all situations. That is, each situation must be judged on its own and the most appropriate action taken for that particular situation. A situation ethicist might argue that killing is moral in some situations, such as the war against Nazi Germany or against the Afghani Taliban harboring al-Qaeda terrorists. Recently, Wolfe (2001) criticized the moral philosophy of the American people as being too situational. Wolfe believes that Americans have rationalized their behavior, behavior that might otherwise be considered immoral, by taking the convenient way rather than the ethical way. He argues that Americans have redefined morality to suit their individual tastes and purposes, using situational ethics as the basis for this action. The result, Wolfe believes, is a lack of accountability and questionable moral behavior. Others would disagree, arguing that flexibility is needed in situations requiring moral decisions. What do you believe?

Health counselors who believe in rule ethics might decide that the use of mood-altering drugs is always immoral. Such counselors might work toward the goal of eliminating such drugs from the behavioral repertoire of all clients. On the other hand, health counselors who are situation ethicists might look at a client's situation and decide that, in some circumstances, the use of mood-altering drugs might be a valid choice. Perhaps the client is in chronic pain and the mood-altering drug provides temporarily relief from that pain. In this case, the health counselor who believes in situation ethics might have the safe use of mood-altering drugs as a goal of the counseling. The counselor would then work with the client to encourage using small doses of the drug, using it with someone else present in case there is a negative reaction, and/or using only the safest drugs and avoiding the physically addictive ones. Admittedly this is a controversial decision on the part of the counselor, but the point being made is that it can be justified as ethical by health counselors with a situation ethicist philosophy.

Ethical Theories of Health Promotion

A further prelude to a discussion of ethical issues in health counseling is the need to understand various ethical theories of health promotion. In a concise summary, O'Connell and Price (1983) describe the ethical theories of natural law, utilitarianism, paternalism, and distributive justice.

Natural Law

This theory is based on the ethical principle of autonomy and states that individuals have the right to choose their own health-related lifestyle without undue influence on the part of the health counselor or health educator. Even in the face of disagreement between the health counselor and the client, it is the client who determines the choice of action and should be supported by the counselor. The only time intervention by the health counselor is warranted is when the client's actions threaten the health and well-being of others. Using the rationale of natural law, cigarette smokers argue they should be free to choose for themselves whether they smoke, as long as their smoking does not adversely affect others. Also, women who believe abortion ought to be between a woman and her physician present a natural-law argument. They are often heard to state that a woman ought to be free to do with her body as she sees fit. One of the most cogent defenses of natural law for the health education/promotion/counseling professions is made by Buchanan (2000) who defines the role of these professions as fostering the *good life* in students/clients. The good life, Buchanan continues, is not using a condom during sexual intercourse or refraining from smoking. Rather, the good life consists of living with integrity, dignity, autonomy, and responsibility. The health counselor advocating this point of view will encourage the client to develop these goals—the good life—by helping the client to process the situation and then decide for him or her self the best course of action.

Utilitarianism

Health counselors believing in utilitarianism feel justified in curtailing or influencing a client's actions if that decision would benefit the society as a whole. As such, utilitarianism is sometimes referred to as *social utility*. Motorcycle or bicycle riders who are required by law to wear helmets are experiencing the results of a utilitarianism point of view. The belief is that since head trauma is a possibility when riding a motorcycle or bicycle, and since these injuries can be serious and costly, it is beneficial to the society to require motorcycle or bicycle riders to wear helmets. With such a law, the health-care system will not be as strained, and the rest of us will not see our health-insurance premiums rise as a result of outlays by insurance companies for the treatment of head trauma. Other examples of utilitarianism theory include automobile seat-belt laws, regulations pertaining to noise levels, and, some would argue, court-required referrals for counseling.

Some advocates of this ethical theory believe there ought to be restraints placed on the use of utilitarianism. They argue that as long as the benefit for society is high, the loss of liberty small, and the practice affected relatively unimportant, a utilitarian approach is justified. Requiring the use of automobile seat belts fits these criteria. However, if the benefit to society is minor, the loss of liberty great, and the practice an important one, utilitarianism is not appropriate to guide health-counseling or health-education decisions. Placing a curfew on a population would, in most instances, be an example of an inappropriate use of utilitarianism.

Paternalism

At the societal level, the paternalism theory refers to the government being able to influence health behavior since it is knowledgeable and acts in the best interests of the individual and the society. Schools, for example, employ a paternalistic point of view when they prescribe the educational experiences for their students based on what they believe is best for those students. At the individual health counselor level, paternalism refers to the health counselor being more knowledgeable than the client and, having the best interest of the client in mind, therefore justified in influencing client behavior. A way of viewing paternalism is that it is designed to protect the individual from his or her self; that is, from risky behaviors. At some point, advocates of paternalism believe, the client will thank the health counselor for intervening in this way.

One of the rationales for intervening in client behavior in this manner is the argument that no behavior is truly voluntary, especially health-related behaviors. The individual is influenced by the media, company advertisements and marketing campaigns, and societal trends, to name a few. To counteract these negative influences, the argument goes, a paternalistic approach by well-meaning, knowledgeable health counselors and health educators is not only warranted, but essential.

Distributive Justice

Based on the ethical principle of justice, this theory states that individuals should get rewards as appropriate, and punishments or disincentives when necessary. To avoid an unfair burden on the *prudent* members of society, insurance surcharges or special taxes (such as "sin taxes" on cigarettes and alcohol) are warranted. Those who use tobacco products should pay more for their health insurance since they draw on the health-care system more, costing the insurance company more than do those who refrain from the use of tobacco. Those who litter the streets should be fined to pay for the cleaning of those streets. Those who drink alcohol should pay a tax on their alcohol purchases that can be used for public-service announcements to discourage others from drinking and to offset the costs associated with drinking and driving.

Those opposed to the application of distributive justice point to the unequal access to health information and health programs. Billboards that advertise cigarette smoking in low-income neighborhoods, and the lack of stress-management programs available to low-income residents are examples of unequal access. Given unequal access, the argument continues, it is unfair to penalize low-income people for their smoking behavior or stress-related illnesses. Furthermore, everyone engages in some unhealthy behaviors. Which of these behaviors should be penalized? Which of them are *imprudent?* Eating too much? Leading a sedentary lifestyle? Driving too fast? Working too hard and too long?

Referring back to the case study presented at the beginning of this chapter, those believing in natural law would give Linda the information she requests to get pregnant since that should be her decision. Those believing in utilitarianism might withhold the information requested. Their rationale might be to help Linda get pregnant would create an undue burden on society that might have to provide financial, counseling, and other support as a result of Linda's domestic situation. Advocates of paternalism might believe that, due to their education and experience, they know what is best for Linda. They might, therefore, withhold the information Linda requests, having her best interests in mind. Lastly, supporters of distributive justice might argue that Linda has a right to the information she requests, but only if she has the resources to manage any complications that might result from having another child.

To Coerce or Not to Coerce

Most Americans intuitively object to coercion, especially when it is they who are being coerced; coercion seems undemocratic. Yet, as described above, several ethical theories justify **coercion**—encouraging, motivating, and influencing clients to behave in certain ways that health counselors believe to be in clients' best interests. Some ethicists even describe many educational practices as coercive. For example, when a health educator selects the textbook to be used in the course, determines which videotapes will be viewed, and what topics term papers will address, the universe of knowledge available to students is limited by the constraints implied in these practices. Call them by whatever name you choose, but many practices in which health counselors engage are coercive. In the scenario described at the beginning of this chapter, the health counselor might be tempted to influence Linda to work on her other problems before becoming pregnant. If the health counselor were to do so, that might be interpreted as coercion since that is not the reason counseling was sought. Coercion becomes even more problematic when the client has not freely chosen to be counseled, such as when a parent brings in a reluctant child for counseling or when the courts refer an offender for counseling.

One expert in health ethics believes that coercion is acceptable if certain conditions are met. Pellegrino (1981) categorizes these conditions as the Principle of Proportionality and the Principle of Self-Determination.

Principle of Proportionality

Coercive measures may be taken only when their effectiveness is unequivocal for large numbers of people and when the control extends over a limited sector of people's lives. In addition, the inconvenience has to be small, the social benefit high, and the economic advantages considerable. Examples of coercive measures consistent with these criteria are requiring immunizations to attend

Coercion. Encouraging, motivating, and influencing clients to behave in certain ways that health counselors believe to be in the client's best interests.

school, enforcing sanitation regulations, posting speed limits, requiring helmets for motorcycle and bicycle riders, fluoridating water supplies, and manufacturing automobiles with built-in seat belts.

However, several questions arise even when attention is paid to these criteria. For example, who determines that the inconvenience is small? Who determines whether the benefits to society are sufficient enough to warrant coercive measures, and what standards are used to make this decision? Motorcycle riders might judge having to wear a helmet a distraction from the joy of the wind rushing their hair. Automobile owners might judge having to pay a higher price for a car due to the inclusion of various safety features burdensome.

Principle of Self-Determination

Coercive measures are acceptable only if voluntary measures have been tried and proven to be inadequate. Even so, coercion should be of the mildest form required to achieve behavior change and should be confined to actions with direct public impact. This latter criterion is designed to prohibit coercive measures for behaviors that are personal and private, lest moralizing take the place of morality. Consequently, coercion is inappropriate when applied to adults in matters of personal sexual preferences, personal family lives, and personal amusements such as drinking alcohol or enjoying pornography.

One form of coercion that is acceptable under the Principle of Self-Determination if the other criteria have been met is providing inducements that encourage the behavior-change goal. For example, health-insurance premiums may be discounted for people who refrain from smoking and who are physically active. This reward for adopting the desired behavior is effective in encouraging and maintaining that behavior. Disincentives might also be effective. When the "sin tax" on cigarettes is raised, for instance, there is usually a decrease in the number of people who smoke. However, disincentives disproportionately affect the poor and, by that standard, one might decide they are immoral. Consider the effect of a tax increase of 50 cents a pack of cigarettes. That increase will mean a higher percentage of income for cigarettes for the poor than it would for the wealthy.

As with the Principle of Proportionality, the Principle of Self-Determination also raises several perplexing issues. For example, who decides which behaviors are public and which are private, and what standards are used to make this decision? Furthermore, who decides whether a sufficient attempt has been made to voluntarily affect the behavior in question and, again, what standards are used to make this decision?

It should be clear from the presentation above that the determination of the morality of health counselors' actions is complex. The judgment regarding the morality of the behavior of health counselors depends on many issues such as the values of the counselor, the ethical theory to which the counselor subscribes, and the comfort the counselor feels with coercive measures. These variables, then, preclude a cookbook approach to ethical issues encountered by health counselors. Each counselor must decide for him or her self what is moral—what is good, what is right. Still, that does not mean that "anything goes." The counselor must be able to justify that actions taken are consistent with ethical theories employed in a democratic society, and with professional ethical standards and professional codes of conduct.

Codes of Ethics

Codes of ethics prescribe standards, state principles regarding responsibilities, and/or define rules expressing duties of professionals to whom the codes apply. Bayles (1981) differentiates between standards, principles, and rules.

> **Codes of ethics.** Standards, principles, responsibilities, and rules expressing the duties of professionals to whom the codes apply.

- **Standards** are intended to guide human conduct and describe desirable traits such as honesty, respect for others, and conscientiousness. Standards may also proscribe undesirable traits such as dishonesty, deceitfulness, and exaggerated self-interest.

- **Principles** prescribe responsibilities but do not specify the required conduct. A code might therefore speak to responsibilities to clients, to employers, to colleagues, to communities, and to the profession.

- **Rules** specify the conduct required to ethically engage in the profession. For example, under some circumstances coercing or manipulating may be proscribed, or inflating one's credentials may be judged contrary to ethical professional practice.

Codes of ethics have many benefits. Clients and students are better able to determine what to expect, and what not to expect, of the professional with whom they are interacting. Furthermore, professional organizations can hold their members accountable for behaving in an ethical manner, and may even be able to initially screen out of the profession those with evidence of past unethical behavior. Lastly, codes of ethics provide professionals with guidelines for their professional conduct when they are confused about the right course of action.

The Code of Ethics for the Health-Education Profession

Recognizing the value of a code of ethics for the profession, health educators have attempted to develop one for many years. The first attempt occurred with the Society for Public Health Education's (SOPHE) publication of a code of ethics in 1976. That code was subsequently revised in 1983. In 1993, the American Association for Health Education (AAHE)—formerly the Association for the Advancement of Health Education—approved a code of ethics for its members. Still,

these codes of ethics were specific to the professional organization, and not to the profession of health education. In 1996, the Coalition of National Health Education Organizations (CNHEO) set about to develop a unified code of ethics for the health-education profession. The code subsequently developed was approved in November 1999 and is known as The Code of Ethics for the Health Education Profession. A more detailed history of the development of a code of ethics for the health-education profession has been published elsewhere (Capwell et al., 2000).

The Code of Ethics for the Health Education Profession is divided into six Articles, with Sections under each Article. The six Articles speak of responsibilities to the public, to the profession, to employers, in the delivery of health education, in research and evaluation, and in professional preparation. Below are listed several Sections of the code that seem particularly relevant to the role of the health counselor (Coalition of National Health Education Organizations, 2000).

- . . . . support the rights of individuals to make informed decisions regarding health, as long as such decisions pose no threat to the health of others

- . . . . accurately communicate the potential benefits and consequences of the services and programs with which they are associated

- . . . . be truthful about their qualifications and the limitations of their expertise and provide services consistent with their competencies

- . . . . protect the privacy and dignity of individuals

- . . . . respect and acknowledge the rights of others to hold diverse values, attitudes, and opinions

- . . . . be sensitive to social and cultural diversity and be in accord with the law, when planning and implementing programs.

- . . . . empower individuals to adopt healthy lifestyles through informed choice rather than by coercion or intimidation

■   . . . . treat all information obtained from participants as confidential unless otherwise required by law

As you read below about specific ethical issues faced by health counselors, keep these sections of the code of ethics in mind.

Ethical Issues Encountered by Health Counselors

There are many ethical issues health counselors are faced with as they perform their counseling duties. Appropriate reactions to some of these are evident, such as when a client reports physical abuse and the law requires the counselor to report that abuse to local authorities. Other issues create more of a dilemma, such as when a client reports abusing drugs and the counselor believes this behavior places the client at risk. Whether to report that behavior to someone else, or to seek help for the client without his or her permission, can be a perplexing decision. The ethical issues presented below present ethical dilemmas that can be resolved a number of different ways. How a health counselor who experiences these ethical issues determines the best course of action depends on the counselor's values, the ethical philosophy to which they ascribe, and their interpretation of the guidelines in their professional code of ethics. Consequently, there are no simple answers to these dilemmas and, therefore, our purpose in presenting them is not to prescribe how to behave in these situations. Rather, these issues are presented to help the health counselor anticipate ethical dilemmas that might be encountered and to have thought of a personal, acceptable, moral response in advance. Having thought about these issues in advance increases the likelihood that the health counselor's response will be a moral right; that is, good and right.

Issue: Who is the Client?

At first glance, it appears obvious that the person sitting across from the counselor is the client. After all, that is the person receiving the counseling. However, the obvious answer is not always the most accurate. When the courts require a student to receive counseling for driving while intoxicated or for being a repeat offender, the client may actually be the court—or society as represented by the court. The goal of the counseling is certainly to serve the person receiving the counseling. However, one might view that as a means to serve society's ends. In fact, in most of these instances, the person being counseled does not even want to be there. That person might even interpret counseling as a punishment. One can imagine the challenges faced by counselors in these situations.

In other instances, a student might be presented for counseling by his or her parents and, also, has no real interest in the counseling goals. In this case, the real client might be the parents. Perhaps a spouse has been directed to attend counseling as a way to avert a divorce. Which spouse is then the client? The importance of this issue becomes clear when we discuss, in the next section, who determines the goals of the counseling.

The counselor needs to decide whether it is moral to counsel someone who has been coerced to attend, and, if so, whether it is moral to direct the counseling to the goals of the person or the goals of the entity who exerted that coercion.

Issue: Who Determines the Outcome of the Counseling?

If it unclear who the client is, it is impossible to determine the goals of the counseling sessions. Counseling theory tells us that the counselor works with the client to facilitate the client's goals. Yet, this is not always such a simple matter. For example, if a strict parent requires a child to receive counseling, is achieving compliance by the child the goal—which the parent would prefer—or is the goal to get the parents to relax their rules and expectations—which the child would prefer? Another possibility is that after viewing the situation, the counselor determines the most appropriate goals of the counseling sessions. So, is it the child's goals, the parent's goals, or the counselor's goals that guide the counseling? If a meeting among parties can iron this all out, and agreement can be reached on the goals of the counseling sessions, the issue is resolved. However, if the parties cannot agree, the counselor has a real dilemma that requires a determination of the moral course of action to take. As a last resort, the counselor may decide that he or she cannot participate in counseling when the client and the goals are unclear, that to do so would be immoral—bad and wrong.

Many years ago, this author wrote of a theory of health education termed "Health Education As Freeing" (Greenberg, 1978). It theorized that people are enslaved by such variables as low self-esteem, high alienation, loneliness, inappropriate loci of control, fear, anxiety, lack of health knowledge, and lack of health skills. The goal of health education then was to free people from these enslaving factors so they could choose health behaviors most consistent with their preferred lifestyles and values. To engage in traditional health education in which the goal is directed to changing specific health behaviors (for example, smoking, drinking, sex) results, I have argued elsewhere, in *iatrogenic disease* (Greenberg, 1985). That is, disease caused by the treatment. Iatrogenic disease resulting from traditional, coercive, manipulative health education is manifested by being dependent, being able to be easily influenced (conformity and peer pressure), and being anxious and fearful about health ("everything causes cancer"). That is certainly not a description of a healthy person.

Iatrogenic disease is also of concern in health counseling. If the goal of health counseling is to influence the student/client to behave in a specific way, it provides a short-term benefit, with long-term harm. The client will not become an independent person with the abilities and skills (problem-solving, decision-making) for resolving subsequent health issues. If one agrees with this argument, the health counselors' role is to facilitate the client's decision by teaching him or her skills that can be applied to resolving the health issue. The health counselors' role is not to determine the best course of action for the client and then attempt to influence the client to adopt that course of action.

Issue: What Role Should the Counselor's Values and Biases Play?

Studies of the mental health of gays, lesbians, and bisexuals find they disproportionately suffer from suicidal ideation, anxiety, depression, low self-esteem, and social alienation as a result of homophobia and social discrimination (Diaz et al., 2001; Gilman et al., 2001; Ryan & Futterman, 2001). Given these data, the health counselor might expect that homosexual students would ask for help in dealing with society's reactions to their sexual orientation. Since all people, health counselors included, have values and biases, it is possible that specific counseling situations occur in which counselors feel uncomfortable providing support. For example, a health counselor may believe that homosexuality is proscribed by religious teachings and, therefore, is a sin. In this case, the health counselor may not be able to provide the unbiased support the student desires and has a right to expect. Replace homosexuality with other health-related issues and the same concern arises. Think of the student who becomes pregnant and is considering an abortion, or the student who engages in sexual behaviors such as coitus or oral-genital sex, or the student who uses mood-altering drugs. In all of these instances, the counselor may try to shift the original purpose of the counseling sessions to what the counselor believes is in the best interest of the client, be that refraining from homosexual activities, refraining from sexual behavior outside of marriage, or not using drugs. If this occurs, the counselor has allowed his or her values and biases to replace those of the client, and this can be considered manipulative. When clients are reluctant to begin a counseling relationship, we term that *resistance* (Brammer & MacDonald, 1996). Perhaps the same term ought to apply to a counselor's reluctance to engage in a relationship with a client whose values are contrary to the counselor's. Think of the choice faced by the health education/counselor in the case study presented at the beginning of this chapter. Some counselors might be reluctant—resistant—to provide Linda information that will help her get pregnant.

One way to respond to situations in which the counselor is uncomfortable with the goals the client has outlined is to discuss this discomfort with the client. This is recommended practice anyhow, whereby the first counseling session should be devoted to engaging the client in a co-operative relationship between the client and the counselor (Lewis, Sperry, & Carlson, 1993). Perhaps such a discussion would result in the counselor describing goals that he or she would accept for the client, with the client agreeing to those goals. Perhaps the client would decide this is not the right counselor for this issue. Alternatively, the counselor might suggest a more appropriate counselor and help the student make arrangements to meet this counselor. Although the counselor may feel assured that his or her moral point of view regarding the presenting issue is the right one, to attempt to manipulate the client to that same point of view may, in and of itself, be considered immoral by others in the counseling profession.

Issue: When and How to Say No

Students/clients may have goals that are contrary to the ethical principles by which the health counselor is guided. For example, a health counselor may not feel comfortable helping a student develop the skill to attract women to his bed. Yet, for a student with low self-esteem issues, that may be the professed goal. Recall that in the case study beginning this chapter, the health educator/counselor wrestled with the decision regarding providing information to help Linda become pregnant or withholding information from her. You probably can think of other examples when a counselor's values are incompatible with a client's desired outcomes for the counseling sessions.

In other instances, the client might wish for the counselor to "do the work" with the client not participating fully in the counseling activities. For example, a student approaches a health counselor with an interest in losing weight. The student asks the counselor for a diet and exercise regimen. The counselor, on the other hand, realizes that the student needs to be a full participant in achieving the counseling goals and, therefore, resists providing

these resources. What is a counselor to do in these situations?

Counseling is a collaborative relationship between the counselor and the counseled. It is not a relationship dictated by the student/client. The counselor need not agree to provide the student with whatever he or she desires. In many cases if that were to occur, it would actually be a disservice to the client. Using the student who wishes to lose weight as an example, one option is to supply that student with resources regarding nutrition and exercise. The student can then read these pamphlets, books, articles, and so on and use the information contained within them to lose weight. At first glance, this appears to be a successful counseling endeavor. However, when that same student wants to stop smoking, study more, or improve communication with other people, he or she will have to rely on the health counselor for other reading material. The result is a dependency on the counselor, rather than the development of research skills that would foster client independence. An old proverb states, "Give me a fish and I eat today, teach me to fish and I eat forever." A counselor believing in the value of fostering client independence—and that should be all health counselors—may have to say *no* to a client's request for reading material that contains information about losing weight. Instead, the counselor and the client should brainstorm ways in which the desired information can be acquired, and devise a strategy for the client acquiring that information. During a subsequent meeting, the client can then discuss with the counselor what he or she found. In this way the client learns an important skill that can be applied to other issues he or she encounters.

This rationale for saying *no* to clients should not be surprising. After all, counselors are taught the skills of active listening, paraphrasing, reflecting, confronting, and other responses that challenge clients to answer their own questions and uncover their own insights. Counselors are advised not to do that for clients, but rather, help clients do that for themselves. The intent of this recommendation is to encourage clients to think about their health issues in a systematic way such that they no longer need the counselor. This strategy means that when the client asks the counselor to answer a question for him or her, the counselor, in effect, says *no*—albeit using one of the many strategies, some of which are mentioned above. Saying *no*, then, can very much be in the client's best interest.

In the case of clients' goals that fly in the face of counselors' views of morality, counselors need to share their concerns with clients. The counselor can identify the problematic nature of the client's goals and attempt to work out a compromise goal they can both accept. Using the example above of a student who wishes to learn skills to "bed down" women, the counselor may not agree to help the student achieve that goal. However, after discussing the counselor's objections and the student's low self-esteem, the counselor and student might agree to work on improving the student's self-esteem and enhancing his communication and interpersonal relationship skills. The student might come to realize that the original goal was on the surface, but the underlying need is to feel better about himself and be able to communicate more effectively so others will value him more which, in turn, will further contribute to his self-esteem.

Recognize, though, that there may be occasions when a compromise is not possible. In that case, the counselor needs to share the ethical concern so the student understands why the counselor refuses to help the student achieve his or her objectives. Depending on the particulars of the situation, the counselor can suggest another counselor who might be willing to work with the student, or suggest the student rethink the goal in terms of the ethical issues raised by the counselor.

Issue: When and How Much to Disclose

A student presents for counseling stating she drinks too much alcohol. Almost every night she is out drinking with friends, and her school work and family life suffer as a result. She earned failing grades on midterm exams in two courses, and has socially withdrawn from her family after several occasions of arguing about her drinking. Coincidentally, the counselor also drank too much when in high school. Should the counselor disclose this information to the student?

On the one hand, **self-disclosure** of this nature fosters empathy with the client. The client thinks, "She really can appreciate what I am going through because she has gone through the same thing." The result can be reciprocal self-disclosure in which the client then discloses even more (Johnson, 1997). Disclosure by the counselor can also result in the student recognizing that others have experienced the same problem and have been able to recover from it. This attitude can encourage the student to work hard toward the counseling goal and contribute to a successful outcome. In addition, disclosure by the counselor can alleviate self-deprecating feelings on the part of the student. "Since she (the counselor) is a good person and she once behaved similar to me, it must be the behavior that is bad, not me." This is not an insignificant insight.

Yet, self-disclosure on the part of the counselor also has its downsides. For one, if the counselor spends too much time discussing his or her own behavior, the student might feel the counselor is not focusing appropriately on the student's issue. In this case, the student may become resentful and sabotage the counseling sessions. Furthermore, disclosure by the counselor might result in the student thinking less of the counselor. "She couldn't control her drinking when she was in high school. What makes me think she'll ever be able to help me control mine?" Lastly, some counselors prefer to present a role model which their clients can emulate. For these counselors, self-disclosure might be seen as interfering with the model of appropriate behavior they wish to present. They may believe that self-disclosure provides the client with a rationale for her own behavior. "She did it when she was young. Why can't I do it when I'm young?"

The issue for the counselor is when is it appropriate to self-disclose and when is it not. Certainly

---

Self-disclosure. When a person shares personal information about him or herself with another person.

this is a matter of counseling skill and strategy. Still, ethical decisions are involved. How is the ethical principle of nonmaleficence to be processed? That is, how might self-disclosure do harm and how can the counselor prevent that from occurring? How is beneficence involved? That is, how can self-disclosure do good and how can the counselor make sure that happens? Does self-disclosure interfere with autonomy by providing the client with an excuse for his or her behavior? "After all, everyone, even the counselor, drinks too much at some time in their lives." Regardless of the resolution of the ethical dilemmas associated with self-disclosure, they need to be processed by health counselors.

Issue: When and How to Make Referrals

As stated in the Code of Ethics for the Health Education Profession, health educators should be truthful about their qualifications and the limitations of their expertise and provide services consistent with their competencies. To do otherwise is to act immorally. In terms of health counseling, **referral** means that when the student presents an issue for which the health counselor is not qualified, the student should be referred to a counselor who is. Yet, a health counselor may believe that since the student came to him or her for help, the student feels comfortable with the health counselor and, therefore, it would be a mistake to refer the student to someone he or she may not even know. With this belief, the health counselor might decide to continue counseling the student even though the issue is beyond his or her capabilities. To demonstrate the absurdity of this point of view, consider a student who expresses the desire to kill himself to his health education teacher. Although the teacher might speak with the student initially, it is clear that someone with more experience and skill in counseling suicidal students needs to be involved. It is obvious in this situation that a

> **Referral.** When a counselor who is not qualified to work with a client's presenting issue refers the client to another counselor.

teacher/health counselor who maintains an exclusive counseling relationship with this student has made a mistake and can be judged as behaving immorally. The ethical principle of nonmaleficence is challenged, and beneficence is questionable at best. This student needs to be referred to someone with the training, experience, and resulting capability to counsel students with suicidal ideation.

Still, ethical issues present themselves when a referral is warranted. First, as mentioned above, the student felt comfortable with the counselor such that he shared his suicidal feelings. To refer the student to someone else, even though necessary, may exacerbate the student's sense of low self-worth. "Ms. Collins doesn't even care enough about me to spend time discussing my thoughts of killing myself. I must really be worthless." Furthermore, the student might not follow through on the referral due to not knowing the person to whom he is referred and feeling uncomfortable discussing such personal issues with a stranger. In addition, the student might feel abandoned by the counselor and the issue may seem even more hopeless.

Yet, there are ways to refer students/clients in a manner that facilitates successful outcomes rather than threatens unsuccessful ones. Brammer and MacDonald (1996) suggest the following when referring clients:

- Explore helpees' readiness for referral. Have they expressed interest in specialized help? Are they afraid of seeing a "shrink"? Do we frighten them with implications of the severity of their problems, such through the connotation we give to "You had better see a psychiatrist!"?

- Be direct and honest about your observations of their behavior that led to your suggested referral. Be honest also about your own limitations. If, after working with them for awhile, you feel that it would be in their best interest to receive more intensive help from a specialist, you might say something like "Let's explore what other possible resources would be available for help with the question." This illustrative statement does not imply they are too disturbed or confused for you to handle and therefore must be in really bad shape.

- It is advisable to discuss the possibility of referral with the referral agency before the problem becomes urgent.

- Determine what other persons have had contact with this helpee, and if you have permission from the helpee, confer with them before suggesting further steps.

- If the helpee is a minor, it is wise to inform the parents of your recommendations and obtain their consent and cooperation.

- Be fair in explaining the services of a referral agency by citing the possibilities and the limitations of that agency. Do not imply that miracles can be performed there.

- Let the helpee or the helpee's parent make their own appointments for the new service, although supportive services such as transportation should sometimes be facilitated.

- Do not release information to any referral source without permission from helpees or their parents in the form of a signed release.

- If you have been having the primary helping relationship with the helpee, it is ethical to attempt to maintain that relationship until the referral is complete and a new relationship is begun.

Adhering to these guidelines can go a long way toward assuring the referral is done in an ethical manner, one in which the client does not feel diminished or abandoned. Recall the case study opening this chapter. Imagine the health educator/counselor decided he or she felt uncomfortable providing Linda with the information she sought. Using the guidelines above, how might the counselor make a referral that is both effective and ethical?

Issue: When and How to Terminate the Counseling Relationship

Luiz has spent the past few months counseling Phil. Initially, Phil presented with a weight problem. He was picked on by the other students, made fun of due to his weight, and was excluded from social activities arranged by the other students in his class. Phil asked Luiz to help him set up a weight-reduction regimen he could follow. Luiz did this and soon Phil was losing 2 pounds a week. Eventually, the counseling sessions turned toward Phil's low self-esteem and his inability to resolve conflicts well. When those issues started to be managed, Phil told Luiz that he had another problem with which he needed help. Luiz suspected that Phil was having difficulty terminating their relationship.

On the one hand, Luiz might feel flattered that Phil believes he is so helpful that he wants to maintain the relationship to have Luiz help him with still other issues. On the other hand, Luiz might suspect that Phil has become dependent on his help and consider that undesirable and unhealthy. The ethical dilemma Luiz faces is whether to terminate their counseling relationship and refuse to help Phil with these other matters, or to continue assisting Phil to wrestle with the issues that affect his life.

When clients become too dependent, and for too long a period of time on health counselors it is probably wise to wean them from the relationship. The danger with **counseling termination** is that, as with referrals, the client may feel abandoned and his or her self-worth diminished. And yet, not to terminate the relationship fosters a pseudodependency that is not in the client's best interest. This issue can be resolved by the counselor following several recommendations for terminating counseling relationships designed to prevent either pseudodependency or feelings of abandonment and diminished self-worth. In terminating counseling relationships health counselors are advised to do the following (Brammer & MacDonald, 1996):

- Either the health counselor or the client should summarize the progress made to date.

Counseling termination. Weaning a client from the counseling relationship if he or she is exhibiting pseudodependency, or if it is in the client or counselor's best interest.

- Keep the conversation at the intellectual level to dissuade exploration of feelings.

- Refer to the previously agreed time limits, if there were any.

- Offer a referral if the client desires to continue a counseling relationship.

- Leave the door open for possible follow-ups to make the termination seem less abrupt.

- Offer to maintain a standby relationship so the client does not feel abandoned.

- Resist expressions of client gratitude since the goal is to have clients feel they resolved their own health issues.

Summary

Health counselors can expect to encounter numerous ethical issues. To best be able to resolve these issues, it is useful to use a systematic approach. *Ethics* is a system to determine whether a course of action is moral or immoral. Something that is *immoral* is bad or wrong, something that is *moral* is good or right. In the system of ethics, *ethical principles* are used as guides to determine whether a course of action is moral or immoral. Examples of ethical principles are nonmaleficence, beneficence, autonomy, justice, honesty, and maintaining confidentiality.

When two or more ethical principles are opposed to one another in any given situation, it is termed an *ethical dilemma*. Ethical dilemmas are resolved by weighting the operative ethical principles—that is, applying one's values— and basing the course of action on the ethical principle(s) deemed most important or valuable. *Values* are estimations of worth and are developed over many years through life experiences. Parents, clergy, schooling, peers, and others with whom we interact influence our values. Since no two people have the same experiences, it is no surprise that people can differ in their values, which will result in their disagreeing about the weighting of the ethical principles that should guide decisions about ethical issues.

Different people with different beliefs may view ethics differently. For example, *rule ethicists* believe there is one rule that governs all situations. On the other hand, *situation ethicists* believe that each situation is unique and, therefore, no one rule can apply to all situations.

There are several ethical theories related to views of ethics. Ethical theories include natural law, utilitarianism or social utility, paternalism, and distributive justice. *Natural law* states that individuals have the right to make their own decisions as long as those decisions do not harm others. *Utilitarianism* states it is justifiable to curtail or influence decisions if society would benefit by such interference. *Paternalism* states that those who know more are able to influence others who are less knowledgeable. That is, those with more knowledge can take a paternalistic attitude—analogous to a parent–child relationship—toward those with less knowledge. *Distributive justice* states that individuals should get rewards as appropriate, and punishment or disincentives when necessary.

Coercion is a controversial area in health counseling. When, if ever, is it moral to use coercion? Two laws can be used to determine if coercion is appropriate: the Principle of Proportionality and the Principle of Self-Determination. The *Principle of Proportionality* states that coercive measures are acceptable when their effectiveness is unequivocal for large numbers of people and when control extends over a limited sector of people's lives. In addition, the inconvenience has to be small, the social benefit high, and the economic advantages considerable. The *Principle of Self-Determination* states that coercive measures are acceptable only if voluntary measures have been tried and proven inadequate. In addition, coercion should be of the mildest form required to achieve behavior change and should be confined to actions with direct public impact.

Codes of ethics are important considerations for health counselors since they provide standards, state principles regarding responsibilities, and/or define rules expressing duties of professionals.

Standards guide human conduct and describe desirable traits. *Principles* prescribe responsibilities but do not specify the required conduct. *Rules* specify the conduct required to ethically engage in the profession. The Code of Ethics for the Health Education Profession was approved in 1999 and includes several sections relevant to health counseling. Among these sections are the rights of individuals to make informed decisions; the responsibility of the health educators/counselors to communicate benefits and consequences; the need for health educators/counselors to be truthful, protect clients' privacy, and respect the rights of others to hold diverse views; and to empower individuals to adopt healthy lifestyles through informed choice rather than by coercion or intimidation.

Examples of ethical issues faced by health counselors include determining who is the client, identifying the counselor's values and biases, deciding when and how to say no, determining when and how much to disclose, knowing when and how to make referrals, and how to terminate the counseling relationship.

Key Terms

autonomy, 40	ethics, 39
beneficence, 40	justice, 40
codes of ethics, 45	morality, 39
coercion, 44	nonmaleficence, 40
counseling termination, 52	referral, 51
ethical dilemmas, 41	self-disclosure, 50
ethical principles, 40	values, 41

Questions for Discussion

1. Consider a social issue you feel strongly about. What ethical principles inform your position on the issue?

2. Consider a social issue or situation in which you find yourself in an ethical dilemma. What ethical principles in friction are causing the dilemma? What are the values and morals that guide your ethical principles?

3. Do you think it is moral to counsel a client who has been coerced to attend counseling? What ethical principles might be operating in your decision whether or not to counsel such a client?

4. Does a counselor need to agree with the goals of the client in order to counsel him/her? How can a counselor respond when his or her ethical principles/values are contrary to the client's goals?

5. When might self-disclosure be necessary or appropriate in the counselor–client relationship? What are the risks and possible consequences of counselor self-disclosure?

Related Web Sites

http://www.amhca.org
The site of the American Mental Health Counselors Association. Provides information about the profession of mental-health counseling, including licensure, scope of practice, practice standards, and ethics.

http://www.judyroberts.net
This site discusses what makes counseling practice ethical. Advice from chairpersons of national counseling associations.

http://www.counseling-usa.com/faq
Counseling-USA. Discusses the American Counseling Association's Code of Ethics and Standards of Practice. "What is the Mental Health Bill of Rights" and other questions are answered.

http://www.counseling.org/resources/codeof
Site features the American Counseling Association's Code of Ethics and Standards of Practice as required by laws, regulations, including courts and health-insurance companies. Includes information on appropriate professional counseling literature.

http://www.nbcc.org/ethics/webethics
The National Board for Certified Counselors. Offers counseling standards of practice based upon the principles of ethical practice embodied in the NBCC Code of Ethics.

Behavioral Analysis, Therapy, and Counseling

LUIS MONTESINOS, PH.D.

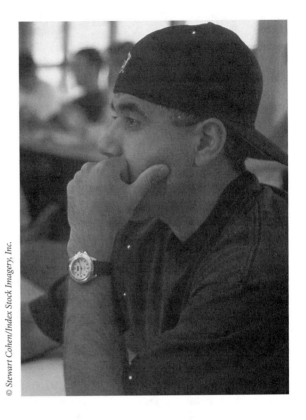

© Stewart Cohen/Index Stock Imagery, Inc.

OBJECTIVES

By the end of the chapter, the reader should be able to:

- Present the rationale for the behavioral approach to changing behavior.

- Describe the most widely used techniques of behavioral analysis and therapy.

- Demonstrate a conceptual and practical understanding of how behavioral strategies can be used to achieve the desired goals in specific target behavior.

Case Study

Amanda was the kind of student who preferred to sit quietly at the back of the class and observe others engaging in lively discussion. Most of the time she got good grades anyway because she always did well on her written assignments, but now she was taking a required class on effective communication for her counseling degree. She knew her own behavior in the class would ruin her performance grade-wise, since everyone else was extroverted and readily engaged with others. The instructor was looking for evidence of clear communication skills that a counselor would need. Amanda was distraught about her shyness and sought the assistance of the school counselor, Jim Thomson, for help in changing her behaviors when in a group of people.

Selection, Definition, and Assessment of the Target Behavior

Behavioral analysis therapy involves the application of learning principles to deviant or abnormal behavior. The first step in any behavioral program is the selection and operational definition of the target behavior. Through interviews, questionnaires, or direct observation the client's complaint is specified in observable, measurable dimensions so it can be properly assessed. The target behavior is defined in terms of frequency, intensity, topography, or time-related dimensions (duration, latency, time elapsed between responses); in other words, it is stated in operational terms. For example, shyness may be defined as the number of times a person avoids talking with others when the opportunity arises, or the time that elapses between when a person is addressed and his/her response. At this point, it should be added that these definitions are always somewhat arbitrary and limited. In spite of being arbitrary, a behavioral definition must still be: objective (observable), clear (read, repeated, paraphrased, and permitted to start observations), and complete (what responses are included or excluded).

A trait must be distinguished from a behavior. A trait refers to what a person is or has and a behavior refers to what a person does. While traits are assumed to be enduring personality characteristics they are not useful in a behavioral approach since they are not specific and they do not help in making predictions or explaining people's actions. To state that someone is always making uplifting comments because he is an optimistic person does not account for the factors that control that specific verbal behavior, it simply labels it. Focusing on what the person does permits attention to be drawn to the factors that are functionally associated with the performance of that behavior. For instance, instead of looking at Amanda's shyness as a general trait, the health counselor using the behavioral approach looked at her specific actions which Amanda perceived as problematic in her life. The essential assumption of the behavioral approach is that behavior is lawful; that is, it obeys certain principles that can be discerned through careful analysis.

> Jim carefully listened and asked questions in his initial meeting with Amanda. He asked her about her physiological response when faced with group situations, and tried to isolate some of her core operating beliefs about herself and others. Then he assessed the pattern of behavior as described by Amanda, from start to finish, including any initial triggers.

Once the behavior has been selected and identified, a goal for the intervention will be specified. This is usually straightforward; however sometimes it is helpful to use specific criteria to select goals (see Table 4.1), such as:

- Assess the client's performance against a normative level; for example, a child might be compared with his/her peers in certain tasks such as talking or reading.

- Determine whether the behavior is dangerous to the individual or others who interact with him/her. Use of verbal or physical violence in intimate relations is an example of this.

- Increase preventative behaviors, such as engaging in safe sexual practices or wearing seat belts while driving.

- Other goals may be related to the promotion of healthy behaviors such as exercising or eating healthy foods; and finally, the goals might be directed by the need to solve a specific clinical problem such as depression or attention deficit disorder.

In addition, the goals should be realistic and the person should be able to achieve them in a reasonable amount of time following well-specified interventions.

Behavioral analysis and therapy. A counseling approach that assumes that behavior is lawful and obeys certain principles that can be discerned through careful analysis; the application of learning principles to deviant (abnormal) behavior.

Table 4.1
Selected Criteria for Identifying Goals

- normative level (peers performance)
- dangerous to self or others (self-injurious, spouse abuse)
- preventative (safe-sex, wearing helmets)
- promotion (exercise, healthy dieting)
- therapeutic (tantrums, attention deficit disorder, depression)

The **behavioral assessment** can be made through interviews, direct observation, and the use of analogue assessment, in several alternative ways. Several of these will be described as follows.

In spite of the behavioral emphasis on observable and measurable targets, less than a third of self-defined behavioral practitioners use direct observation as their main mode of assessment. This is most likely due to cost and the practical issues involved in conducting such assessments. Interviews are by far the most widely used, albeit less researched, method of assessment. After building rapport the counselor will try to discover the problem, including when, where, and how often it occurs (trying to discern the conditions that maintain the behavior). The counselor will then educate the client in the behavioral approach. The antecedents and consequences of the behavior will also be explored. It is important to keep in mind that the antecedents might be setting events or predisposing factors and that the consequences may not be clear or immediate. A person might react angrily at a comment made by an office mate either because he had an argument with his significant other in the morning before leaving the house or because he is running a fever.

> **Behavioral assessment.** Initial gathering of client's behavioral information that may be done through interviews, direct observation, self-monitoring, analogue assessment, study of antecedents and consequences, and so on.

Due to the retrospective nature of the data obtained through interviews, the validity of information obtained this way may be questionable. The person may (willingly or with no awareness) selectively retrieve some material and not others, or report whatever is most accessible to his/her awareness. Using structured interviews can help control this tendency.

Direct self-report inventories might be useful in initial screenings. However the information must be taken at face value. Several problems can occur with the self-report inventories: the client might want to present him or her self in a better light; she/he might overestimate or underestimate the problem; and there may be an inconsistency between verbal and actual behavior.

> For instance, in the case of Amanda, most of the time she did not feel that her shy behavior affected the outcome of her classes or her perceived intelligence by others, although she did feel limited by it. It seemed probable to Jim that she was overestimating the extent of her introverted behavior, as opposed to her feelings of introversion or shyness. They determined together that the most problematic behavior that Amanda felt was limiting her was her tendency to not speak up even when she had something valuable to add to the class. This left her feeling frustrated and unappreciated by others, even though it was she who was not speaking up. This would be the target behavior their strategy would focus on modifying.

Checklists and rating (frequency, intensity) scales might be completed by someone other than the client who has information regarding his/her behavior. The reliability and observer bias issues involved in this type of assessment make it more useful as a complement to other primary assessment strategies.

During self-recording (self-monitoring), the client observes and records his or her own behavior. This strategy has obvious advantages in that it is time-efficient, and both overt and covert behaviors can be assessed while protecting the client's privacy. However, it relies heavily on the ability and motivation of the client to engage in the recording process.

Jim had Amanda keep a journal of her next class session, in which she as usual sat in the back and observed. She jotted down notes each time she had an inclination to speak and didn't—then she recorded the first feeling/thought that kept her from speaking up. She was instructed to notice her commentary on what others had to offer and any judgments that might occur. She also was asked to distinguish those specific instances where she really wanted to add something to the class from those times when she felt she *should* add something. This would provide her insight into what caused her specific behaviors and help her to see herself more objectively.

Systematic naturalistic observations can be done continuously or using time sampling, in which a number of observations are divided into brief intervals. In this case, problems of interobserver reliability, reactivity, practicality, time factors and costs must be considered.

Two types of analogue assessment are:

- **Simulated observations.** This refers to setting up conditions that closely resemble the natural environment in which the client behavior is occurring. It has proven useful in the observation of interactions among couples.

- **Role-playing,** where the client and the counselor will engage in the acting out of specific target behaviors. The main problem with analogue type of assessment deals with "external validity"—How representative of real-life situations are the observations?

Finally, physiological measurement can be used to assess the target behavior. This is an important strategy due to the growing recognition of the need to assess the physiological element in psychological problems such as anxiety and depression. However, in spite of technological advances, issues of validity, cost-efficiency, and practicality continue to be important factors in the widespread use of these strategies.

Stage and Decision to Change

Besides selecting, defining, and assessing the target behavior it is also important that the history of the problem be reviewed: Have there been any previous attempts to change the behavior? What have

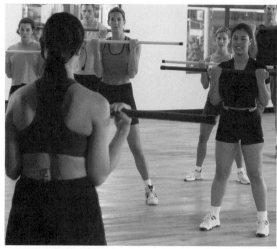

© *PhotoDisc*

Behavioral therapies assist many people in making lasting lifestyle change.

they consisted of and what where the results of those attempts?

At this point, the client's stage of change must be assessed, using the Transtheoretical Model Dimensions developed by Prochaska and DiClemente (1984) (see Chapter 6 for more in-depth discussion). Is the client in the precontemplation (not ready for change), contemplation (thinking about change), preparation (ready to change), action (initiating change), or maintenance (continuing change) stage? The answer to this question will indicate what intervention strategies would be the most appropriate to use with that particular client.

Finally, the issue of decisional balance (the pros and cons) of changing the target behavior and the level of self-efficacy of the client must be also assessed. In a program to increase exercise, for example, the cons of exercising might outweigh the pros for a particular client. This dynamic will be reversed in the action stage. Likewise, the level of self-efficacy of the client often increases as he or she moves from the early stages to the action and maintenance stages of the program. In fact, a study on exercise relapse in a college population found that subjects who relapsed had significantly lower self-efficacy scores than those who maintained their exercise levels (Sullum & Clark, 2000).

Date/time	Target Behavior	Place	Antecedents	Consequences	Thoughts/feelings

Figure 4.1
Sample self-monitoring record-keeping form

Baseline and Functional Analysis

Once the behavior has been operationally defined and the goal has been specified, a direct observation and recording of the behavior takes place. Generally, when this is done by the client it is termed *self-monitoring* and the phase of the program is called *baseline*. During the baseline phase the client is asked to observe and record his/her behavior without intervening. Questions regarding where, when, antecedents, consequences, and accompanying cognitions and emotions of the behavior are explored.

Self-monitoring involves observing, recording, and evaluating one's own behavior, and the antecedent and consequent conditions associated with it. The accuracy of self-monitoring varies considerably, depending on the client's skill, the behavior being observed, the situation in which the observation is taking place and the specific self-monitoring procedures used (Carver & Scheier, 1990).

Self-monitoring is usually the first step in developing a self-management program and it is a continuous process throughout the intervention so that progress, or lack of it, can be assessed. The process involves three steps:

- discriminating when the target behavior occurs

- recording the response in a systematic and consistent way

- interpreting or evaluating the information obtained

For example, someone trying to change his or her eating habits may want to keep a log of every-thing he eats (including meals and snacks) during three days (see Figure 4.1). It is recommended that a weekend day be included since those days tend to be different in terms of eating behaviors. The recording log will also contain information on the way the food was prepared, the circumstances where eating occurs, and how much serving was ingested.

The systematic observation of one's own behavior is not something people usually do on a regular basis; thus, when they do, dramatic changes can occur. In those instances, the mere act of observing oneself may cause reinforcing or prohibitive effects affecting the behavior that is being observed. It is presumed that in the case of behaviors that the client wants to decrease, a mechanism of avoiding negative (aversive) consequences (technically, negative reinforcement) through simply having to record instances of target behaviors is responsible for the change in behavior. In the case of behaviors that the client is trying to increase it is believed that the recording serves as a reinforcer, thus increasing its likelihood of occurrence. For example, a person trying to increase their exercise might be positively influenced by data reflecting her progress in weekly jogging. However, such reactive changes in behavior tend to be short-lived, therefore other methods must be applied as well.

The information gathered through the baseline should provide the information required to conduct a functional analysis. **Functional analysis**

Functional analysis. The process of testing hypotheses regarding the functional relations among antecedents, target behaviors and consequences; used in the behavioral approach.

refers to the process of testing hypotheses regarding the functional relations among antecedents, target behaviors, and consequences. After defining the target behavior and conducting observations and other kinds of assessment a counselor can hypothesize what is causing the behavior. This should predict antecedents associated with the behavior, how different consequences maintain the behavior, and why the behavior does not occur when it is expected. In essence, it answers the question of what the function (purpose) of the behavior is. Of course, a functional analysis could also be conducted based on information obtained through interviews or other assessment means, but the information would not be as reliable; thus the preferred means should always be direct observation (Pellios et al., 1999).

In terms of antecedents and consequences the following questions should be addressed:

Antecedents

- When does the problem behavior usually occur?
- Where does the problem behavior usually occur?
- Who is present when the problem behavior occurs?
- What activities or events precede the occurrence of the behavior?
- What do other people say or do immediately before the behavior occurs?
- Does the person engage in any other behavior before the problem behavior occurs?
- When, where, with whom, and under what circumstances is the problem behavior least likely to occur?

Consequences

- What happens after the problem behavior occurs?
- What do you do when the problem behavior occurs?

- What do other people do when the problem behavior occurs?
- What changes occur after the problem behavior?
- What does the person get after the problem behavior occurs?
- What does the person avoid or escape from after the behavior occurs?

By suggesting antecedents and consequences that are specifically and consistently associated with the occurrence of the behavior, a functional analysis helps the counselor select the most appropriate treatment beyond what might have been intuitively chosen as the appropriate intervention.

Intervention Strategies

Once the functional analysis has been completed, then the hypothetically most appropriate intervention should be implemented. It is highly likely that several different techniques will be needed. Following is a description of some of the behavioral techniques that can be implemented.

Environmental Changes (Antecedents, Stimulus Control)

The target behavior is frequently controlled by events that signal the opportunity for that behavior to occur. The person who smokes usually lights up a cigarette when she gets into the car, or the individual who engages in exercise finds that the presence or absence of a significant other in the gymnasium makes all the difference. In order for those antecedents to gain control over the behavior, they must have been associated repeatedly with the performance of the target behavior, followed by reinforcing consequences. Once the presence of the antecedents reliably predict the performance of the behavior then it is said that the behavior is under stimulus control; that is, the presence of those specific antecedents increase the likelihood of occurrence of the behavior. Antecedents not only establish the conditions necessary for the behavior to occur but can also influence its occurrence by generating expectations (that certain consequences will follow the performance of those behaviors).

If the functional analysis determines that antecedents exert a great control (or fail to exert control) over the behavior then changing those antecedents might be all that is needed to change the behavior.

The notion here is that it is possible to change problem behaviors that are maintained by environmental stimuli by precisely altering the stimuli that increase the likelihood of occurrence. That is, to alter the antecedent stimuli (these can be physical, social, and/or private such as cognitions and emotions) will have an effect on the occurrence of the behavior. Thus, interventions will focus on changing the physical environment, modifying social interactions, and attending to internal dialogues respectively.

The more general antecedents of behavior are setting events and stimulus events. Setting events refer to aspects of the situation, the task, levels of deprivation or satiation, and the presence or behavior of others. For example, if someone is trying to control their eating of unhealthy foods, he or she might engage in drinking lots of liquids before going to a place where those kinds of foods will be served.

Some of these setting events are separated in time from the occurrence of the behavior but their presence (via cognitions) will alter the likelihood of certain behaviors to occur. An example of this would be when someone is mentally rehearsing a particular skill that will be performed some time later or when a person attempts to be in a focused mood when having to participate in an athletic event.

Stimulus events refer to the fact that some stimulus will increase the likelihood of occurrence of some behaviors while other stimulus will decrease the likelihood of occurrence. The process known as differential reinforcement refers to a procedure by which a response is reinforced in the presence of one stimulus (Sd) but not in the presence of another (S^). Once the person has learned to respond (to discriminate) differently in front of the stimuli it is said that the response is under stimulus control. Some individuals will engage in specific unhealthy practices (smoking for example) only while in the presence of other smokers or while driving; the conspicuous presence of healthy foods makes its consumption more likely. When dealing with unhealthy behaviors the association between those stimuli and the behavior needs to be broken. That can be done either by avoiding the situation (or persons) associated with smoking or by changing the value of engaging in the behavior (increasing the cost of engaging) of it.

Prompts are specific types of antecedents that can control the occurrence of a response and that might facilitate its initiation and maintenance. Prompts might be verbal (as in instructions), gestures (pointing to), and modeling or physical guidance. Once the prompt has been associated several times with the consequence, it will acquire its properties and thus can control the occurrence of the behavior with no reinforcement. Prompts have been used successfully in different health-related behaviors. Lombard et al. (1995) reported its successful use in the establishment and maintenance of exercise (walking for at least 20 minutes, three times a week).

Fading refers to the gradual elimination of prompts while the response occurs at an acceptable level in the situation. If a person has used some prompts such as posting signs to remind her to eat healthy during the first months, she might want to start fading them out by gradually eliminating them first from one room, then from another, until they have disappeared (faded) completely. This process assumes that antecedents that occur normally in the environment will help in the maintenance of the newly acquired behavior.

Use of Consequences/Reinforcers (Positive, Negative Reinforcement)

Reinforcement is probably the most widely known and used set of behavioral techniques. Consequences will influence the likelihood of future occurrence of the response; if consequences

> **Reinforcement.** A behavioral technique that uses consequences to increase the likelihood of future occurrence of a behavior; can be positive or negative.

are reinforcing the likelihood will increase, if they are punishing the likelihood will decrease.

When consequences increase the likelihood of future occurrence of behavior they are called reinforcers, and they can be either positive or negative. Both will increase the likelihood of occurrence of the behavior they follow. The difference resides in that in the case of positive reinforcement an event is delivered (introduced) into the environment while in the case of negative reinforcement the consequence of the behavior an event (stimulus) is removed. In order for reinforcers to be effective they need to be delivered immediately after the behavior occurs and in a consistent manner.

Epstein et al. (1997) found that positive reinforcement affected the physical activity levels and preferences of obese children. Children who were given positive reinforcement for choosing less sedentary activities increased their physical activity and were less likely to prefer sedentary activities in the future.

A related concept is the one of extinction; it simply refers to the removal of the reinforcing consequences. Obviously in order for extinction to work the reinforcer has to be correctly identified and the capacity to control its delivery is crucial. It is expected that because of this operation the rate of the response will decrease and eventually disappear. For example, it is not uncommon that a person who verbally abuses others is frequently reinforced by the unassertive or submissive response of those whom he aggresses. In this case, what is maintaining (reinforcing) the behavior is the other's response. Assuming there is some degree of control over another's response, it could be replaced by a more assertive response which would not only decrease the aggressor's response by eliminating the reinforcer but would also act as a punisher.

Punishment is the opposite of reinforcement, and technically, it does not necessarily entail pain, coercion, or retribution. Simply, it refers to any event that when delivered or removed results in the weakening of the response that precedes it. Responses that are followed by punishing consequences will be less likely to occur in the future in similar situations. Someone trying to increase ex-

ercising might design a point system whereby which she would lose a point for each minute spent engaging in sedentary activities. For this strategy to work it is essential that the points have a certain value for the person. This is done by making sure that the points will result in access to certain activities or events known to be reinforcing. This brings up the issue of how to determine what is reinforcing.

One of the greatest difficulties of this method is how to discover the events that would serve as reinforcers. There is evidence that those activities that are performed with a greater frequency when the person is free to engage in (or select from) any number of activities can serve as reinforcers for low-frequency activities. This is known as the Premack Principle (Premack, 1959). If you are trying to increase the number of manuscript or assignment pages you write on a daily basis you might want to follow the completion of a page by watching TV for 15 minutes (this is assuming that watching TV is a high-frequency behavior in your repertoire). The other condition for effective reinforcers is that they be contingent on the behavior; this means that access to the reinforcing event is dependant upon the performance of the desired behavior. In the example given above, the person would have access to TV viewing only after performing the behavior (writing a page) and not under any other circumstance.

Sometimes the target response may be too complex or the elements making it up might not exist in the person's behavioral repertoire. In those instances, procedures such as shaping might be utilized. In fact, most if not all behavior change processes follow a shaping pattern. Shaping refers to the reinforcement of successive approximations (responses increasingly similar to the target behavior). These are reinforced while those dissimilar (or that do not approximate) the target behavior are extinguished. Typical examples of shaping are language development (and a great number of other behaviors learned during childhood) and animal training.

Preston et al. (2001) compared cocaine-using methadone-maintenance patients to a standard contingency-management (abstinence) group using a shaping procedure. Both groups earned vouchers based on the results of their urinalyses. The abstinence group earned vouchers for cocaine-negative results only, while the shaping group received vouchers for specimens with a 25 percent or more decrease in cocaine metabolite during the first 3 weeks. During the last 5 weeks, both groups received vouchers for negative urine tests only. During the last 5 weeks, readings were lower for the shaping group, suggesting that the procedure might have prepared the patients better for total abstinence.

Cognitive Behavioral Therapies

Cognitive behavior therapies refers to a group of procedures based on the assumption that behavior change can be achieved by altering cognitive processes, since maladaptive cognitive processes are the main factors responsible for maladaptive behaviors. It is further assumed that cognitions (beliefs, assumptions, expectations, attributions, and attitudes) can be modified directly (teaching clients to modify their maladaptive thoughts) or indirectly (helping clients to change their overt behaviors which in turn will change their cognitions). For instance, with a client who would like to stop smoking, a maladaptive thought might be "when I'm stressed I need a cigarette to get me through." The client could directly address this thought, or could prove it to him or her self through testing. If the client can get through a stressful situation without smoking, then their action disproves for them that maladaptive thought.

There are essentially two different groups of techniques that are subsumed under cognitive behavioral therapies (see Table 4.2). The first group, labeled cognitive restructuring therapies, focuses on erroneous cognitions (maladaptive thoughts)

> **Cognitive behavior therapy.** A grouping of techniques which are based on the assumption that behavior change can be achieved by altering cognitive processes, since maladaptive cognitive processes are the main factors responsible for maladaptive behaviors.

Table 4.2
Cognitive Behavioral Therapies

Cognitive Restructuring Therapies
Focuses on erroneous cognitions (maladaptive thoughts); seeks to change them directly.

Cognitive Behavioral Coping Skills
Teaches more adaptive responses; focuses on the deficits of adaptive cognitions.

---

and seeks to change them directly. The second group, labeled cognitive behavioral coping skills, focuses on deficits of cognitive processes and attempts to establish more adaptive responses.

Cognitive Restructuring. Broadly, cognitions are defined behaviorally as self-talk (internal verbalizations) and, in spite of including sensory images (visual, auditory, tactile), the main research and applied focus has been on self-talk. Usually the first step is for the counselor to make the client become aware of these processes, since for the most part thinking is a process with no awareness of itself. Self-talk seems especially important when new healthy behaviors are being initiated (starting an exercise program, for example). There is a need to identify the blocking statements and replace them with ones that are more positive. Cognitions are relevant not only as antecedents but as consequences to the behaviors in question as well. Whatever self-verbalizations followed the performance or nonperformance of the target behavior might serve a reinforcer or a punisher in the future.

> In the example of the shy student, Amanda, one of the strategies that the health counselor utilized was replacing negative self-talk. After identifying the negative thoughts/fears that occurred when Amanda felt the desire to speak up in class, Jim suggested more positive affirmative statements that promoted a feeling of self-acceptance and empowerment. Amanda was to think of it as a duty for her to share her wisdom with others, not as some need for reward or attention, which clearly caused a conflict for her. In addition, she was going to practice letting go of the need to judge her own statements and the statements of others, which caused undue

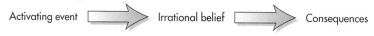

Figure 4.2
Rational emotive therapy

pressure and anxiety about speaking at all. Jim helped her to see how risk-taking could be seen as a positive thing for her, a development of courage and character. She liked to challenge herself and seemed ready to confront her habitual patterns of relating. In her next class, Amanda had a list of affirmative statements she would use as guidance, and an objective to take a risk she normally wouldn't, and then let go of judgment of whatever happened as a consequence.

Thought Stopping. This technique is usually used to deal with obsessive, anxiety-provoking, or self-defeating thoughts that the client might feel are uncontrollable. In this technique, the maladaptive thought pattern is interrupted abruptly by first the counselor or therapist and then the client yelling STOP! The thought is then replaced by other more adaptive thoughts (usually of a pleasant nature) that compete with the disturbing ones. It is an easily learned self-control technique. Although its results have not received wide empirical support it can be important in building in the client a sense of self-efficacy and control. A person wanting to quit smoking for example might be constantly repeating to herself that she has no willpower to overcome her addiction. By interrupting those kind of thoughts and replacing them with more positive ones she can set the stage for engaging in more healthy behaviors.

In the case study above, the health counselor might have instructed Amanda to mentally command herself to "STOP!" when she noticed through self-recording how a fear or negative thought prevented her from speaking up. If she suddenly felt a worry over how she would be seen, she could simply interrupt this line of thinking or feeling before it could control her action.

Rational Emotive Therapy (RET). This approach was developed by Albert Ellis and its goal is to change the irrational thoughts (implicit self-verbalizations) believed to cause psychological disturbances such as anxiety, depression, anger, and guilt. According to RET it is the interpretation of the events and not the events themselves that causes the disturbed emotions or behaviors.

According to this view, an activating event triggers some irrational cognitions (beliefs) and these cause the consequences, psychological problems such as anxiety, depression, anger, and guilt (see Figure 4.2). These irrational beliefs arise from problems in reasoning or logical errors such as absolute thinking, overgeneralizing, or catastrophizing.

Ellis suggests that there are two basic themes that underlie all irrational beliefs. The first has to do with the notion of personal worthlessness (a specific generalization associated with failure, self-denigration) and the second with a sense of duty or low frustration tolerance (must, have to, should, and ought to). The process of RET consists first of identifying the thoughts based on irrational beliefs, secondly of challenging them through an active disputing, and thirdly, of replacing them with more rational, adaptive beliefs (Ellis, 1997).

Had Jim decided to apply the Rational Emotive approach to Amanda's problem, he would help her identify the irrational beliefs that were controlling and causing her behavior in a group situation. For instance, if she felt that she didn't have the right to speak (that is, Why should anybody listen to me?) he could help her penetrate to the underlying assumption forming that belief: Did she feel unworthy, incapable, or unsafe among others? Once they identified the underlying controlling and irrational belief Amanda could challenge it and replace that belief or set of beliefs with more rational freeing beliefs. These might be something like, " I am a valuable person with valuable things to say," or "I am a worthy intelligent person whether people like me or not," or simply, "I love myself and honor myself through speaking my truth." Then in the future whenever she noticed those irrational beliefs creating her thoughts/feelings she could recognize the dynamic and reference her situation from a more rational emotional standpoint.

Ellis (1997) has reported the effective use of his approach (which he lately labels Rational Emotive Behavior Therapy to emphasize the use of behavioral strategies within the approach) with people with disabilities and when confronting fatal diseases (Ellis & Abrams, 1994).

Cognitive Therapy. This approach developed by Aaron Beck assumes that psychological disorders are maintained by distorted cognitions. The client is taught to view his/her beliefs as tentative hypotheses and is encouraged to test their validity by gathering evidence that supports or rejects them. Cognitive therapy's primary area of application has been on depression.

Beck refers to irrational/maladaptive cognitions as automatic thoughts because clients report that these thoughts appear as if they were reflexes. There are six common cognitive distortions:

1. Arbitrary inference
2. Overgeneralization
3. Selective abstraction
4. Personalization
5. Dichotomous thinking
6. Magnification or minimization

Cognitive Therapy attempts to correct the client's faulty information processing, modify the client's dysfunctional beliefs, and provide clients with skills and experiences that create adaptive thinking. First, empathy is built and the client is then engaged in a Socratic dialogue (encouraging client's reflection). The client is encouraged to view automatic thoughts as hypotheses and through collaborative empiricism to test these hypotheses (usually through homework assignments). Sometimes these tests reveal that the belief is valid. The task then is to help the client avoid the maladaptive reaction.

There are different techniques used to achieve the treatment goals in this approach. The three-column technique is a homework assignment that asks the client to identify errors in thinking. In the first column the client describes the situation, in the second the automatic thoughts, and in the third the logical errors.

Then some direct and indirect methods are used to change the dysfunctional beliefs and encourage more adaptive thinking. Among the direct methods are the following:

- generating alternative explanations (modeling and rehearsal)

- reattributing and assigning responsibility (when clients believe they have more control than what they really do)

- decatastrophizing (specific reattribution when client imagines terrible things will happen)

Among the indirect methods the following interventions are used:

- Overt behavioral interventions; clients are encouraged to engage in behaviors that may help them to challenge/reconstruct their thoughts. The more severe the problem, the more reliance is put on this behavioral homework.

- Activity schedule; plan of daily routine, useful for depression or high anxiety.

- Mastery and pleasure rating; sense of accomplishment and enjoyment.

- Graded task; small sequences that lead to a goal (shaping).

Cognitive therapy has been used successfully with patients being treated for early-stage cancer (Antoni et. al., 2001).

Cognitive Behavioral Coping Skills. As mentioned above, these groups of techniques are used when it is assumed the problem is maintained by a deficit of adaptive cognitions and the treatment goal is to train the client in obtaining those skills.

Self-Instructional Training. This technique focuses on specific statements that the person makes (self-talk) and that guide him/her to behave, think, or feel in specific ways. It was originally used to help children who exhibit impulsive behavior, to think and plan before acting (Meichembaum, 1977). It is assumed that self-instructions will permit the person to focus more on what the specific task entails, while guiding the behavior, providing encouragement and reducing anxiety. The training in self-instruction consists of three steps:

1. identifying the problem and defining what are the most appropriate behaviors for that situation
2. identifying the self-instructions that will be most effective in the problem situation
3. using behavioral skills training to learn the self-instruction process

In this last step the following strategies are used:

- **cognitive modeling**—The counselor or therapist performs the task while verbalizing aloud the instructions while the person observes.

- **cognitive participant modeling**—The client performs the task as the therapist verbalizes the self-instructions aloud.

- **overt SI**—The client performs the task and verbalizes self-instructions aloud.

- **fading of overt SI**—The client performs the task while whispering.

- **covert SI**—The client performs the task while "talking to him/herself."

This technique could be particularly useful to someone who is trying to stop smoking or indulging in the consumption of other drugs.

Problem-Solving Therapy (Skills Training). This strategy is recommended when the client presents a deficit of skills related to social situations (interpersonal problems). This is a systematic process by which the client will generate several potentially effective solutions to a problem, then will rationally select the most appropriate solution and will then implement and assess its effectiveness. The training is intended not only to deal with the immediate problem but also to provide the person with skills that he/she can use to confront possible future problems.

The training proceeds in different stages:

- Stage 1: Adopting a problem-solving orientation.
  a. identify the problems as they occur
  b. acknowledge that problems are part of our daily life
  c. assess alternatives that would be effective in solving the problems

- Stage 2: Defining the problem and setting the goals
  a. a precise definition is needed in order to generate specific solutions
  b. a precise definition permits one to formulate goals:
    - **situational focused**—those aimed at changing the situation itself.
    - **reaction focused**—those aimed at changing emotional and cognitive reactions to the situation.

- Stage 3: Generating alternative solutions
  Brainstorming

- Stage 4: Deciding on the best solution
  - Examine potential consequences, practicality of alternatives
  - Create a rating scale of solutions

- Stage 5: Implementing and evaluating

Stress Inoculation Training (SIT). This technique is designed to help the client cope with situations where anger, anxiety, or pain is present. Making an analogy with the medical approach to certain diseases, it pretends to inoculate clients against stressful situations by presenting them with small or manageable doses of the event so that they do not feel overwhelmed. The client is trained in specific coping skills (analogous to antibodies) such as cognitive restructuring, desensitization, behavioral rehearsal, and relaxation. After the client has learned those skills, they are then exposed to the stressful events (Meichenbaum, 1977; 1985). The training involves three phases:

1. The first phase, **conceptualization or educational phase,** is based on the notion that before starting the actual training the client has to have a receptive conceptual framework, has to understand the approach in theory. This phase is subdivided into three steps:

   a. Assessment, where the client is asked to list the stressors and their thoughts and feelings regarding them. The client is made aware of the fact that these thoughts and perceptions can create stress.

   b. Reconceptualization of stress as the interaction between the stressor and the person's thoughts and perceptions.

   c. The goals of training are described in language that is relevant to the trainee.

2. In the second phase, **skill acquisition and rehearsal,** the client learns relaxation, cognitive restructuring, and problem-solving. Once this has been achieved, rehearsal of the skills through role playing, modeling, and imagery rehearsal proceeds. Imagery rehearsal refers to the process by which certain skills are rehearsed in the client's mind to confront the stressful events in a graded fashion. The assumption is that if the person rehearses the skills in his/her imagination, performance will be enhanced.

3. In the third and final stage, **follow-through,** the client will actually try to use the coping skills taught in the real situations in a gradual way (from less stressful to more stressful).

SIT has been used successfully with senior high school students preparing for graduation from high school. Participants underwent a 6-week training program after which they evidenced significantly higher scores than a control group in self-efficacy and rational beliefs. They demonstrated a higher use of cognitive restructuring strategies than controls when presented with a scene depicting a potentially traumatic transition at the end of the program (Jason & Burrows, 1983).

Hains and Szyjakowski (1990) reported that young males who received SIT to help them cope with stress, when compared to a control group, showed significant reductions in levels of anxiety and anger, improvement in self-esteem, and an increase in the number of reported positive cognitions in response to a hypothetical situation. Treatment gains were maintained at a 10-week follow-up.

A program designed by Kiselica et al. (1994) might be useful as a guide for those interested in applying this approach. During the *conceptualization stage,* a discussion of stress, stressors, anxiety, and anxiety-related symptoms was conducted and members were asked to generate three examples of anxiety-provoking situations, which would be used in future sessions.

In the second session the *skill-acquisition phase* started, relaxation was introduced both conceptually and through exercises of progressive muscle relaxation. Participants were encouraged to practice at least twice a day and keep a log of their experiences with relaxation training.

During the third session a *cue-controlled relaxation procedure* was introduced, consisting of associating the relaxation response with a word or phrase and then learning to elicit relaxation by repeating the cue word or phase in actual anxiety-provoking situations. Group members were encouraged to continue using progressive muscle relaxation and to incorporate the cue-controlled relaxation to their daily routine.

Skills acquisition and rehearsal phase were combined with the *application follow-through phase* during the following sessions. Every new skill that was taught in the training sessions was encouraged to be transferred to the real world.

In the fourth, fifth, and sixth sessions, the students were introduced to the notion of *cognitive restructuring* through a handout describing how self-defeating thoughts can lead to self-defeating behaviors and the need to replace self-defeating thoughts with self-improving thoughts. Possible applications of the procedure to the anxiety-provoking situations provided in the first session were discussed. The session ended by encouraging group members to continue using progressive muscle relaxation and cue-controlled relaxation.

Assertiveness training was conducted during the fifth, sixth, and seventh sessions. The concept was introduced, discussed, and rehearsed through role-playing.

The eighth session was used to *review and assess the experience* as well as to inform students of the different resources available for them.

Compared with controls, those who participated in the program showed significantly greater improvements on self-report measures of trait anxiety and stress-related symptoms at post-test. Differences in these measures were still significant at a 4-week follow-up assessment. No significant differences were found between the two groups in either academic achievement at either post-test or follow-up (Kiselica et al., 1994).

Social support refers to the recruitment of significant others to help in the efforts to change the target behavior and is an important part of any self-management program. A recent study found that low social support was independently associated with several unhealthy behaviors (alcohol consumption, lack of physical activity, irregular sleep hours, and not using a seat belt) in both men and women (Allgoewer et al., 2001). It has also been reported that the supportive presence of spouses can influence the outcome of a smoking-cessation program (Mermelstein et al.,1983)

The active participation of significant others will be important not only in the initiation of change but also in its maintenance. These persons will be asked to participate in different ways, providing antecedents or consequences or acting as models for the client. For example, if one person would like to start an exercise program he might arrange things so as to meet a friend at the gymnasium, or if another individual wants to cut down on her drinking she might want to increase her interactions with her nondrinking friends (Miltenberg, 2001).

Behavioral contract refers to a written document usually signed by the individual and one or more persons by which both parties commit themselves to the program. The document will explicitly identify and define the target behavior, specify the data-collection method, the level that the target behavior should achieve in a certain period of time, the contingencies involved, and who will deliver those contingencies. This is considered to be a self-management technique because the signing of the contract is assumed to serve as control for the target behavior.

The clear identification of the target behavior and the statement of a clear objective is characteristic of any behavioral intervention. The target behavior will be something that needs to be initiated, increased, or eliminated, something relevant for the individual that, when changed in the direction desired, will make a difference in his/her quality of life. For example if you wanted to increase your time of study, you might want to state a certain amount of time per week as the target behavior.

The measurement of the behavior is essential to provide objective evidence of the occurrence of the target behavior. It should resolve any ambiguity or conflict that might arise. There are several ways (dimensions) in which behavior can be assessed. Permanent product for example, refers to the outcome of a behavior. This might mean the number of cigarettes that remain in a pack at the end of the day. Other ways are direct observation, recorded either by others or by the person him/herself.

The third element of the contract stipulates clearly when the behavior must be performed or at what time the outcome of its performance will be assessed. Someone trying to increase exercise might want to stipulate in the contract that swimming will occur on Mondays, Wednesdays, and Fridays at 7:00 A.M. in the Recreation Center.

The contingency to be applied is the fourth element in the contract. It should be clearly stipulated under what circumstances the reinforcing or punishing consequences will be applied. Finally,

---

Social support. The assistance received by the others in one's life, which may be emotional, financial, spiritual or informational in nature.

Behavioral contract. A written document usually signed by the individual and one or more persons by which both parties commit to a particular behavioral program.

the person responsible for applying the contingency will be clearly identified.

Behavioral contracts have been used successfully in helping people to reduce weight (Kramer et al., 1986), increase the amount of exercise (Wysocki et al., 1979), and improve academic performance (Miller & Kelley, 1994).

Maintenance/relapse prevention. Any behavior change program faces the likelihood of failing if appropriate measures are not taken to ensure the changes will transfer and be maintained in everyday life. Besides including specific strategies during training, special attention has to be given to situations that can precipitate relapse once the training phase has ended. Marlatt & Gordon (1985) have devised a specific procedure to deal with this problem with clients who are trying to overcome their addictive behaviors. The model is applicable to other problems as well.

The idea is to prepare the person in advance for the possibility of a lapse by teaching the client coping skills that can be directly used in high-risk situations. Problem-solving skills, relaxation training, and cognitive restructuring might be employed. If lapses do occur they are conceptualized as single events, not as a sign of complete failure. In some cases, lifestyle changes might be needed to reduce or eliminate high-risk situations. For example, a person who has been released from an inpatient drug and alcohol treatment program is often taught new coping skills to reduce the chance of relapse. However, if he or she does (which is often the case) experience a relapse into former behavior, it is crucial that the person view the lapse as an isolated event and not see the total rehabilitation effort as a failure. A certain amount of cognitive restructuring is needed so that the person does not "give in" to old thought patterns and their consequent behaviors. This is why lifestyle changes are so important in preventing relapse. Avoiding high-risk situations is much easier than the perception of having to start over after a relapse occurs.

A person involved in an exercise program might want to prepare for high-risk situations by first defining clearly what will be considered a lapse or a relapse and under what conditions might these occur. In a study conducted by Simkin and Gross (1994), lapse was defined as failing to participate in cardiovascular exercise during one week of the 14-week assessment period. Relapse was defined as at least 3 consecutive weeks without any exercise.

Perhaps one of the most relevant aspects of **relapse prevention** is to change the evaluation of it from negative to positive. The view that individuals who relapse will recycle back into various stages is suggested by the transtheoretical model. It has been suggested that the relapsing experience might facilitate future attempts at initiating behavior change.

Conclusions

In closing, this chapter has presented different behavioral strategies that can be used to achieve behavior change. Target behavior might be excesses (smoking, eating junk food) or deficits (exercise, studying, social skills) and the strategies should be adapted to the goal. It is desirable to use the techniques within a self-management program since this would take care of the issues of maintenance and transfer. In addition, it has been suggested that continuous assessment be utilized since this provides empirical support for any claim. At the same time it permits one to review what is being implemented to determine if the desired results are occurring. Finally, it must be emphasized that in order for the techniques to be effective they have to be applied in a systematic and valid way; that is, the technique applied must follow the principles on which it is based and be implemented accordingly.

Relapse prevention. Measures taken to ensure that behavior changes made will be maintained in everyday life; preparing a client for a lapse by teaching the client coping skills that can be directly used in high risk situations.

Summary

Originally, the field of behavioral analysis and therapy was defined as the application of learning principles (mainly operant and respondent) to deviant (abnormal) behavior. Since then, the approach has evolved to include phenomena previously considered unsuitable for scientific study (that is, cognitions). Today the behavioral approach is a well-respected and established, complex field. What was regarded as nonscientific some decades ago today is accepted as the legitimate focus of assessment and intervention.

It has also become apparent that the term *behavior modification* does not accurately describe the approach, since it refers to any method by which behavior is modified or changed, including surgery or drugs. In fact, as early as 1973 Krasner and Ullmann suggested that the term be replaced. Similar considerations led other practitioners to call the area *applied behavior analysis,* emphasizing the need for the understanding (analysis) of behavior for applied (practical) ends (Baer et al., 1968; 1987). In consequence, throughout the chapter the terms *behavior analysis* and *therapy* are used because they encompass the full range of activities and conceptual approaches that coexist in the field and do not have any of the negative connotations that the label *behavior modification* carries.

The behavioral approach focuses on specific behaviors and/or cognitions, on the current determinants of behavior (as opposed to remote events) and strongly advocates continuous assessment and evaluation of interventions based on scientific psychological principles (Miltenberg, 2001; Kazdin, 2001).

This chapter described the different behavioral strategies and techniques available for professionals involved in helping people to change their health-related behaviors. Self-management is the final goal of every behavior intervention and it is a likely scenario to be encountered by counselors and other health professionals working with ambulatory clients.

Key Terms

behavior analysis and therapy, 56

behavioral assessment, 57

behavioral contract, 68

cognitive behavior therapy, 63

functional analysis, 59

reinforcement, 61

relapse prevention, 69

social support, 68

Questions for Discussion

1. Describe the basic characteristics of the behavioral approach. What are the strengths of the behavioral approach for health counselors? What are its limitations?

2. Explain the difference between reinforcement and punishment. Provide one example for each of the possible arrangements and their effects on behavior.

3. Explain the difference between cognitive restructuring and cognitive behavior coping skills. Select one technique of each group and describe when it would be appropriate to apply them.

4. Discuss relapse prevention and describe how you would plan for it in the treatment of a specific problem.

5. Discuss what kind of information is recorded during the practice of self-recording. Why is self-recording a powerful behavioral tool?

Related Web Sites

http://www.envmed.rochester.edu/wwwrap/behavior/jaba/jabahome
The site of a journal that publishes research about applications of the experimental analysis of behavior to problems of social importance.

http://www.wmich.edu/aba/
The Association for Behavior Analysis is dedicated to promoting the experimental, theoretical, and applied analysis of be-

havior. It encompasses contemporary scientific and social issues, theoretical advances, and the dissemination of professional and public information.

http://www.behavior.org/

Provides information to the public about a range of practical applications of behavioral technology. You will find information about a number of different resources, from autism to behavioral safety, where behavior analysis has made a positive difference in the lives of people: improving education, helping to promote positive parenting, promoting workplace safety and satisfaction, guiding people to make decisions about their lives which provide maximal adjustment in their environments.

http://www.rebt.org/

Site of Dr. Ellis' institute to promote his vision of therapy which emphasizes individuals' capacity for creating their emotions; the ability to change and overcome the past by focusing on the present; and the power to choose and implement satisfying alternatives to current patterns.

http://www.aabt.org/

The site of a professional, interdisciplinary organization that is concerned with the application of behavioral and cognitive sciences to understanding human behavior, developing interventions to enhance the human condition, and promoting the appropriate utilization of these interventions.

Health-Enhancing Behaviors

MICHELE M. FISHER, D.P.E.,
AND SHAHLA WUNDERLICH,
PH.D., R.D.

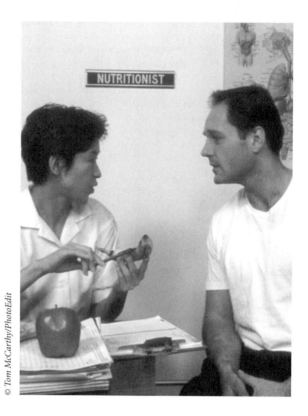

© *Tom McCarthy/PhotoEdit*

OBJECTIVES

By the end of the chapter, the reader should be able to:

- Identify health benefits associated with regular physical activity

- Discuss recent recommendations for physical activity

- Design an exercise program to enhance physical fitness

- Apply strategies to change activity-related behavior

- Describe healthy nutrition

- Identify the components of body composition

- Identify factors that regulate energy intake and body weight

- Compare and contrast various types of weight-maintenance management strategies

As has been mentioned in previous chapters, the concept of health is multidimensional, including physical, emotional, mental, social, environmental, and spiritual aspects of well-being. Hence, there are a multitude of health-enhancing behaviors within each area such as physical activity, healthy eating, stress management, social involvement, and abstinence of smoking. Many of these behaviors are related to more than one dimension of health. For example, physical activity and optimum nutrition have been shown to have a positive effect on physical, emotional, and mental aspects of wellness. The focus of this chapter will be primarily on the physical component of health, regarding two specific, but related health-enhancing behaviors: exercise and nutrition. The information presented in this chapter will be helpful for health counselors working with clients who: (1) wish to lose weight, (2) are interested in starting an exercise program, (3) would like to eat healthier, and (4) are interested in reducing their risk for cardiovascular disease. The behavior of exercise will be discussed first, followed by information on healthy nutrition. Both exercise and nutrition are important factors in weight management, which will conclude this chapter on health-enhancing behaviors.

Exercise

Physical Activity and Health

Over the past century the average life span of Americans has jumped from 47 to 76 years, with a dramatic rise in those living beyond 85—the fastest-growing segment of the U.S. population. In the early 1900s infectious diseases such as smallpox, polio, and tuberculosis were the primary sources of mortality. Since then, advances in environmental and medical technology have all but eradicated many of the most-feared illnesses. Today, chronic diseases evolving over a period of time have replaced communicable illnesses as the leading causes of death. Currently, heart disease is the number-one killer of Americans, followed by cancer, stroke, and chronic respiratory disease. Detrimental choices in lifestyle, particularly those related to diet and physical activity, have been implicated as contributing factors in the development of cardiovascular disease and some forms of cancer.

Exercise-related terminology. Prior to reviewing the association between activity and health, it is important to define a few exercise-related terms. **Physical activity** is defined as any body movement that is brought about through contraction of skeletal muscles and results in an increase in

> **Physical activity.** Any body movement that is brought about through contraction of skeletal muscles and results in an increase in energy expenditure.

Table 5.1
Health-Related Components of Physical Fitness

Cardiorespiratory endurance: the ability of the body to engage in large-muscle, dynamic exercise for a prolonged period of time

Muscular strength: the maximum force that can be exerted by a muscle group in a single effort

Muscular endurance: the ability of a muscle group to exert force repeatedly or sustain a contraction for a period of time

Flexibility: the range of motion at a joint

Body composition: the relative percentage of fat and fat-free tissue (muscle, bone, and water) in the body

energy expenditure. This term encompasses a fairly wide range of pursuits from low-intensity activities such as walking, boating, and gardening to the higher-intensity activities of karate and tennis. **Exercise** is a subset of physical activity that is characterized as planned, structured, repetitive movement designed to improve one or more aspects of physical fitness. Physical fitness can be defined as a set of attributes that enables the body to perform physical activity without undue fatigue. There are several components of physical fitness, some related to general health and others related to performance in sport. The components most important for promoting health include cardiorespiratory endurance, muscular strength, muscular endurance, flexibility, and body composition. Definitions for the health-related components of physical fitness are presented in Table 5.1.

Health Benefits of an Active Lifestyle. The benefits of a physically active lifestyle on health are well established. An inverse relationship between physical activity and cardiorespiratory fitness with all-cause mortality has been documented in a number of epidemiological studies, such that

> **Exercise.** Planned physical activity designed to improve physical fitness.

higher levels of activity and fitness are associated with a lower risk of death (Blair et al., 1996; Kushi et al., 1997). Many of these studies are based on a single evaluation of fitness or habitual activity with subsequent follow-up for mortality. Further evidence for the beneficial role of an active lifestyle is seen in previously sedentary adults who increase physical activity or fitness levels and show a reduction in the risk of death (Blair et al., 1995; Paffenbarger et al., 1994). The value of exercise in promoting longevity is maintained even when other contributing factors such as age, gender, and health status are taken into account. In other words, exercise is beneficial for people of all walks of life, including children, adults, and older adults.

A longer life is certainly an attractive prospect for most individuals, however of equal or greater importance is quality of life. An active lifestyle has also been linked to a lower risk for several chronic diseases. Substantial evidence exists for reduced incidence of coronary artery disease, high blood pressure, colon cancer, type-2 diabetes, obesity, and osteoporosis in those who regularly participate in physical activity. Additional research is necessary to delineate the role of exercise in cerebral vascular disease and some forms of cancer (breast, prostrate). Physical activity also seems to have a positive impact on mental health, particularly in relieving symptoms of anxiety and depression, as well as in the management of daily stress. The health benefits of physical activity are summarized in the Surgeon General's Report on Physical Activity and Health (Table 5.2). On a related note, physical activity is not only implicated in the prevention of chronic illness, but is also an important component in the management of established health conditions such as cardiovascular disease, hypertension, diabetes, and arthritis. Additionally, physical activity serves as an adjunct to dietary and behavioral modification in long-term weight management. Health counselors should be knowledgeable about the specific benefits of exercise on health, as many clients start an exercise program over concerns about their personal health. For example, a client who has recently been diagnosed with high blood pressure may have questions about what he or she can do to avoid being put on

Table 5.2
Health Benefits of Regular Physical Activity

- Reduces the risk of dying prematurely from all causes
- Reduces the risk of dying prematurely from heart disease
- Reduces the risk of developing diabetes
- Reduces the risk of developing high blood pressure
- Helps reduce blood pressure in people who already have high blood pressure
- Reduces the risk of developing colon cancer
- Reduces feelings of depression and anxiety
- Helps control weight
- Helps build and maintain healthy bones, muscles, and joints
- Helps older adults become stronger and better able to move about without falling
- Promotes psychological well-being

Source: United States Department of Health and Human Services (1996). Physical Activity and Health: A Report of the Surgeon General. Atlanta, Georgia: U.S. Department of Health and Human Services, Public Health Service, CDC, National Center for Chronic Disease Prevention and Health Promotion.

medication. Modifications in diet as well as a mild exercise program could be recommended to help reduce blood pressure.

Recommendations for physical activity. In response to overwhelming evidence in support of the health-promoting effects of exercise, several organizations have released statements recommending regular physical activity for the general public. A joint recommendation was issued in 1995 by the Centers for Disease Control and Prevention (CDC) and the American College of Sports Medicine (ACSM) stating that "Every U.S. adult should accumulate 30 minutes or more of moderate-intensity activity on most, preferably all, days of the week" (Pate et al., 1995). A year later, the Surgeon General concluded that: "Significant health benefits can be obtained by including a moderate amount of physical activity (e.g., 30 minutes of brisk walking or raking leaves, 15 minutes of running, or 45 minutes of playing volleyball) on most, if not all, days of the week. Through a modest increase in daily activity, most Ameri-

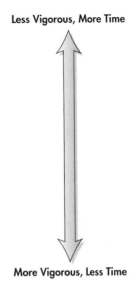

Washing and waxing a car for 45–60 minutes
Washing windows or floors for 45–60 minutes
Playing volleyball for 45 minutes
Playing touch football for 30–45 minutes
Gardening for 30–45 minutes
Wheeling self in wheelchair for 30–40 minutes
Walking 1¾ miles in 35 minutes (20 min/mile)
Basketball (shooting baskets) for 30 minutes
Bicycling 5 miles in 30 minutes
Dancing fast (social) for 30 minutes
Pushing a stroller 1½ miles in 30 minutes
Raking leaves for 30 minutes
Walking 2 miles in 30 minutes (15 min/mile)
Water aerobics for 30 minutes
Swimming laps for 20 minutes
Wheelchair basketball for 20 minutes
Basketball (playing a game) for 15–20 minutes
Bicycling 4 miles in 15 minutes
Jumping rope for 15 minutes
Running 1½ miles in 15 minutes (10 min/mile)
Shoveling snow for 15 minutes
Stairwalking for 15 minutes

Less Vigorous, More Time

More Vigorous, Less Time

Figure 5.1
Examples of moderate amounts of physical activity
Source: United States Department of Health and Human Services, 1996. Physical
Activity and Health: A Report of the Surgeon General.

cans can improve their health and quality of life." Both of these recommendations are considerably different from the previous emphasis on physical fitness, through more vigorous exercise of at least 20 minutes for three times per week. Many believed that anything less than this was not beneficial. Subsequently, many people chose to do nothing at all. The new message is that any activity is better than no activity. Health benefits have been documented at levels of activity below the threshold for enhancing cardiorespiratory endurance.

Moderate intensity can generally be defined as activity performed well within a person's capacity and can comfortably be sustained for a prolonged period of time (approximately 45 minutes). One way of quantifying intensity is through the use of metabolic equivalents (METs). The amount of energy expended at rest is equivalent to 1 MET. Therefore, an activity at 4 METs would represent four times the resting energy expenditure. For most adults, activities at 3 to 6 METs fall into the moderate category. Alternatively, more intense activities (> 6 METs) such as bicycling uphill or stair climbing, present a significant cardiorespiratory challenge and would be classified as "vigorous" in-

tensity. The Surgeon General's Report suggests a minimum goal of expending 150 calories per day or 1,000 calories per week to achieve health benefits. For any given target caloric expenditure, the duration of the activity session is inversely related to the relative intensity. Moderate activities such as brisk walking or raking leaves should be performed for 30 minutes, whereas more intense activities (running, jumping rope) could expend 150 calories in as little as 15 minutes. Examples of "moderate physical activity" are presented in Figure 5.1.

Another departure from the traditional exercise prescription is that the activity does not need to be performed as a single continuous exercise session. Rather, it may be accumulated throughout the day as multiple short bouts of activity (of at least 10 minutes). Therefore the recommendation to incorporate physical activity into one's daily lifestyle could be met by activities such as walking the dog, parking the car farther away from a destination, riding a bicycle to run simple errands, or taking the stairs rather than the elevator. Endeavors such as these may not appear to be significant, however the accumulation of added steps throughout the day is what could make the difference in promoting health. Although not an exercise specialist, a health counselor is certainly in the position to suggest ways a client may incorporate more activity into his/her lifestyle, and therefore meet the Surgeon General's recommendation for physical activity and improve health.

It seems clear that moderate intensity physical activity performed on a regular basis is sufficient to yield significant health benefits. However, one might ask, "If some is good, is more better?" There does appear to be a dose-response relationship between physical activity and health. As a follow-up to the recommendation for a daily dose of moderate physical activity, the Surgeon General states: "Additional health benefits can be gained through greater amounts of physical activity. People who can maintain a regular regimen of activity that is of longer duration or of more vigorous intensity are likely to derive greater benefit." This amount of physical activity is also likely to improve cardiorespiratory endurance. According to the ACSM the threshold for improving cardiorespiratory endurance is exercise performed at 50–85 percent of maximum oxygen consumption for 20 to 60 minutes, 3 to 5 times per week. Of course, there is such a thing as too much exercise. The incidence of injuries and chronic fatigue rises sharply in those engaged in vigorous exercise 6 to 7 times per week.

Cardiorespiratory fitness is the most commonly cited aspect of physical fitness when discussing the health-promoting effects of exercise. Hence, many fitness programs in the 1970s and 1980s (commercial, corporate, and clinical) focused primarily on exercise to improve cardiorespiratory endurance. Over the last decade or so a more comprehensive approach to exercise programming has been adopted to include activities that enhance/maintain muscular fitness and flexibility. Both of these indices of physical fitness contribute to quality-of-life issues with respect to musculoskeletal health and the capacity to perform routine daily activities. This is particularly important for older adults.

Exercise Programming

Preliminary Considerations. Prior to initiating a significant increase in activity level, it is wise to conduct some form of health appraisal to ensure that the activity is safe. The Physical Activity Readiness Questionnaire (PAR-Q) was developed by the Canadian Society for Exercise Physiology (1994) to identify those who might be at risk during exercise, and should consult their physician before starting an exercise program (Figure 5.2). This tool is an easy-to-use self-administered questionnaire that consists of seven questions regarding signs and symptoms of cardiovascular disease, and orthopedic history. A positive answer ("Yes") to any of the questions necessitates follow-up with the client's physician for medical clearance. Apparently healthy adults under the age of 70 years, who pass the PAR-Q, can participate in moderate physical activity without a medical evaluation. The PAR-Q is recommended as the minimum standard of health assessment for individuals starting a program of moderate-intensity exercise

A more extensive health evaluation may be warranted for those who intend to engage in more vigorous exercise. The ACSM recommends a medical examination for older men ($\geq$45 years of age) and women ($\geq$55 years of age) who wish to begin a vigorous exercise program. Of course, anyone with documented cardiovascular, respiratory, or metabolic disease should obtain medical clearance prior to any exercise program, regardless of intensity (Balady et al., 1998).

Fitness Assessment. A preliminary assessment of physical fitness is often conducted to determine initial levels of cardiorespiratory endurance, muscular strength/endurance, flexibility, and body composition. Information obtained through fitness assessment can be used to: (1) educate participants on their personal fitness levels in comparison to health-related standards, (2) develop reasonable fitness goals, (3) design an individualized exercise program tailored to the needs of the participant, and (4) evaluate progress toward fitness goals. Numerous assessments have been published for each of the health-related fitness components. Some are fairly simple field tests that require little time or equipment, while others involve more complicated techniques in the laboratory. It is beyond the scope of this text to provide a detailed description of assessment protocols.

PAR-Q & YOU
(A Questionnaire for People Aged 15 to 69)

Regular physical activity is fun and healthy, and increasingly more people are starting to become more active every day. Being more active is very safe for most people. However, some people should check with their doctor before they start becoming much more physically active.

If you are planning to become much more physically active than you are now, start by answering the seven questions in the box below. If you are between the ages of 15 and 69, the PAR-Q will tell you if you should check with your doctor before you start. If you are over 69 years of age, and you are not used to being very active, check with your doctor.

Common sense is your bets guide when you answer these questions. Please read the questions carefully and answer each one honestly: check YES or NO.

YES	NO		
❑	❑	1.	Has your doctor ever said that you have a heart condition <u>and</u> that you should only do physical activity recommended by a doctor?
❑	❑	2.	Do you feel pain in your chest when you do physical activity?
❑	❑	3.	In the past month, have you had chest pain when you were not doing physical activity?
❑	❑	4.	Do you lose your balance because of dizziness or do you ever lose consciousness?
❑	❑	5.	Do you have a bone or joint problem that could be made worse by a change in your physical activity?
❑	❑	6.	Is your doctor currently prescribing drugs (for example, water pills) for your blood pressure or heart condition?
❑	❑	7.	Do you know of <u>any other reason</u> why you should not do physical activity?

If

You

Answered

YES to one or more questions

Talk with your doctor by phone or in person BEFORE you start becoming much more physically active or BEFORE you have a fitness appraisal. Tell your doctor about the PAR-Q and which questions you answered YES.
- You may be able to do any activity you want—as long as you start slowly and build up gradually. Or, you may need to restrict your activities to those which are safe for you. Talk with your doctor about the kinds of activities you wish to participate in and follow his/her advice.
- Find out which community programs are safe and helpful for you.

NO to all questions

If you answered NO honestly to <u>all</u> PAR-Q questions, you can be reasonably sure that you can:
- start becoming much more physically active—begin slowly and build up gradually. This is the safest and easiest way to go.
- take part in a fitness appraisal—this is n excellent way to determine your basic fitness so that you can plan the best way for you to live actively.

<u>Informed Use of the PAR-Q:</u> The Canadian Society for Exercise Physiology, Health Canada, and their agents assume no liability for persons who undertake physical activity, and if in doubt after completing this questionnaire, consult your doctor prior to physical activity.

DELAY BECOMING MUCH MORE ACTIVE:
- if you are not feeling well because of a temporary illness such as a cold or a fever—wait until you feel better; or
- if you are or may be pregnant—talk to your doctor before you start becoming more active.

Please note: If your health changes so that you then answer YES to any of the above questions, tell your fitness or health professional. Ask whether you should change your physical activity plan.

Figure 5.2.
Physical activity readiness questionnaire.
Source: Reprinted with permission from the 1994 revised version of the Physical Activity Readiness Questionnaire (PAR-Q and You). The PAR-Q and You is a copyrighted, pre-exercise screen, owned by the Canadian Society for Exercise Physiology.

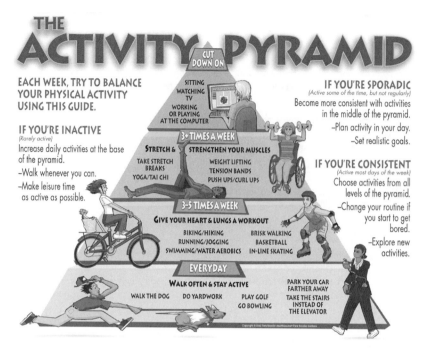

Figure 5.3
The activity pyramid
Source: Copyright © 2002 Park Nicollet *HealthSource*® Park Nicollet Institute. Reprinted by permission.

Professionals in exercise science who have been trained in the various fitness appraisal protocols should conduct fitness testing.

The Exercise Program. An exercise program is prescribed as a combination of **F**requency, **I**ntensity, and **T**ime. Also known as the FIT formula, this set of variables specifies how often one should exercise, how hard the exercise should be, and how long the exercise should last. *Frequency* is usually expressed as the recommended number of exercise bouts per week. The description of exercise *intensity* varies according to the type of activity. Exercise targeting the cardiorespiratory system is generally quantified as a percentage of cardiorespiratory endurance (maximum oxygen consumption) or maximum heart rate, whereas activities stressing muscular strength or endurance are characterized as a combination of load (amount of weight to be lifted), number of repetitions/lifts per set, and number of sets to be performed. In contrast, intensity for flexibility exercises would be in-

struction on how far one should stretch, generally to "a point of mild discomfort." *Time* refers to the duration of an exercise bout, usually denoted as minutes per session. The manner in which the FIT formula is applied to the exercise prescription will vary depending upon the targeted aspect of fitness.

Recommendations regarding daily moderate activity, and exercise to promote various aspects of physical fitness are summarized in The Activity Pyramid (Figure 5.3). This is an excellent educational tool that can be used with clients to help them understand how to incorporate a variety of exercises into a comprehensive exercise program that touches many of the health-related components of physical fitness.

The base of the pyramid represents recommendations from the Surgeon General to incorporate physical activity into your daily routine. Essentially, clients should try to incorporate more "steps" in their daily lifestyle, as described earlier in the chapter. Those who are currently inactive should start at the base of the pyramid, before moving on to the upper levels.

The second tier reflects formal recommendations from the ACSM to develop cardiorespiratory endurance. Aerobic activities, whether classified as traditional exercise or recreational, generally involve the large muscle groups of the body and are continuous in nature. Examples of aerobic activities are numerous and include, but are not limited to, the following: walking, biking, jogging, rowing, swimming laps, skating, stair climbing, cross-country skiing, dancing, jumping rope, racquet sports, and basketball. The recommended training frequency for improving cardiorespiratory endurance is three to five sessions per week. Beginners should start at three workouts per week, and gradually progress up to 5 days per week. The intensity at the second tier is somewhat higher than that at the base of the pyramid. A range of 50–85 percent of maximum oxygen consumption is suggested by the ACSM, although individuals of low fitness may initially show gains in fitness at intensities as low as 40–50 percent of maximum oxygen consumption. Generally, a target heart rate zone is prescribed (by an exercise specialist) at a specific intensity range (that is, 60–70 percent maximum oxygen consumption) based on the client's initial fitness level. The recommended time for the exercise session is between 20 to 60 minutes.

Activities promoting muscular fitness are the focus of the third tier in the Activity Pyramid. The suggested frequency for this type of exercise is two to three times per week. Muscular strength and endurance can be enhanced with resistance training involving free weights, calisthenics, variable resistance machines, or elastic tubing. A regimen of moderate load and repetition will result in modest gains for both muscular strength and endurance. The ACSM advises the following for apparently healthy adults:

- a program of 8–10 exercises that trains the major muscle groups

- a minimum of 1 set of 8–12 repetitions, performed to the point of fatigue (or 10–15 repetitions for older clients [>50–60 years])

- a training frequency of 2–3 sessions per week, alternated with days of rest to allow for ample recovery.

It is important for clients to adhere to safety precautions regarding proper lifting technique and breath control (avoid holding breath by maintaining rhythmical breathing pattern). Supervision by an exercise specialist is advisable for clients who are unfamiliar with this type of exercise. Another aspect of musculoskeletal fitness is flexibility, which is important for maintaining joint health and reducing the incidence of low back pain. A stretching routine, stressing the major muscle groups, should also be performed at a frequency of two to three times per week to achieve and maintain a healthy level of flexibility. The stretches should be performed as a gradual movement to the point of mild discomfort and held 10 to 30 seconds. The ASCM recommends that each stretch be repeated for a total of three to four repetitions with a rest period of 30 to 60 seconds between stretches. At the top of the pyramid, the emphasis turns to reducing the amount of time spent in sedentary pursuits. This could be accomplished informally by taking an activity-based break like a short walk, while engaged in a sedentary task.

Exercise Safety. The following guidelines should be considered as clients undertake an exercise program to ensure safety.

Warm-up. A 5–10 minute warm-up should be performed prior to any activity (cardiorespiratory exercise, weight training, stretching). Warming up enables the body to gradually prepare for the exercise and may reduce the risk for musculoskeletal injury. The warm-up should incorporate dynamic, low-intensity exercise that mimics the primary activity. For example, a slow walk would be an appropriate warm-up for a session of brisk walking. If planning a bout of weight training, the dynamic warm-up should be followed by a light set of resistance exercise. Stretching exercises may be included in the warm-up, but should follow the dynamic portion of the warm-up period.

Cool-down. The exercise session should be concluded with a 5–10 minute cool-down, performed at lower intensity. Cooling down allows the body to gradually return to a resting state and reduces the risk of cardiovascular complications, such as low blood pressure and dizziness. This is also an excellent time to include the flexibility component of the program.

Progression. The exercise program should be progressed gradually. Progression can be divided into three phases: initial conditioning, improvement, and maintenance (American College of Sports Medicine, 2000). The goal of the initial phase is to allow the individual to adapt to the increase in activity through low to moderate exercise, while at the same time preventing muscle soreness or injury that might discourage adherence to the exercise program. An increase in physical fitness is the primary objective during the improvement phase. This phase is characterized by periodic upgrades in workload to promote continued development of physical fitness. Once fitness goals have been achieved in the improvement phase, the client can move on to the maintenance phase, continuing with a similar workout routine.

Additional information regarding exercise programming and prescription is summarized in the ACSM Position Stand on "The Recommended Quantity and Quality of Exercise for Developing and Maintaining Cardiorespiratory and Muscular Fitness, and Flexibility in Healthy Adults" (1998). Clients interested in starting a formal exercise program to enhance physical fitness should be encouraged to work with a fitness professional with expertise in the area of fitness assessment and exercise prescription.

Changing exercise-related behavior. Despite the numerous benefits of regular exercise on health, a large proportion of the general population (40 percent) reports no participation in leisure-time physical activity. Furthermore, the percentage of individuals not engaged in leisure-time physical activity is higher in select groups such as women, minorities, older adults, individuals with disabilities, and those with lower achieved educa-

tion level (CDC, National Center for Health Statistics, 1998–1999). Similar trends in the opposite direction are noted for these specific populations with regard to participation in various forms of exercise (moderate exercise, vigorous exercise, strengthening exercise, stretching exercise). For example, rates of participation in "30 minutes of activity 5 or more days per week" are higher in males than females, Caucasians compared to minorities, youth compared to elders, and in college graduates as opposed to those with less education. A summary of percentages for those who report no leisure activity, as well as those who engage in regular exercise is presented in Table 5.3.

Among the goals of the "Healthy People 2010: Understanding and Improving Health" document is to increase levels of physical activity (United States Department of Health and Human Services/CDC, 1998–1999). Specific objectives regarding physical activity include the following:

- Reduce the proportion of adults who engage in no leisure-time physical activity
  (40 percent → 20 percent).

- Increase the proportion of adults who engage regularly, preferably daily, in moderate physical activity for at least 30 minutes per day
  (15 percent → 30 percent).

- Increase the proportion of adults who engage in vigorous physical activity that promotes the development and maintenance of cardiorespiratory fitness 3 or more days for 20 or more minutes per occasion
  (23 percent → 30 percent).

- Increase the proportion of adults who perform physical activities that enhance and maintain muscular strength and endurance
  (18 percent → 30 percent).

- Increase the proportion of adults who perform physical activities that enhance and maintain flexibility
  (30 percent → 43 percent).

Health counselors may play an important role in encouraging sedentary adults to adopt a more active lifestyle. The social learning–social cognitive theo-

Table 5.3
Percentage of Individuals Engaged in Physical Activity from Select Populations

	No Leisure-Time Physical Activity (1997)	30 Minutes of Activity 5 or More Days per Week (1997)	Vigorous Physical Activity (1997)	Strengthening & Endurance Exercises (1998)	Stretching Exercises (1998)
Total	40%	15%	23%	18%	30%
Gender					
Female	43%	13%	20%	14%	30%
Male	36%	16%	26%	21%	30%
Ethnicity					
African Am	52%	10%	17%	16%	26%
Hispanic	54%	11%	16%	13%	22%
White	38%	15%	24%	18%	30%
Education					
<9th grade	73%	7%	6%	4%	16% (<H.S.)
H.S. grad	46%	14%	18%	11%	23% (H.S.)
College grad	24%	17%	32%	26%	36% (>H.S.)
Age					
18–24 yr	31%	17%	32%	28%	36%
25–44 yr	34%	15%	27%	21%	32%
45–64 yr	42%	14%	21%	14%	28%
65–74 yr	51%	16%	13%	10%	24%
≥75 yr	65%	12%	6%	7%	22%
Disability					
Yes	56%	12%	13%	14% (1997)	29% (1995)
No	36%	16%	25%	20% (1997)	31% (1995)

Source: Modified data from the National Health Interview Survey as presented in Centers of Disease Control and Prevention, National Center for Health Statistics, Healthy People 2000 Review, 1998–1999.

ries are often used for clients with a desire to change their behavior regarding physical activity. A client is more likely to achieve and maintain an increase in activity level if the exercise program is individualized, taking into account personal, behavioral, and environmental factors (King & Martin, 2001).

The program should be personalized by linking physical activity to specific concerns and goals. In other words, the outcomes of the behavior change must be relevant to the lifestyle of the individual. A health counselor can provide information about how an exercise program would improve specific health issues and enable a client to perform certain activities at home with greater ease. For example, a walking program combined with some moderate resistance exercise would help a 62-year-old woman with concerns over osteoporosis, maintain bone density, and pick up her toddler grandson when baby-sitting. The health counselor may also be in a position to dispel some of the myths regarding exercise. Many clients grew up with the "no pain, no gain" adage, and believe that exercise must be difficult and painful to attain health benefits. We now know that even light to moderate exercise can yield positive effects on various health issues.

There are several behavioral and environmental factors to consider when adopting a change in physical-activity behavior. Some of the common barriers to exercise include lack of time, lack of confidence in ability to exercise, lack of social support, lack of internal motivation, and lack of resources (safe and convenient exercise facilities). A health counselor may help a client to identify personal barriers to exercise and subsequently develop strategies to overcome these hurdles to behavior change. There are a number of strategies that address the issue of lack of time. One suggestion is that the client monitor his or her schedule for a period of a week and identify at least three time slots of 30 minutes for exercise. A client could also be advised to take 10 to 15 minutes during his or her lunch hour and in the morning/evening to take a walk. In this case it is particularly important to select activities that are convenient and require minimal preparation time (United States Department of Health and Human Services, 1996).

Approximately 50 percent of those who start an exercise program drop out within six months of initiating the program. One step toward ensuring adherence to the program is to consider potential barriers to exercise as discussed above. The exercise plan should incorporate strategies to overcome perceived barriers, as well as focus on personal goals to achieve desired outcomes. Clients who believe that the benefits of the exercise outweigh the negative aspects (such as time commitment) are more likely to stick with the program. Additional tips to promote compliance to

an increase in physical activity level include the following:

- Incorporate a variety of activities that the client enjoys to reduce boredom.

- Start with low to moderate exercise and progress gradually to minimize muscle soreness and risk of injury.

- Involve family and friends in physical activity for social support or consider group exercise.

- Periodically reassess progress toward personal goals and modify the program accordingly (note that goals must be attainable, measurable, and relevant to client).

Case Study

Recommending an Exercise Program

A 20-year-old college student has experienced a 15-pound weight gain since he entered school 3 years ago. He tries to fit in some mild resistance training twice a week, but does not perform any regular cardiorespiratory exercise. Recently he joined an intramural basketball team, and finds that he becomes winded after a few minutes of play. The student would like to drop a few pounds and get into shape so that he can feel better about participating in recreational activities. Discuss your recommendations for how he might change his behavior and incorporate exercise to meet his personal goals.

Answer. The student should incorporate moderate physical activity into his daily routine between classes. This could be done through walking, taking the stairs, and playing informal games that are somewhat active (such as Frisbee, catch). These simple activities could be implemented in relatively short blocks of time and could also be done in a social context if he so desires. The added expenditure of calories would help contribute to weight loss. He should also be directed to see a fitness professional on campus, to obtain a formal exercise program to raise his cardiorespiratory endurance so that he does not become so easily winded when playing basketball. He would likely be advised to select from a variety of cardiorespiratory activities such as walking/jogging, cycling, swimming, rowing machine, or in-line skating. The exercise program should start at a moderate intensity (50–65 percent of maximum oxygen consumption) for 20 to 30 minutes three to four times per week. He would then be advised to gradually progress to a program at 60–75 percent of maximum consumption for 30 to 40 minutes 4 to 5 times per week. Of course, dietary modifications would also play a critical role in achieving his goal-related weight loss.

Nutrition and weight-management issues will be discussed in the next section.

Nutrition and Weight Management

Healthy Weight Management

Epidemiological research indicates a J-shape relationship between body weight and mortality. This means that being either underweight or overweight increases the risk of a premature death. Therefore, the definition of healthy weight is a weight within the range associated with good health and longevity. In the United States healthy weight guidelines were historically established by the insurance industry, in part based on longevity. These guidelines gave healthy weight ranges for adults based on height. Today healthy weight ranges are given based on Body Mass Index (BMI), which will be defined later in this chapter.

Body weight in adults is regulated by several internal and external factors, which makes it a complex system to control. Internal factors, such as the endocrine and nervous systems, physiologic, genetic, and metabolic factors maintain the balance between energy intake and energy expenditure under normal circumstances. The external factors are the ones that can be managed by lifestyle modification. The two external factors, which are emphasized in many health textbooks, are exercise and nutrition. The 1996 Surgeon General's Report on Physical Activity and Health states that the sedentary lifestyle in the U.S. population is a contributing factor to increase in body weight. Excess energy intake is another contributing factor. The American Dietetic Association's position on weight management for adults (1997) states that it "requires a lifelong commitment to healthful lifestyle behaviors emphasizing eating practices and daily physical activity that are sustainable and enjoyable." The management of energy intake and physical activity can influence body weight significantly and can lead to a healthy body weight throughout a person's life.

Body composition. Weight alone does not reflect the amount of adipose tissue in the body; hence **body composition** is more critical in determining heath risks than just body weight. The human body consists primarily of fluid, muscle, organs, bone, and adipose tissue. The three main components of the body are fluid, fat, and lean body mass. Lean body mass is defined as the total weight of the body minus the weight of the fat content. Lean body mass represents the active tissue that is involved in metabolic activities whereas fat tissue or adipose tissue represents the less active component in the human body. However, a certain amount of body fat, usually referred to as percentage of fat, is necessary for the body's vital functions. These functions include protection of internal organs, insulation, production of some hormones and bile for the digestion of fat, and assistance in the digestion, absorption, and transport of the essential fat-soluble vitamins (A, D, E, and vitamin K). Age and physical condition can change the proportion of some or all these components. Approximately 60–65 percent of body weight is water and the fluid content is much higher in infants and young children than in adults. Likewise, the variation in physical activity changes the state of hydration and muscle-mass contents. For example, muscular athletes may be classified as overweight because of a large amount of muscle mass or lean body mass rather than an excess of adipose mass or fat tissue. Body fat ranges from 20 to 25 percent in adult women and from 12 to 20 percent

Body composition. The relative percentage of fat and fat-free tissues (muscles, bone, and water) in the body.

in adult men. The essential body fat, the fat necessary for normal physiologic functions, is about 12 percent for women and approximately 3 percent for men. The remaining fat in the body is storage fat, which accumulates in adipose tissue. The loss of body fat below the level of essential fat is not compatible with good health. At the same time, body fat more than 30 percent in women and 25 percent in men is considered unhealthy.

The distribution of fat on the body may be more critical than the amount of fat alone. Intra-abdominal fat that is stored around the abdominal organs or upper body is referred to as central obesity, "android" or "apple-shaped," which is associated with elevated risk for cardiovascular disease and some types of cancer (Whitney & Rolfes, 2002). This distribution is very common in men and in women after menopause. Fat distribution around hips and thighs is referred to as lower-body fat, which presents fewer health risks. This is more common in women during the reproductive years and is also called "gynoid" or "pear-shape."

Methods to Assess Body Composition. There are several methods to assess body fat and body composition. The most common ones are described below:

- Skinfold—This method measures subcutaneous body fat by using a caliper to gauge the thickness of a fold of skin. The basis for this estimate of body fat relies on the assumption that almost half of the body fat is subcutaneous. Several measurement sites have been identified as most reflective of body fat, such as the back of the arm, below the shoulder blade, upper chest, abdominal, hip, thigh, and calf. The selection of sites is based on the population tested and the particular formula chosen to compute percent fat from the sum of skinfolds.

- Hydrodensitometry—In this method the body density is estimated by weighing the person first in air and then weighing them again while submerged under water. The estimate of body density can in turn be used to predict percent body fat.

- Bioelectrical Impedance—A low-intensity electrical current is applied through electrodes attached to the feet and hands. Normally, electrolyte-containing fluids, which are primarily found in lean body tissues, readily conduct an electrical current. Fat tissue does not conduct electricity as well. The measurement of electrical resistance through the body is then used in an equation to estimate the overall percentage of body fat.

Regulation of Energy Intake and Body Weight. Foods and their components—carbohydrates, protein, and fat—all contribute to the total energy (Kcal or kilocalorie) one consumes. Total energy intake must be regulated for achieving an optimal weight and a healthy lifestyle. One of the popular misconceptions regarding diet is that only fat intake must be regulated in order to balance energy intake. Moreover, food consumption is regulated by internal factors such as hunger, a physiological drive for food, and satiety, a feeling of satisfaction. Both of these internal stimuli are generated by the nervous system and hormonal interaction, which operate as feedback mechanisms within the body. External environmental factors such as sensory inputs, emotions, habits, and cognitive behavior influence food consumption as well. Therefore, eating is a complex behavior regulated by psychological, social, metabolic, and physiological factors (Levine & Billington, 1997). Because of this complexity, it is difficult to determine specific factors that lead to overeating and weight abnormalities.

Achieving a balance between energy expenditure and energy intake is the key factor in maintaining healthy body weight under normal conditions. To achieve this **energy balance** the body must meet its energy needs without going over or under its energy expenditure. To estimate the body's total energy need (total energy expendi-

Energy balance. When a person's energy consumed (calories) per day closely matches his or her energy expenditure.

Table 5.4
Sample Computation of Caloric Intake and Expenditure

Susan is a 21-year-old college student weighing of 59 kg*. She reports an activity level of light to moderate. She also recorded her food intake for one day estimating a consumption of 100 g fat, 200 g carbohydrate (CHO), and 100 g protein.

Caloric Intake	Caloric Expenditure
100 g of fat $\times$ 9 Kcal/g = 900 Kcal	REE = 59 $\times$ 0.9 $\times$ 24 = 1274 Kcal
200 g of CHO $\times$ 4 Kcal/g = 800 Kcal	Activity = 1274 $\times$ .45 = 573 Kcal
100 g of protein $\times$ 4 Kcal/g = 400 Kcal	TEF = (1274 + 573) $\times$ .10 = 185 Kcal
Total caloric intake = 2,100 Kcal	Total = 1274 + 573 + 185 = 2,032 Kcal

* To convert kilograms (kg) to pounds (lb): 1 kg = 2.2 lbs. Therefore, 59 kg $\times$ 2.2 = 129.8 lbs. To convert pounds to kilograms divide the weight in pounds by 2.2.

ture, TEE), three main components of energy expenditure must be calculated.

1. Basal metabolic activities (resting energy expenditure, REE) compromise about two-thirds of the energy needed to sustain normal body functions. Resting energy expenditure may be computed with one of the following formulas:
   - Females:
     REE = weight (kg) $\times$ 0.9 Kcal/kg $\times$ 24 hr
   - Males:
     REE = weight (kg) $\times$ 1.0 Kcal/kg $\times$ 24 hr

   There are other methods for estimating REE such as Harris and Benedict's formula which takes into account a person's weight, height, and age (Mahan & Escott-Stump, 2000).

2. Physical activity is the most variable component and depends on the type, duration, and intensity of activity, body weight, and muscle mass. The expenditure for physical activity is calculated as a percentage of energy expenditure (REE). It may range from 10 percent in a person who is confined to bed to 50–60 percent for an athlete. In the case of nonathletes participating in exercise, 30–45 percent of REE is used for light activities and 45–60 percent of REE is computed for moderate intensity activities.

3. The thermic effect of food is the energy needed for food to be utilized by the body. This is computed as 10 percent of the sum of REE and physical activity expenditure.

Estimation of food intake in Kcal can be done in one of two ways. First, the fat, protein, and carbohydrate quantities in each food can be estimated from food-composition labels or a standard food database such as those issued by the U.S. Department of Agriculture. Caloric equivalents for a single gram of fat, carbohydrate, and protein are 9, 4, and 4 kcal/g respectively. A second option is to use a computer program, which has the food composition tables built in. The standard approach to food-intake surveys is usually to obtain a daily average from 3-day or 7-day food records, 24-hour recall, and food frequency data. A sample computation of caloric intake and expenditure is presented to Table 5.4.

In the table, Susan's caloric intake was computed for each nutrient by multiplying her consumption in grams by the respective caloric equivalent. A total caloric intake was then calculated as the sum of Kcals for all three nutrients. Resting energy expenditure was obtained by entering Susan's body weight (kg) to the formula for REE. Activity and thermic effect of food expenditures were computed as 45 percent and 10 percent of REE respectively. The total energy expenditure was ascertained as the sum of these three components. Susan's energy balance is: energy consumed (2,100 Kcal) vs. energy expenditure (2,032) Kcal. Her energy intake for this day exceeded slightly her energy output by 68 Kcal. From the practical perspective this is close to an energy balance. Energy imbalance is typically a difference of 200

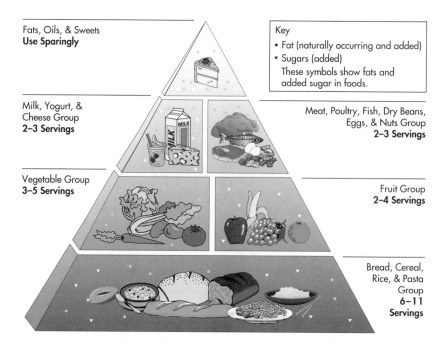

Figure 5.4
Food guide pyramid
Source: The United States Department of Agriculture, 1992.

or more Kcal per day or 10 percent or more of the total Kcal requirement.

The body receives its energy needs from foods in chemical form. This means that foods are made up of many chemical molecules (nutrients) such as proteins, carbohydrates, fat, vitamins, and water. When these nutrients metabolize in the cells, this chemical energy is transformed into other forms of energy such as mechanical, chemical, heat, and electrical energy for the body's health maintenance. Nutritional management can do the regulation of this energy intake from foods intentionally by regulating either the quantity or the nutrient density of the food consumed. Foods that provide more nutrients per unit of energy are called nutrient-dense foods. Nutrient-dense foods are important because they enable a person to obtain all the essential vitamins and minerals required for good health without eating too many Kcal. Examples of nutrient-dense foods are most fruits and vegetables. Nutrient-dense foods make up a significant part of the Food Guide Pyramid, a

dietary guide to the kinds and amounts of foods one should eat daily (Figure 5.4).

The Food Guide Pyramid divides foods into the five major food groups and the amounts are given in terms of "servings." Each food group provides some, but not all, of the nutrients one needs. All food groups are important sources of nutrients and for good health they need to be included in daily meals. When the diet is planned to include a wide variety of foods in each group, the result is a diet that is adequate in all nutrients. The Food Guide Pyramid emphasizes that the intake of the plant-based foods such as grains, vegetables, and fruits should be almost 75 percent of a day's intake. The recommended number of servings is in ranges in order to accommodate the energy requirements for all ages. For example, the lower number of servings from each food group provides enough energy for older adults or sedentary women who need about 1,600 Kcal. The upper level provides about 2,800 Kcal for active young men, very active women, and teenage boys. The middle range, about

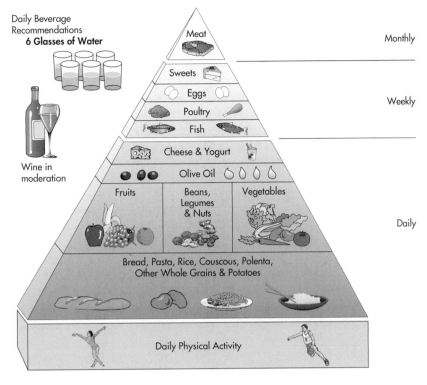

Figure 5.5
The Mediterranean diet pyramid
Source: ©2000 Oldways Preservation and Exchange Trust. http://oldwayspt.org

2,200 Kcal meets the needs for most children, teenage girls, active women and sedentary men.

To address the needs of a diverse population, the U.S. Department of Agriculture has translated the Food Guide Pyramid into many languages and they are available on the USDA Food and Nutrition Information Center Web site at: http://www.usda.gov. There is also a Food Guide Pyramid for young Children (USDA Center for Nutrition and Policy Promotion, 1999) and a Modified Food Guide Pyramid for 70+ adults which focuses on the nutritional needs of older adults (Russell, Rasmussen, & Lichtenstein, 1999). Some regions of the world have developed their own food-guide pyramids based on the cultural practices and availability of certain foods in those regions. Figure 5.5 illustrates the Mediterranean Diet Pyramid as an example (Oldways Preservation and Exchange Trust, 2000).

These food guides can be effective educational tools for teaching and promoting healthy eating habits by motivating clients to change their food behaviors. Encouraging high consumption of natural plant-based foods such as whole grains, fruits, vegetables, and other nutritious foods is the main purpose of these guides.

Healthy Weight. Healthy weight means not being overweight or underweight. Being overweight is more prevalent than being underweight, but being underweight also presents health risks. Healthy weight also must indicate the appropriate proportions (percent) of the body's components, namely fluid, muscle mass, fat, bone, and others. Body Bass Index (BMI), an index of a person's weight in relation to height, is a common formula for classifying body weight, but it does not reflect body composition and/or the percentage of body fat.

Table 5.5
Body Mass Index Table (BMI)

Body Mass Index Table

To use the table, find the appropriate height in the left-hand column labeled Height. Move across to a given weight. The number at the top of the column is the BMI at that height and weight. Pounds have been rounded off.

BMI	19	20	21	22	23	24	25	26	27	28	29	30	31	32	33	34	35
Height (inches)	Body Weight (pounds)																
58	91	96	100	105	110	115	119	124	129	134	138	143	148	153	158	162	167
59	94	99	104	109	114	119	124	128	133	138	143	148	153	158	163	168	173
60	97	102	107	112	118	123	128	133	138	143	148	153	158	163	168	174	179
61	100	106	111	116	122	127	132	137	143	148	153	158	164	169	174	180	185
62	104	109	115	120	126	131	136	142	147	153	158	164	169	175	180	186	191
63	107	113	118	124	130	135	141	146	152	158	163	169	175	180	186	191	197
64	110	116	122	128	134	140	145	151	157	163	169	174	180	186	192	197	204
65	114	120	126	132	138	144	150	156	162	168	174	180	186	192	198	204	210
66	118	124	130	136	142	148	155	161	167	173	179	186	192	198	204	210	216
67	121	127	134	140	146	153	159	166	172	178	185	191	198	204	211	217	223
68	125	131	138	144	151	158	164	171	177	184	190	197	203	210	216	223	230
69	128	135	142	149	155	162	169	176	182	189	196	203	209	216	223	230	236
70	132	139	146	153	160	167	174	181	188	195	202	209	216	222	229	236	243
71	136	143	150	157	165	172	179	186	193	200	208	215	222	229	236	243	250
72	140	147	154	162	169	177	184	191	199	206	213	221	228	235	242	250	258
73	144	151	159	166	174	182	189	197	204	212	219	227	235	242	250	257	265
74	148	155	163	171	179	186	194	202	210	218	225	233	241	249	256	264	272
75	152	160	168	176	184	192	200	208	216	224	232	240	248	256	264	272	279
76	156	164	172	180	189	197	205	213	221	230	238	246	254	263	271	279	287

Source: Adapted from Clinical Guidelines on the Identification, Evaluation, and Treatment of Overweight and Obesity in Adults: The Evidence Report. National Institute of Health Obesity Evaluation Initiative (1998).

BMI is therefore appropriately supplemented with a body fat measurement.

BMI is determined by the following formula:

$$(BMI) = \text{weight (kg)/height (m)}^2 \; or$$
$$\text{weight (lb)/ height (in)}^2 \times 705^*$$

Table 5.5 illustrates the weight classifications based on BMI. Healthy weight ranges from a BMI of 18.5 to 24.9, with underweight being below 18.5 and overweight being above 25.

Overweight and **obesity,** BMI more than 25 and 30 respectively, continue to rise dramatically

---

* The NIH Practical Guide for Identification, Evaluation, and Treatment of obesity and Overweight in the US uses 703 rather than 705 for calculating BMI (NIH, 2000)

Obesity. Excessive fat deposits in adipose tissue, having a Body Mass Index (BMI) of 30 or more.

in the United States. The average BMI of adults in the United States is about 26.5. Over half of the adults in the United States are considered overweight and the problem is so widespread that some refer to it as an epidemic (Koplan & Dietz, 1999).

The excessive fat deposits in adipose tissues can cause overweight and obesity. There are some theories and mechanisms that may explain the fat cell development and metabolism in humans. Basically, if the energy intake is more than the energy spent, the excess energy will be stored in the fat tissue (adipose). The enzyme lipoprotein lipase (LPL) promotes fat storage. Therefore, people with high LPL activity store fat more efficiently. Obese people, who have more fat cells, also have more LPL activity and even modest excesses in energy intake have a more significant impact on them than on lean people (Kern, 1997). The activity of LPL is partially regulated by gender hormones such as testosterone in men and estrogen in women. Set-point theory, which states that a body tends to maintain a certain body weight by means of its internal control, explains why it is difficult for underweight persons to maintain weight gains and for overweight persons to maintain weight losses.

Underweight is having a body weight that is too low, BMI less than 18.5, and has adverse health effects. The causes of underweight conditions are as diverse as those leading to overweight conditions. Underweight could be due to internal factors such as heredity, hunger, satiety irregularities, metabolic, or psychological factors or excessive physical activity without providing enough calories for this expenditure. An extreme underweight condition known as anorexia nervosa is a major eating disorder, which must be treated by health professionals. Weight-gain strategies emphasize eating foods that provide many Kcals (kilocalories) in a small volume (energy-dense foods) and exercising to build muscles.

Weight-Loss (Management) Techniques

An estimated 30–40 percent of American women and 20–25 percent of American men are trying to lose weight at any given time (NIH, 1992). The American Dietetic Association's position is that "the goal of obesity treatment should be refocused from weight loss alone to weight management, which means achieving the best weight possible in the context of overall health" (American Dietetic Association, 1997). There are many weight-management strategies, but they can be effective only if they include healthy and sustainable eating and exercise. Effective strategies can be placed into the following categories:

- **Dietary modification**   A restricted energy diet is the most common method of weight management.

- **Physical activity**   A combination of cardiovascular and resistance exercise can serve as an important adjunct to dietary modification.

- **Behavior modification**   Instituting an overall change of behavior by manipulation of environmental factors which may trigger a given behavior and its consequences.

- **Pharmacotherapy**   For persons with a BMI of 30 or above, pharmaceutical agents in addition to a diet and exercise program can be helpful.

- **Surgery**   In case of morbid obesity, with BMI of 40 or higher, surgical procedures may be considered.

Dietary Modifications. Dietary modification should take into consideration that while the energy levels are reduced, the diet needs to continue to be nutritionally adequate. The energy level required varies with the individual's size and activities and can be classified as: (1) moderate energy deficit diet having daily 1,200 calories (women) to 1,400+ calories (men), (2) a low-calorie diet containing 800–1,200 calories/day (women) and 800–1,400 calories/day (men), (3) and a very-low-calorie-diet (VLCD) containing 800 or fewer calories per day. Healthy eating habits and physical activity should be emphasized at all levels of energy-reduction programs (Shape Up America! American Obesity Association, 1998). Low-energy diets should be prescribed and monitored by physicians and registered dietitians.

Numerous commercial diet programs are also available. However, the long-term effectiveness of these programs is not clear (Mahan & Escott-Stump, 2000). Fad diets and practices should be examined very carefully and not used unless under the supervision of a physician or registered dietician. To evaluate weight-loss programs, several publications are available. The Institute of Medicine published *Weighing the Options*, which describes a set of criteria that could be used to evaluate and treat the problem of obesity. A report from The Federal Trade Commission (FTC), which for the first time included representatives of the weight-loss industry, scientific community, state, federal government, and consumer groups, also addresses issues regarding weight-loss products and programs (Gross & Daynard, 1997). A year later, the NIH released *Clinical Guidelines on the Identification, Evaluation, and Treatment of Overweight and Obesity in Adults—The Evidence Report* (NIH, 1998). The guidelines provide evidence for the effects of the treatment of overweight and obesity.

Physical activity. Physical activity combined with moderate caloric restriction is one of the most commonly recommended strategies for achieving and maintaining a healthy weight. The relative contribution of exercise to short-term weight loss in combined diet and exercise programs appears to be minimal; however, exercise is an important factor in the maintenance of weight loss over time. Individuals who are overweight have special needs, which should be considered when designing an exercise program. The primary goal in this population is to maximize energy expenditure, while minimizing the risk of injury. The ACSM recommends a target activity-related energy expenditure of 300–400 Kcal per day for those trying to lose weight. Sedentary clients should start at 150–200 Kcal and work up to the target energy expenditure gradually over time. A list of common activities with corresponding MET values is presented in Table 5.6. Caloric expenditure can be estimated from the MET value with the following formula: (METs $\times$ 3.5 $\times$ body weight in kg)/200 = Kcal/min. Therefore, a participant weighing 100 kg would expend 6.1 Kcal/min if walking at a moderate pace (3 mph) on level ground. One

of the keys to success in a long-term weight-management program is adherence to a routine of regular physical activity. Selected activities should be convenient and fun, based on the client's interests. Low-impact activities such as walking, stationary cycling, and swimming are often chosen to reduce stress on joints and risk of injury. Incorporation of a variety of activities in the exercise program will also help to minimize boredom and promote compliance. The FIT formula is applied with a greater emphasis on moderate intensity (50–70 percent of

Table 5.6
Common Activities and Corresponding MET Values

Activity	METs Used
Aerobic Dance—low impact	5.0
Basketball—shooting baskets	4.5
Bicycling—general/leisure, <10 mph	4.0
Bicycling—stationary, 100 Watts	5.5
Canoeing—for pleasure, general	3.5
Dancing—general	4.5
Gardening—general	5.0
Golf—pulling clubs	5.0
Ice skating—general	7.0
Mowing lawn—walk, hand mower	6.0
Raking lawn	4.0
Rowing—stationary, 100 Watts	7.0
Tennis—doubles	6.0
Tai Chi	4.0
Skiing—cross country, 2.5 mph, slow or light effort	7.0
Snow shoeing	8.0
Swimming laps—freestyle, slow, moderate or light effort	8.0
Walking—2.5 mph, firm surface	3.0
Walking—3.0 mph, level, moderate pace, firm surface	3.5
Walking—3.5 mph, level, brisk pace, firm surface	4.0

Source: Selected activities taken from Ainsworth et al. (1993). "Compendium of physical activities: classification of energy costs of human physical activities," in *Medicine and Science in Sport* 1, 1993, 71–80. Reprinted by permission.

maximum oxygen consumption) performed over a longer duration (40–60 min/ day) than in the general population (American College of Sports Medicine, 2000). A relatively low-moderate intensity is advised, as it is tolerated better with lower risk of injury, and is associated with higher rates of adherence. The combination of a lengthy duration and high frequency (five to seven times/week) should yield adequate energy expenditure to achieve a negative caloric balance. A recently published ACSM Position Stand on strategies for weight loss recommends an accumulation of 200 to 300 minutes of exercise per week for successful weight management (Jakicic et al., 2001). Moderate resistance training might also be incorporated to help maintain lean body mass and enhance muscular strength, needed for an active lifestyle.

Behavior modification. Behavior modification can play an important role in supporting efforts to achieve and maintain appropriate body weight. The first step in this process is to become aware of certain behaviors, for example consuming high-fat foods and not engaging in enough physical activity. The next step would be developing strategies to change these behaviors such as selecting nutrient-dense and low-fat foods and including an exercise routine in the daily schedule.

Pharmaceutical management. Pharmaceutical management can be helpful in individuals with high body-mass indexes of 30 and above, or 27 and above with other risks, in addition to a diet and exercise program. These medications can affect the brain to suppress appetite, increase metabolism, and selectively interfere with fat absorption. However, these medications may have side effects, and the benefits and risks must be evaluated carefully and consultation with a physician is strongly recommended before taking any diet medications.

Surgery. Surgery should be considered the last option for weight management. This option is reserved for individuals for whom all other options have failed and whose BMI is 40 or higher or 35 with other risk factors. These procedures decrease the amount of food entering and/or being absorbed from the gastrointestinal tract. Some of these procedures include esophageal banding, gastric restrictive surgery, and jejunal bypass among others. Postoperative follow-up and evaluation at regular intervals by the surgical team and registered dietitian is recommended (NIH, 1998).

Healthy Nutrition/Dietary Modification

Nutrition counseling is based on individual lifestyle modification. All aspects of healthy behavior must be taken into consideration to achieve the optimum results. For example, balancing energy expenditure and energy intake by combining a nutritionally balanced dietary regime with exercise could be the principle for a successful and healthy weight-loss program. At the same time reasonable expectations about health and weight goals and how long it will take to achieve this goal are also very important. Healthy weight that reduces health risks for cardiovascular disease, diabetes, high blood pressure, and cholesterol should be a preferable goal rather than focusing on the weight loss alone. Realistic goals for successful weight-management program need a reasonable time frame. For example, a 200-pound person losing 10–20 pounds in a year is more likely to maintain the losses than if he/she tries to lose 70 pounds in a year. Rapid weight loss may mean the excessive loss of essential body components, such as fluids and lean tissue, and a rapid weight gain to follow (Whitney & Rolfes, 2002).

Determination of ideal body weight (IBW) and target body weight can be useful when developing weight-management goals. Ideal body weight may be calculated with the Hamwi formula (Miller, 1985). In this method, 106 pounds are allowed for the first 5 feet of height for men plus 6 pounds for

Nutrition. A well-balanced meal plan that includes nutrient-dense foods, fruits, vegetables, grains, lean meats or meat alternatives, and low-fat dairy foods which supply no more than 30 percent of calories as fat.

every additional inch over 5 feet. For women, 100 pounds is allowed for the first 5 feet plus 5 pounds for each additional inch. This applies to persons with a medium frame size. Up to 10 percent can be added for a large frame and up to 10 percent can be subtracted for a small frame. For example, a large-frame-size woman who is 5'3" tall, would have an IBW of 126.5 pounds [(100 pounds + 15 pounds) + 10 percent (115 pounds)].

The term *ideal body weight* may reflect the variations between all individuals, but it provides a valuable point of reference. Unfortunately, for many obese individuals, IBW based on height may not be realistic; nor does it take into account body composition. A target body weight (TBW) aimed at reducing the percent fat by a moderate amount may be quite effective in reducing health risks, even if the IBW is not reached. A simple formula for computing TBW is to divide the fat-free weight by the desired percentage (decimal form) of lean body mass. For example, the 5'3" woman above may have a percent body fat of 33 percent and weigh 160 pounds. She could start with a reasonable goal of reducing her percent body fat to 27 percent. Her desired percentage of lean body mass would be obtained by subtracting 27 percent from 100. This value of 73 percent would be expressed in decimal form as .73 and plugged into the denominator of the formula. The amount of fat in the body is determined by multiplying the current body weight by the current percent body fat in decimal form (160 pounds × .33 = 53 pounds of fat). Fat-free weight can then be ascertained by subtracting the amount of fat in the body from the total body weight (160 − 53 = 107 pounds). Target body weight would be calculated as follows: 107 pounds/.73 = 146 pounds. The resultant weight-loss goal of 14 pounds is much more realistic for long-term weight loss than 34 pounds to achieve IBW. Once the client has lost and maintained this initial goal for at least 6 months, she could consider additional weight loss.

In planning a healthy nutrition program for weight management, all foods should be included. There is no need to exclude or include specific foods, as most fad diets suggest. Diet modification should be based on the following concepts:

- **Energy**—Energy should be limited but provide nutritional adequacy. The total energy intake should not go below 1,200 calories a day for women, 1,400 for men and energy expenditure should exceed energy intake. In other words, an adult needs to increase activity and reduce food intake enough to create a 500-Kcal deficit/day. This will result in a weight loss of about 1 pound per week, which is considered a reasonable weight-loss rate (NIH, 1998).

- **Nutritional adequacy**—Nutritional adequacy should be a high priority even with limited energy intake. A well-balanced meal plan will allow individuals to lose weight and meet their nutrient needs. This meal plan includes nutrient dense foods, fruits, vegetables, whole grains, lean meats, or meat alternates, and low-fat dairy foods, which supply no more than 30 percent of kilocalories as fat.

- **Carbohydrates**—Carbohydrate-rich foods should be the base of a balanced meal plan. Plant-based foods such as whole grains, fruits, vegetables, and legumes provide complex carbohydrates and fiber. They are also good sources of many vitamins and minerals and are low in fat. These foods are considered nutrient-dense.

- **Fats**—The American Heart Association recommends that 30 percent or less of calories should be from fat. Recent studies on the effects of leptin, a protein produced by fat cells that decreases appetite and increases energy expenditure, indicates that high-fat meals tend to lower blood leptin. The low level of blood leptin causes hunger and therefore causes a person to overeat (Chapelot et al., 2000). The advice is to limit high-fat foods and choose fat sensibly, including unsaturated fat in the meal plan.

- **Protein**—Protein-rich foods provide satiety and 10–20 percent of kcals should be from protein foods such as lean meats, eggs, dairy, and plant-based protein foods such as legumes and nuts.

- **Portion sizes**—Small portions of all foods should be included in a balanced meal plan.

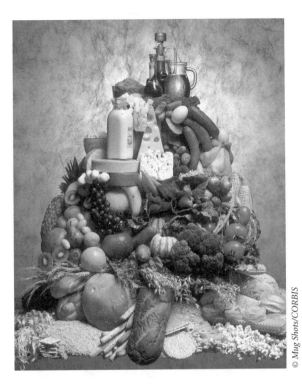

© *Mug Shots/CORBIS*

Good nutrition means eating from all the food groups in a healthy portion.

Even no-fat and low-fat foods can provide sufficient kilocalories if they are eaten in large enough quantities.

- **Concentrated sweets and alcoholic beverages**—Consider limiting empty kcal foods such as alcoholic drinks and concentrated sweets and include plenty of water throughout the day.

The lifelong "eating plan for good health" rather than a "diet for weight loss" is more likely to keep lost weight off for a long time (Whitney & Rolfes, 2002).

Nutrition Counseling and Behavioral Changes. Health counselors must understand the importance of the multidimensional and holistic nature of health and wellness. This means that there are many aspects to health that interact with one another. Dietary modification or healthy eating be-

havior is one of these many aspects. Nutrition counseling should facilitate positive dietary change, which in turn will lead to a successful and satisfying health outcome. Health counselors have to motivate their clients to change through self-managed behaviors and by setting some achievable dietary goals. For example: reducing the fat content in the diet by 2 teaspoons a day is achievable. Demonstrating the resulting reduction in total energy intake, that is, that 2 teaspoons of fat equal 90 Kcal (2 × 5 grams of fat/tsp × 9 Kcal/g of fat = 90 Kcal), will motivate clients to change their eating behavior. Once the client achieves this goal, the next step is to double the reduction until the overall dietary goal is met. In facilitating nutritional change, counselors should tailor strategies to their client's stage of change and their willingness to change (Sigman-Grant, 1996). Overall dietary goals should be set with the help of professional nutrition counselors. Motivated individuals could achieve and maintain these goals with successful eating-behavior modification.

Case Study
Making Dietary Recommendations

A 37-year-old schoolteacher would like to lose some weight and feel more energized. She was advised to complete a 3-day food diary, which was entered into the computer for analysis. Her diet was found to be high in overall Kcal, fats, and simple sugars. Body-composition analysis revealed a BMI of 31.44 kg/m^2 and percent body fat of 34 percent. Aside from her job, her only consistent activity revolves around walking the dog each morning for 5–10 minutes. Discuss your recommendations regarding dietary modification and physical activity to enable this client to achieve weight-loss goals.

Answer. The client should make moderate changes to her diet to reduce her caloric intake. She could start by eating smaller portions of nutrient-dense foods, such as whole grains, vegetables, fruits, and lean meats. Limiting her fat intake to less than 30 percent of her diet would also help to reduce overall caloric intake. She should refrain from snacking or eating high-fat fast foods, and substitute with sliced vegetables or low-fat crackers. Avoiding an excessive intake of soda or sweets, which may be low in fat but high in calories, would also be an important step. In addition to dietary modification, the client should also try to incorporate more physical activity into her daily routine. Perhaps she could walk the dog both in the morning and evening. She could also do more walking while running errands and make a habit of taking extra steps. It is important for her to realize that even activities such as housework, gardening, and dancing contribute to her daily energy expenditure. Once she is successful in accumulating 30 minutes of daily moderate activity, she might consider a more formal exercise program of moderate intensity for 40–50 minutes 5–6 days per week.

Behavioral-modification techniques should be applied for both changes in diet and exercise, taking into account triggers for overeating/eating high-fat snacks as well as barriers to physical activity.

Summary

An active lifestyle is associated with numerous health benefits including the prevention and management of many chronic diseases. Regular exercise is also attributed to optimizing quality of life and extending independent living in older adults. As a result the Centers for Disease Control, American College of Sports Medicine, and Surgeon General recommend daily moderate physical activity for all American adults. Additional health benefits can be obtained with exercise that meets the threshold for improving cardiorespiratory endurance. Guidelines for physical activity and developing various components of physical fitness are summarized in the Activity Pyramid (see Figure 5.3). As with exercise, good nutrition and weight management are also associated with health and longevity. Body composition and particularly fat distribution are more influential in good health than weight alone. Weight management ultimately comes down to achieving a balance between caloric intake and energy expenditure. The majority of weight-loss techniques focus on reducing caloric intake while increasing energy expenditure. Common weight-loss methods include dietary modification, physical activity, pharmacotherapy, and as a last resort, surgery. Behavior-modification techniques should be applied in developing appropriate personal goals and strategies for overcoming barriers that might prevent adoption and maintenance of healthy diet and exercise patterns. Successful weight management revolves around a lifelong program of healthy eating and regular physical activity. The changes in these health-enhancing behaviors are sometimes gradual, but the main objective is to make a permanent change.

Key Terms

body composition, 83	nutrition, 91
energy balance, 84	obesity, 88
exercise, 73	physical activity, 73

Questions for Discussion

1. Describe the health benefits associated with regular physical activity and optimum nutrition.

2. Explain strategies utilized to promote adoption of a more healthful behavior (that is, regular physical activity, optimum nutrition).

3. Discuss the role of physical activity and diet in successful weight management.

4. Develop an exercise plan that would address each tier in the Activity Pyramid.

5. Develop a sound dietary program that incorporates the tenants of the Food Guide Pyramid.

Related Web Sites

http://www.acsm.org
Web site of the American College of Sports Medicine. Promotes research and education in the areas of sports medicine and exercise science, including publications, certifications, career center, and health activity updates.

http://www.americanheart.org

Site of the American Heart Association. Provides information on warning signs, diseases, conditions, CPR and ECC, Healthy Lifestyles, advocacy, publications, Heart and Stroke Encyclopedia, science and professional links.

http://www.nutrition.org/

Site of the American Society for Nutritional Sciences. Features the *Journal of Nutrition* current issue and archives online.

http://www.cdc.gov/nccdphp/phyactiv.htm

Centers for Disease Control Physical Activity Information. Shares CDC's Physical Activity Efforts, the Surgeon General's Report on Physical Activity and Health, guidelines for school and community programs, nutrition, Report to the President.

http://www.health.gov/healthypeople/

Healthy People 2010. The Web site of this important government publication in user-friendly format, exploring health promotion in individuals, communities, and the nation.

Addiction and Health-Compromising Behaviors

ARDEN GREENSPAN-GOLDBERG,
M.S.W., A.C.S.W., B.C.D, AND
ISABEL BURK, M.S., C.P.P., C.H.E.S.

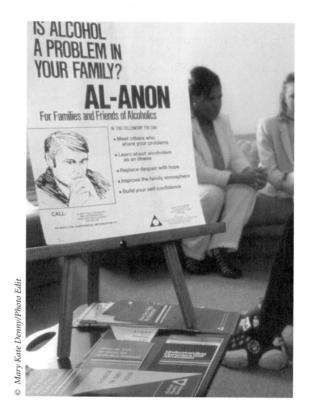

© *Mary Kate Denny/Photo Edit*

OBJECTIVES

By the end of the chapter, the reader should be able to:

- Identify and define key terms related to substance abuse and eating disorders

- Describe the impact of substance abuse on the individual, family, workplace, and society

- Utilize the transtheoretical model for stages of change

- Explain the etiology (causes) of eating disorders: anorexia nervosa, bulimia, binge eating, dual addictions

- Explain the process of recovery for substance abuse and eating disorders

- Identify and implement the U.S. Public Health Service guidelines for tobacco intervention (5 As).

- Discuss the latest research and trends in the field of eating disorders and internet addictions

Health-Compromising Behaviors

Health educators and counselors know a lot about choice. Although some people have been known to declare "I'm only hurting myself," it's not so simple. Personal choices and behaviors, such as drinking alcoholic beverages or eating disorders, have consequences to the self and to others.

An individual who uses tobacco products, for instance, risks immediate and long-term health problems, including bad breath, stained teeth and fingers, burns and fires, breathing difficulties, cardiovascular diseases, cancers of the mouth and lung, and so on. Secondhand (sidestream) smoke presents health issues for others in the same room or area as a smoker. These health risks impact not

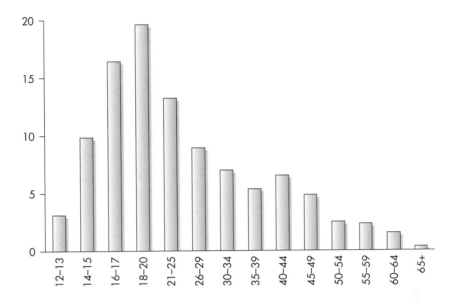

Figure 6. 1
Illicit drug use by age—last 30 days
Source: 1999 U.S. Department of Health and Human Services, National Household Survey of Drug Abuse—SAMHSA.

only the individual but also the family and the community.

Health-compromising behaviors are never simple, never totally straightforward, and are often linked with shame and guilt. Because of the complicated nature of human behavior, health educators and counselors may find themselves treading lightly, listening carefully to what is said and what is *not* said, reflecting and discussing nuances, tone of voice, body language, and so on.

This chapter will provide an overview of behaviors that seriously affect individuals, families, and communities, with case studies for application.

Drug-Use Patterns

Substance use exists in a continuum from **abstinence** (absolutely no use) to daily use, with countless permutations. Any amount of alcohol or other

Abstinence. To refrain completely from a substance or activity.

drug produces immediate effects on the body, the brain, and behavior.

Because of the widespread presence of alcohol, tobacco, and other drugs, health educators should always be prepared to recognize and address these issues. Some people seek advice because they are concerned about a family member, friend, colleague, or peer; others may have a clear problem to discuss, but it may turn out to be associated with an unmentioned alcohol or drug problem.

How widespread are these problems? In 1999, a national survey estimated that 15 million Americans used illicit drugs at least once within the past 30 days (U.S. Department of Health and Human Services, 1999). Males are more likely to use illicit drugs than females (8.7 percent males vs. 4.9 percent of females). The majority of users are under age 30 (see Figure 6.1).

Substance Abuse and Dependence

The 1998 National Household Survey on Drug Abuse reported that approximately 8 million

Americans were dependent on alcohol, almost 4 million were dependent on illicit drugs, and 1.5 million were dependent on both.

The Diagnostic and Statistical Manual of Mental Disorders, Fourth Edition (DSM-IV) lists two categories of serious problems: drug abuse/misuse and drug dependence (see also Chapter 10). Drug **dependence** means that a person continues to drink or use drugs despite experiencing significant substance-related problems and cognitive, behavioral, and physiologic symptoms, such as physical **withdrawal** or the need to use increasingly large amounts (U.S. Department of Health and Human Services, 2000). The main component of dependence is compulsive and uncontrollable drug use (Leshner, 1999).

Table 6.1 lists the seven criteria related to substance dependence, as defined by the DSM-IV. When someone meets *three or more criteria during a 12-month period,* he/she is considered dependent.

Substance abuse is the choice to continue substance use despite adverse effects on family or work, trauma, or negative health or legal consequences (U.S. Department of Health and Human Services, 2000). Table 6.2 defines the criteria given in the DSM-IV for the Diagnosis of Substance Abuse.

Medical Consequences

Alcohol abuse contributes to more than 100,000 deaths each year in the U.S (Schneider Institute, 2001). As a point of reference, about 105 million Americans consumed alcohol within the past 30 days (U.S. Department of Health and Human Services, 2000).

Consumption of alcoholic beverages during pregnancy exposes the developing fetus to the risk of Fetal Alcohol Syndrome (FAS) (U.S. Department of Health and Human Services, 2000). FAS-

---

Dependence. Compulsive and uncontrollable use of a substance or practice of a behavior.

Withdrawal. A psychological and/or physical syndrome experienced when one addicted to a substance for a prolonged period does not ingest the substance.

Table 6.1
DSM-IV Criteria for Substance Dependence

1. Tolerance, as defined by either:
   (a) need for increased amounts of the substance to achieve the desired effect
   (b) Markedly diminished effect with continued use of same amount of the substance

2. Withdrawal, manifested by either the characteristic withdrawal syndrome for each specific substance, or a similar substance is taken to relieve or avoid withdrawal symptoms.

3. The substance is often taken in larger amounts or over a longer period than was intended.

4. Persistent desire for substance, or unsuccessful efforts to cut down or control use.

5. Much time is spent to acquire the substance, use the substance, or recover from its efforts.

6. Important social, occupational, or recreational activities are given up or reduced because of substance use.

7. Substance use continues despite physical or psychological problems related to the substance.

Source: From Diagnostic and Statistical Manual of Mental Disorders, Fourth Edition, Text Revision. Washington, D.C., American Psychiatric Association, 1994. Reprinted with permission from the Diagnostic and Statistical Manual of Mental Disorders, Fourth Edition. Copyright 1999 American Psychiatric Association.

Table 6.2
DSM-IV Criteria for Diagnosis of Substance Abuse

Substance abuse is defined as "a maladaptive pattern of substance use leading to clinically significant impairment or distress, as manifested by one (or more) of the following, occurring within a 12-month period:

1. Recurrent substance use resulting in a failure to fulfill major role obligations at work, school, or home

2. Recurrent substance use in situations in which it is physically hazardous

3. Recurrent substance-related legal problems

4. Continued substance use despite having persistent or recurrent social or interpersonal problems caused or exacerbated by the effects of the substance

Source: From Diagnostic and Statistical Manual of Mental Disorders, Fourth Edition, Text Revision. Washington, D.C., American Psychiatric Association, 1994. Reprinted with permission from the Diagnostic and Statistical Manual of Mental Disorders, Fourth Edition. Copyright 1999 American Psychiatric Association.

related birth defects include low birth weight and facial abnormalities such as wide eyes and small head circumference. Other prenatal defects may involve brain abnormalities, including reduced cognitive function, poor verbal and reasoning skills, poor balance, and motor and spatial disabilities.

Referral

It's easy to imagine that family and friends would be concerned about people who drink or use drugs and want to discuss their concerns with a health educator or counselor. Perhaps a teenage girl is concerned that her boyfriend drinks and then drives to the movies, or a father worries about his son's pot smoking. Maybe a tennis player notices that her doubles partner can't run as far or as fast since she started smoking.

Sometimes people work together to arrange an **intervention** to benefit the person they are worried about. Each person makes a list of his/her specific concerns, and they arrange to meet in a group, along with the person they are concerned about. They each discuss their fears or worries, not to create guilt, but to explain how the drinking or drugging affects them. Some individuals enter counseling or substance abuse treatment after an intervention, but some don't.

On the other hand, a traumatic or dangerous event, or perhaps a close call, might precipitate a visit to the counselor's office. Or he/she may wake up with a hangover or feel ill. Whatever the impetus, people who come to discuss these issues should be welcomed.

Screening

A health counselor should always be alert to problems or issues related to alcohol or other drugs, even if it isn't the stated cause for the meeting. In general, counselors need to find out about the client and his/her problems to make appropriate referrals. Do not rush; listen to responses and feel-

---

Intervention. When a health counselor makes suggestions, observations, assessment or referral to aid another person.

---

ings. This is important because it lays the foundation for collaboration and behavior change.

Be calm, hopeful, and confident, and answer questions as they arise. It may be helpful to offer information about alcohol and drug issues. Explain the chronic nature of substance-abuse problems, how problems progress, how alcohol and drugs can impact many facets of a person's life.

The next section describes the Transtheoretical Model of Behavior Change, which can be used with issues related to substance abuse.

Transtheoretical Model of Behavior Change

Changing behavior is a complex undertaking. It takes time, energy, and effort. In fact, any activity that a person initiates to help modify their thinking, feeling, or behavior is part of the process of change (Prochaska et al., 1994).

Although many people wish to change their behaviors, they may not know how to go about it. The transtheoretical model can be applied not only to substance abuse, but to any health-compromising behavior (see Chapter 4 for an in-depth discussion of behavioral analysis and therapy).

Not all clients arrive ready to make dramatic changes in their behaviors. In fact, some clients may consult a counselor to clarify if there is a need to change. Others return to counseling to resume or revive their process of change. Progressing just one stage can improve the chances that an individual will work on an identified problem such as substance abuse (Prochaska et al., 1994).

Researchers have identified six stages of change in the transtheoretical model: precontemplation, contemplation, preparation, action, maintenance, and termination.

1. In the **precontemplation** stage, the individual is not even considering the possibility of change. An individual in this stage is not actively considering treatment or recovery and is very resistant to change. He/she may not consider tobacco, alcohol, or other drug use to be a problem for him/her at all, despite what others think or say. He/she may think that other people have a problem when they bring it up. In this stage it is important to raise awareness of the problem, especially related to the individual.

2. The **contemplation** stage can be ambivalent. A person may waiver between seeking treatment and rejecting the idea. In this stage, the individual learns more, tries to understand the situation, and considers the possibilities of change. This can be an emotional, hopeful time as people open their minds to the potential for change.

3. An individual in the **preparation** stage is seriously considering taking action within the next month or so. In this stage, people make firm resolutions and adjustments, and engage in personal planning for the anticipated change in behavior. They may have some reservations, but will be likely to convince themselves of the need to change and the possibilities of success. Drawing up a detailed plan for action in this stage enhances the process.

4. Individuals in the **action** stage are committed to imminent change. This is a busy time, a time of effort and energy. During this stage the motivated individual is consciously adhering to new behaviors, to new beliefs and patterns, and interpersonal support and reinforcement can be very helpful. Expect occasional slips, and plan for renewed efforts toward the desired behavior.

5. The **maintenance** stage features working to sustain new behaviors. Individuals are proud of their achievements and work consciously to prevent **relapse** (returning to previous behaviors). Slips can occur, but individuals may be more conscious of the events and situations that can trigger a relapse. This stage reflects success, but still requires time and energy to maintain positive behaviors. Maintenance can be a lifetime experience for some people.

6. The sixth stage is the **termination** stage. In this stage, behavior change has become deeply ingrained with no fear of relapse. Can people really achieve this stage? After all, it can be questioned whether temptation is ever gone.

Relapse. A temporary setback, a lapse, a return to unhealthy coping that can occur in the recovery process.

Table 6.3
Stages of Change

Stage	Characteristics
Precontemplation	No consideration of change
Contemplation	Study of possibilities, potential rewards of change; look at alternatives
Preparation	Specific planning for behavior change
Action	Initiation of change activities
Maintenance	Struggle to prevent slips and relapse; planning for continued success; ongoing vigilance
Termination	Cycle complete, relapse possibilities remote

According to Prochaska et al. (1994), four criteria help define the possibility for termination: (1) A radical change in self-image, redefining the self as healthier and stronger; (2) When situations that used to trigger relapse no longer tempt the individual to revert to the old behaviors, that is a strong indicator of successful, permanent change; (3) Solid confidence in the success and endurance of the change, translated into belief in self-efficacy; (4) Lifestyle modifications that support success and promote continuing personal growth. When all four criteria intersect in an individual, it is less likely that he/she will be returning to maintenance. Table 6.3 summarizes Stages of Change.

Why are these "stages of change" so important for a health counselor? Prochaska (1994) says, "The key to success is the appropriately timed use of a variety of coping skills." A health counselor can be very helpful in guiding the client toward awareness and personal insight that will move him/her to the next stage—or helping the client understand the barriers to that progress.

Most important, the counselor needs to match the client with an appropriate intervention. For instance, it is unrealistic to expect a smoker in the precontemplation stage to agree to sign up for stop-smoking hypnosis. Instead, it may be useful for someone in this stage to become more aware of his/own personal vulnerability to the documented effects of tobacco use. Gentle questions about respiratory conditions, shortness of breath, and so on, can help elucidate how smoking affects his/her life. The more personal the impact, the better the chance that an individual will contemplate behavior change.

The next section discusses health-counseling suggestions for tobacco **addiction,** a health-compromising problem shared by millions of Americans.

Tobacco Addiction

Tobacco use contributes to 430,000 deaths in the United States each year, the number-one cause of preventable death and disease in this country (National Institute on Drug Abuse, National Institute of Health, Research Report on Nicotine Addiction, 1998).

Nicotine is addictive. Recent studies (National Institute on Drug Abuse, 1998). reveal that nicotine activates the brain circuitry regulating feelings of pleasure. Each "puff" stimulates the brain a little. Immediately on entering the body, nicotine stimulates the adrenal glands to release adrenaline. This increases blood pressure, respiration, and heart rate, and sends more glucose to the bloodstream.

Medical Consequences

Cigarette smoking has been linked to about 90 percent of all lung cancer cases (National Institute on Drug Abuse, 1998). Smoking increases the risk of heart attack, stroke, and cardiovascular diseases, and contributes to emphysema, chronic bronchitis, and asthma (Schneider Institute, 2001). Pregnant women who smoke are at greater risk for giving birth prematurely, and their infants may weigh less than nonsmokers' babies.

Health counseling can help tobacco users understand risks to themselves and others, look ahead, and plan and implement a personalized program for quitting (**cessation**).

Assessment/Intervention

Tobacco dependence is a chronic condition that often requires repeated intervention. About 70 percent of the 50 million smokers in the United States have made at least one attempt to stop smoking (Schneider Institute, 2001). Most smokers make several attempts before they successfully quit.

In October 2000, The U.S. Public Health Service released updated guidelines for working with tobacco users. The document recommends the **5 As:**

Ask, Advise, Assess, Assist, Arrange

Ask: Systematically Identify Tobacco Users at Every Visit. When an individual presents himself/herself for health counseling or for any reason, ask about tobacco use. Discuss their patterns of use: how often and how much, when, where, and how. Describe a typical day's tobacco use.

Advise: Strongly Urge All Tobacco Users to Quit. State some positive effects of quitting tobacco, personalized if possible. For instance, if the individual mentions that it's hard to climb stairs, remind him/her that smoking taxes the heart during exertion.

Assess: Determine Willingness to Make A Quit Attempt. Ask the tobacco user if he or she is willing to make a quit attempt at this time or in the next 2–3 weeks. If the answer is negative, offer hope for the future. If the answer is positive, work out a tentative plan.

Addiction. When one feels dependent, controlled, or negatively influenced by a behavior or substance.

Cessation. The stopping or "quitting" of a particular behavior.

Assist: Aid the Patient in Quitting. Ask the client to set a quit date and to tell family, friends, and coworkers about quitting. Discuss withdrawal symptoms, including irritability, shorter attention span, or problems sleeping. Help the client anticipate triggers such as meal time, morning awakening, and bedtime. Discuss a range of options, including "cold turkey" cessation, nicotine gum, nicotine patch, and so on.

Arrange: Practical Cessation Counseling and Support. Help the client identify events, feelings, or activities that increase the risk of smoking, and discuss coping skills for each.

Case Study

Cassandra

Cassandra was a 23-year-old woman, 4 months pregnant with her first child. She had smoked 10–12 cigarettes daily for 7 years. At her first visit, her obstetrician told her she should quit smoking. Cassandra immediately cut down to six cigarettes a day, but she didn't quit entirely.

The doctor referred Cassandra to a patient educator, John, for assistance. Knowing about the Stages of Change, he reaffirmed her decision to quit (Preparation). Using the 5 As model, it was clear that due to her pregnancy and her physician's advice, coupled with her decision to try, Cassandra was prepared to quit and to use John's assistance to move from Preparation to Action to Maintenance.

John helped her learn more about her smoking patterns, discussed previous attempts to quit, and highlighted positive points. He told Cassandra to set a date to quit and write it down.

He suggested she tell her family and friends, asking for their encouragement. John prepared her for withdrawal from nicotine, and discussed her dependence on cigarettes to cope with stress. He recommended that she chew sugarless gum whenever she felt edgy and remind herself of the gift of health for herself and her baby. After a month without tobacco she proudly called herself a nonsmoker. After 8 weeks, the urge to smoke reduced and her confidence soared. At 4 months smoke-free, John told her that she was firmly in the Maintenance Stage.

Cassandra had a healthy baby boy and brought him to the patient educator's office, showing off her "tobacco-free" accomplishment. Months later, she rarely felt the urge to smoke, and said her baby kept her so busy that she didn't have time to light up.

Substance-Abuse Treatment

Early recognition and intervention for substance-abuse problems saves lives, enhances productivity, and reduces personal and societal health risks. The health educator has a key role in identifying potential problems and educating individuals about health-compromising behaviors such as substance abuse. This may mean education about substances, effects, addiction, and treatment. Or it may mean a referral to a treatment specialist or addiction counselor.

Substance-abuse addiction is a chronic disease requiring long-term management. Almost 3 million people received treatment for drug or alcohol problems in the past year (U.S. Nat. Inst. on Drug Abuse, Nat. Inst. of Health 1999). On any given day, more than 700,000 people in the United States receive treatment for alcoholism (Fuller & Hiller-Sturmhofel, 1999). Males are twice as likely to be in drug or alcohol treatment as females (NIDA NHS 1999).

The initial task of treatment is to regain control over drug craving, drug seeking, and drug use (Leshner, 1999). Although treatment helps stop health-compromising behaviors, most people need consistent support to continue their recovery.

Addiction treatment services include **assessment,** treatment planning, therapy, medications when appropriate, behavioral counseling, monitoring for substance use, support groups, case management, and continuing care (Leshner, 1999).

Assessment. An initial estimation of the patient's understanding of the need for treatment, the treatment regimen, and the degree of mastery of any requisite skills necessary for compliance.

Twelve-Step and Self-Help Groups

The 12-step philosophy developed by Alcoholics Anonymous (AA) (see Table 6.4) offers people a new way of living to help break the cycle of addiction and maintain abstinence (Alcoholics Anonymous Twelve Steps and Twelve Traditions, 1986). While some people utilize self-help as their sole treatment protocol, other people find that self-help groups complement and extend the effects of

---

Table 6.4
Twelve Steps of Alcoholics Anonymous

1. We admitted we were powerless over alcohol—that our lives had become unmanageable.

2. Came to believe that a Power greater than ourselves could restore us to sanity.

3. Made a decision to turn our will and our lives over to the care of God as we understood Him.

4. Made a searching and fearless moral inventory of ourselves.

5. Admitted to God, to ourselves, and to another human being the exact nature of our wrongs.

6. Were entirely ready to have God remove all these defects of character.

7. Humbly asked Him to remove our shortcomings.

8. Made a list of all persons we had harmed, and became willing to make amends to them all.

9. Made direct amends to such people wherever possible, except when to do so would injure them or others.

10. Continued to take personal inventory and when we were wrong promptly admitted it.

11. Sought through prayer and meditation to improve our conscious contact with God as we understood Him, praying only for knowledge of His will for us and the power to carry that out.

12. Having had a spiritual awakening as the result of these steps, we tried to carry this message to alcoholics and to practice these principles in all our affairs.

Source: The Twelve Steps are reprinted with permission of Alcoholics Anonymous World Services, Inc. (A.A.W.S.) Permission to reprint the Twelve Steps does not mean that A.A.W.S. has reviewed or approved the contents of this publication, or that A.A.W.S. necessarily agrees with the views expressed herein. A.A. is a program of recovery from alcohol only—use of the Twelve Steps in connection with programs and activities which are patterned after A.A., but which address other problems, or in any other non-A.A. context, does not imply otherwise.

---

professional treatment (NIDA Principles). Some organizations have adapted the 12-step philosophy for other problems, such as Narcotics Anonymous, Overeaters Anonymous, Gamblers Anonymous, and so on.

Self-help groups are very valuable. Becoming part of a group helps people develop a support network, teaches and reinforces skills for recovery and healthier living, and encourages responsibility. The group provides a sense of belonging and helps establish an individual's identity as a nonuser.

Weiss et al. (1996) found that self-help attendees who went to at least one meeting per week were more likely to abstain from drug use than those who did not attend. Weight Watchers® is another well-known example of the positive effects of group membership.

Relapse

Change is a complex and time-consuming process and changing behavior can be stressful because the learning process is not linear, but fluid. Naturally, changing behavior will include slips and relapses into previous behavior. For instance, stress may lead to a slip back to drinking or drug use. But a slip doesn't mean failure; it is part of the change process.

Health educators can help people prepare for slips. What precipitated the slip? What can be learned from the slip? How did it feel? What happened? Use a slip as a learning experience to help create coping strategies that can prevent future slips and strengthen recovery.

Case Study

Mike

Mike, age 19, was in his second year in college, rooming in the fraternity. He started to drink beer with his friends at the fraternity house and at local bars on the weekends. He didn't drink during the week.

The fraternity brothers had vodka-shot competitions and Mike could hold his own. Sometimes he drank more than a dozen beers and five or six shots in a night.

One evening, Mike blacked out. Later he was told he threw up in his fraternity brother's new car. Mike admitted perhaps he had a little too much to drink, just this once. His girlfriend Mary started to notice a change in Mike's behavior. He came late to Monday-morning classes. He didn't pay attention and wasn't prepared for work due in class.

Mary became concerned and confronted him. She said, "You have a drinking problem, and unless you get some help, I will stop seeing you."

Initially Mike was defensive. "I only drink on weekends. I'm not an alcoholic like my father, who drinks every day," he replied. Mike was still in the Precontemplation stage.

Reluctantly, he let Mary make an appointment with a counselor at school. Mike was shocked when the counselor told him that he was a binge drinker. The counselor defined this as drinking five or more drinks at one sitting for a male, and four or more drinks at a sitting for a female. The counselor was friendly and understanding. He referred Mike to an alcohol-treatment specialist and suggested he join Alcoholics Anonymous. After taking some time to think things over, Mike went to see the treatment specialist. Later he attended his first meeting of Alcoholics Anonymous. With the support of his girlfriend and counselors, he progressed through the stages to the Action stage, committing himself to work on this health-compromising behavior.

Prevention

Counselors should be aware that the earlier the initiation into substance use, the more likely a person is to become dependent on a substance later in life. Youth who begin drinking alcohol before age 14 are five times more likely to become dependent on alcohol as adults than people who begin drinking after age 20 (Grant & Dawson, 1997). And those who start using illicit drugs (such as marijuana) before age 14 are much more likely as adults to be dependent on an illicit drug (U.S. Department of Health and Human Services, 1999).

Therefore prevention efforts aimed at youth can have wide-reaching implications for the individual and for society. Delaying the first use of substances greatly reduces the risk of later abuse and/or dependence (Grant & Dawson, 1997). Ideally, prevention should begin early and continue throughout life, with frequent and consistent pro-health messages. But prevention starts at home.

What can parents do? To begin with, they should make sure their children feel their love. A landmark national study showed that youth in grades 7–12 who felt close to their parents, who felt their parents and family members cared about them, and who were satisfied with their family relationships were much less likely to become involved in risky behaviors such as alcohol and other drug use (Resnick et al., 1997).

Parents should clearly state their values related to substance use, and reinforce these views several times a year. Youth who said they never talked with their parents about drugs were almost twice as likely to have used drugs, when compared with youth whose parents talked about drugs on a regular basis (Partnership, 1999). Parents can use opportunities such as a television show or song to discuss alcohol, tobacco, or other drugs.

Consider prevention a continuation of good parenting practices: know where your children are, know their friends, set guidelines, and follow through (Partnership, 1999). In addition, children need to rehearse for the day when they will be confronted by a friend: "Hey, want a drag off my cigarette?" "Join me in a beer!" Children who are prepared are better able to resist substances.

It's also important for parents to help their children understand the short-term consequences of substance use. For instance, cigarette smokers' breath and clothing smells, and it can be an expensive habit. Youngsters who perceive that they may be adversely affected socially or financially by substances are much less likely to use them.

Most important, parents must reinforce that alcohol, tobacco, and drug use is not the norm! Although media and hype might lead young people to think otherwise, the fact is that most people are *not* involved with substances.

Health counselors play an important role in strengthening positive messages and correcting the misperceptions that clients may present. Keep up with the local trends and be prepared to share the data with clients, parents, and the community.

America's Culture of Being Slim: The Myth of the Barbie Doll and the Man of Steel

Health educators and counselors need an understanding of the external pressures and cultural expectations related to self-image and body image, for instance, the "Beauty Myth": "You can't be too thin, too beautiful, or too rich (Wolf, 1991)." Unfortunately for those who do not debunk, question, and resist the myth, people can be caught up in the vicious cycle of fitting in or pleasing others, submerging their sense of self and identity.

Overweight people face prejudice, and seeing body fat as something repulsive is part of that problem. Think of comments such as, "Gained some weight lately?" "You could stand to lose a few pounds." "You'd look so much more attractive if you lost weight." These comments can trigger self- and body-hatred and dangerous cycles of dieting.

Our massive cultural disturbance is the contemporary preoccupation with body image and body weight (Wolf, 1991). The scale's "magic number," can make a day that's full of hope, or can beat down one's self esteem. When a female's worth is linked solely to her appearance, this leaves her vulnerable to body dissatisfaction and finding means to fit into the culture's and media's vision of beauty. At this point, beauty is truly only skin deep.

Barbie, once a "harmless" little girls' doll, has not significantly changed its shape since the 1950s. If Barbie were to be stretched out to her full height, she'd be "Anorexic Barbie." A physical anomaly! Consider this:

A five-year-old girl wanted a "My Size Barbie" for Christmas. Her mom tried to dissuade her, but couldn't. "Barbie is too skinny," Mom insisted. "Why don't you get a doll that looks more normal?" But the girl wanted Barbie. She told her mother that the television said the doll was made for 3- to 5-year-olds. Mom reluctantly gave in. With a rush of excitement the girl tried on Barbie's bridal outfit, only to come to her mother with a look of sadness and disappointment. "The outfit doesn't fit me. I'm too fat."

Mom told the daughter "They lied on television." She hugged her. "I love you, all of you, and you're not fat." In the mother's eyes, the advertising hurt her daughter.

If this 5-year-old child was impacted, can you imagine the impact on a female reaching puberty when the body redistributes fat! Is Barbie the ideal? No, but a vulnerable teen who sees very skinny rock stars, actresses, or fashion models often believes she should fashion herself in their likeness.

Now let's look at the male side of the spectrum. There are two meanings to a "six pack": a case of beer or an extremely lean, muscular torso. Where the trend toward muscularity used to be a small segment of the population (Mr. Universe, Jack Lalane), now health clubs and weight rooms have become havens for teens and young men trying to create a "perfect physique." Self esteem is elevated according to who has the biggest muscles and a "cut," fat-less torso. Some males have substituted liquid-protein drinks, vitamin supplements, and other substances like creatine for food, hoping to pump their bodies up.

Innocent diets or body toning, when taken to an extreme, can become obsessive. When people get caught up in this vicious cycle, it sometimes leads to an eating disorder.

Eating Disorders on a Continuum

At first glance it's hard to imagine obesity, anorexia nervosa, bulimia, and binge-eating disorder as having features in common. But all four groups of people can become obsessed with their weight. Some obese people go on numerous diets only to find themselves yo-yoing up and down. Yo-yo dieters can end up at a higher weight, straining their heart. Anorexic people restrict their food intake to an extreme and can utilize the bulimic strategies of binging (uncontrollable eating) and purging (vomiting, laxative abuse).

Bulimia and binge eating disorder involves compulsive, uncontrollable overeating. These people utilize food as a coping mechanism to punish, deprive, self-soothe, and regulate oneself through one's body, or, similar to a druglike substance, to deal with feelings of low self-esteem, pain, anger, rage, depression, emptiness, anxiety and despair to name just a few.

The bulleted descriptions below, adapted from the American Psychiatric Association Diagnostic and Statistical Manual of Mental Disorder, Fourth Edition, aid in defining, screening, and assessing whether a person is suffering from anorexia nervosa or bulimia.

Eating Disorders

Health educators and counselors must be aware of early warning signs, prevalence, medical conditions, causes, and consequences of **eating disorders,** and make timely interventions.

Anorexia Warning Signs

Anorexia is an eating disorder characterized by extreme underweight.

- Refusal to maintain body weight at or above a minimally normal weight for age and height. (Weight loss leading to maintenance of body weight less than 85 percent of that expected: or failure to make expected weight gain during period of growth, leading to body weight less than 85 percent of that expected.) Intense fear of gaining weight or becoming fat even though underweight.

- Disturbance in the way in which one's body weight or shape is experienced, undue influence of body weight or shape on self-evaluation, or denial of the seriousness of the current low body weight.

- In postmenarcheal females, amenorrhea, that is, the absence of at least three consecutive menstrual cycles.

Eating disorder. When a person uses food as a coping mechanism to punish, deprive, or self-soothe in order to deal with feelings of pain, depression, and so on. These include anorexia nervosa, bulimia, and binge eating.

Table 6.5
Anorexia Nervosa's Warning Signs

- Sudden severe drop in weight
- Denial of hunger
- Refusal to eat certain foods
- Avoidance of situations that involve food
- Fanatical counting of calories or fat grams
- Frequent comments that one feels fat
- Terrified with real or imagined weight gain
- Withdrawal from some activities and friends
- Exercising to an extreme

Medical Complications. The body is starved and deprived of food, vitamins, and nutrients. Common symptoms include extreme fatigue, blackouts, slow heart rate, low blood pressure, heart attack, dehydration, dry skin, hair loss, and a growth of body hair called lanugo. Bone density decreases, leading to osteoporosis and muscle weakness (Eating Disorders Awareness and Prevention Incorporated web site).

Prevalence/Incidence. Anorexia nervosa is one of the most common psychiatric diagnoses in young women (Hsu, 1996). Between 1 and 2 percent of American women suffer from anorexia nervosa. Between 5 and 20 percent of individuals struggling with anorexia nervosa will die and the probability of death increases within that range depending on the length of the condition (Zerbe, 1995; Eating Disorders Awareness and Prevention Incorporated web site).

Etiology—Causes. The development of anorexia nervosa is multidetermined. A biopsychosocial-familial understanding gives the flavor of the complexity of this disorder. Counselors often learn of a history of dieting behavior in first-degree relatives, as well as a preoccupation with thinness. Counselors look for psychiatric disorders, or alcohol or substance abuse in the family of origin. A recent divorce, illness, death, or separation, or some other life trauma may actually set this disease in motion. Affective states not easily articulated—

such as rage, sadness, hurt, confusion, worthlessness, and helplessness, among others—may complicate the situation.

The onset of puberty, when the body is in a physiological and emotional upheaval and there is a redistribution of body fat, can also trigger these disorders. "Researchers are also beginning to understand how dieting, exercise, semi-starvation and amenorrhea may actually be used to avoid or inappropriately cope with the developmental demands of adolescence and young adulthood" (Bulik & Johnson, 2001).

Case Study

Amy

Here is a case study of a young woman who severely restricted her food intake—a classic case of anorexia nervosa.

Amy was 18 years old and going off to college in a few months. She was both excited and nervous. She recently had lost 25 pounds and was looking unhealthily thin to her father. Her father suggested she talk to a psychotherapist who was also an eating-disorder specialist.

At her initial interview, Amy shared her father's concern with her recent dramatic weight loss of 25 pounds. She described herself as "pleasing and a perfectionist." Amy spoke proudly of her ability to diet and said that as a chubby child she was frequently teased by children at school and by an older sister.

She had been on many unsuccessful diets since early childhood. She believed her mother once had an eating disorder, and her father's sister had suffered from anorexia at a younger age.

Amy felt out of sync with other teens her age. She did not have a boyfriend. Amy did not report any physical or sexual abuse. She became more restrictive with her food intake and began to eat only fruit and vegetables. Food was no longer her friend, but her foe.

The therapist referred her to a medical doctor for a full medical evaluation, to a nutritionist, and to a psychiatrist. By the time she left for college, Amy had lost 10 more pounds. Her therapist seriously doubted she could adjust to all the academic and social challenges of college life.

At Thanksgiving, Amy called her father to bring her home. She was crying, homesick, and unable to eat. Her blood pressure and heart rate were low; she looked terrible. Amy knew she needed help to stop the secretive, addictive, compulsive behavior. She desperately wanted to get better and agreed with the recommendations of her physician and therapist to be hospitalized at an eating-disorder unit.

After a 2-month hospitalization, she entered an intensive outpatient treatment program. Amy regained some weight, and through psychotherapy, realized she needed to stay at home and attend a local college. She learned to eat when she was hungry (demand feeding) and stop when she was full. Amy became clearer about the function and purpose of her eating disorder.

Slowly Amy learned to accept herself and her body, joining a support group and attending weekly meetings. She made cognitive and behavioral changes that helped her refocus her energy in a more positive manner. She is on the road to recovery.

Bulimia Warning Signs

Bulimia is characterized by recurrent episodes of binge eating and, generally, purging. Binge eating is characterized by the following:

- Eating, in a discrete period of time (for example, within any 2-hour period), an amount of food that is definitely larger than most people would eat during similar time and circumstances.

- A sense of lack of control over eating during the episode (for example, a feeling that one cannot stop eating or control what or how much one is eating).

- Recurrent inappropriate compensatory behavior in order to prevent weight gain, such as self-induced vomiting; misuse of laxatives, diuretics, enemas, or other medications; fasting; or excessive exercise

- The binge eating and inappropriate compensatory behaviors both occur, on average, at least twice a week for 3 months.

- Self-evaluation is unduly influenced by body shape and weight. See Table 6.6, next page.

Table 6.6
Bulimia Nervosa Warning Signs

- Obsessed with dieting and weight loss
- Evidence of binge eating and purging behaviors
- Large quantities of food missing
- Frequent and lengthy bathroom usage
- Withdrawal from activities and friends
- Yellowing and thinning of teeth from purging
- May exercise to an extreme

Source: Levine, 1994.

Medical Complications. Bleeding and rupture of the esophagus from vomiting are possible complications arising from bulemia. Electrolyte imbalance can lead to lowering of blood pressure, irregular heartbeats, and possibly trigger a heart attack. Laxative abuse can lead to kidney and ulcer complications.

Prevalence. Approximately 80 percent of bulimia nervosa patients are female (Gidwani & Rome, 1997). Estimates of the incidence of bulimia run as high as one-fifth of all college-age women (Pipher, 1994, p. 170).

Etiology—Causes. Refer to Etiology–Causes of Anorexia Nervosa, above. In addition, Pipher says "while anorexia nervosa often begins in junior high, bulimia tends to develop in later adolescence. It's called the 'college girl's disease' because so many women develop it in sororities and dorms. While anorexic girls are perfectionist and controlled, bulimic young women are impulsive and they experience themselves as chronically out of control. Bulimic women come in all shapes and sizes" (Pipher, 1994).

Binge-Eating Disorder (Compulsive Overeating)

A person diagnosed with BED does not utilize bulimic compensatory or purging behavior to rid themselves of the excess calories accumulated during the binge. Rather they frequently binge uncontrollably, rapidly consuming food without tasting it, eating not necessarily based on physical hunger, with little or no sense of fullness. Some people who suffer from BED may develop a medical condition such as diabetes, heart complications, or high blood pressure. Estimates indicate that about 60 percent of people struggling with binge-eating disorder are female, 40 percent are male (National Institute of Health, 1993). About 25 percent of obese people suffer from BED (Fairburn, 1993). Many people who suffer from BED have a history of depression (National Institute of Health, 1993).

Obesity

Experts debate whether obesity is considered an eating disorder. Most researchers believe it is not, based on genetic predisposing variables (Brownell & Foreyt, 1986). Not every obese person has medical complications. In fact, those who are more physically fit put less stress on their heart and health than those who continually go on and off numerous diets.

Davis (2001) cites multiple studies that suggest physical health is more closely related to physical fitness than to weight itself. In an overview of weight management research, Gaesser (2001a, 2001b) states that 95 percent of diets fail and that diets can cause eating disorders. According to Gaesser (2001a, 2001b) the majority of dieters regain more weight than they lost, and intentional weight loss can cause weight problems.

Obesity seems to protect against osteoporosis, a leading cause of disability among North American women (Bulik & Johnson, 2001). Future research dedicated to examining the risk for obesity will no doubt lead to the understanding of multiple genes and environmental variables that may influence obesity, such as sedentary lifestyle, high-fat diets, and overeating.

Dual Diagnosis

Dual diagnosis is a term commonly used when two distinct medical disorders exist within an individual. Most recently the term describes the co-existence of a mental-health disorder and substance-abuse problems (U.S. Dept. of Health and Human Services, 1995, TIP report #9).

In real life, a psychotherapist who is a trained eating-disorder specialist has to be able to treat not only an eating disorder, but also drug addiction, alcoholism, binge drinking, plus a most complex symptom and ineffective coping strategy, cutting, also known as self-mutilation.

"Self-mutilation is more of a problem than has been thought, especially with people who have eating disorders. In fact, individuals with eating disordered behavior, especially bulimic behavior, are at a high risk for self-mutilation and are likely to do so the longer they have had the eating disorder." (Favazza, DeRosear & Conterio, 1989; Farber 1998, 2000).

According to Farber, "Self-cutting is only part of a spectrum of self-mutilating behavior, the infliction of injury to one's body resulting in tissue damage or alteration. Other forms of self-mutilation include burning, scratching, needle-sticking, hair-pulling, severe nail/cuticle biting and chewing."

With the person who cuts, a team approach is most important. A physician must treat and see the cuts, and a psychiatrist must administer appropriate medication, usually antidepressants or a mood stabilizer. If the conditions become extremely dangerous and/or life-threatening, a hospitalization may be indicated, either in a detoxification facility or a residential treatment setting where the person can begin to heal.

Levenkron (1999) sees the therapeutic relationship as one where the patient has a second chance to learn to "trust, attach and depend." Most of these patients have suffered major traumas in their short lives, and have utilized cutting as a means of numbing their pain, expressing anger and rage, mostly directed at themselves, and wiping out undesirable thoughts and other feelings. These feeble attempts at self-regulation serve to disconnect and isolate themselves from meaningful relationships and communication with significant others in their lives.

Case Study

Barbra

Barbra is now a 22-year-old college student who works part-time in a day-care center. She was referred by her mother. Barbra is in recovery for binge drinking, anorexia, bulimia, and abusing amphetamines. Her most persistent symptom, self-mutilation (cutting), has been pervasive, entrenched, and ritualistically enacted once a day, mostly before bedtime. Barbra saw an eating-disorder specialist against her will and spent most of the sessions in absolute silence.

The therapist felt her discomfort and anger, which Barbra denied. Through her mom, who periodically saw this therapist, a traumatic history was tearfully shared. Barbra's father had been diagnosed with cancer and quickly became weak, bedridden, and unable to do simple tasks. Ten-year-old Barbra had no clue how ill her father was. He did not let on, nor did her mother. When he died, Barbra withdrew, held in her grief, and did not let anyone comfort her. In time she became even more private and guarded. She first evidenced anorexic symptoms at age 16, became bulimic and abused marijuana at 17, began to abuse amphetamines, and cut herself at the age of 18.

Barbra briefly attended college, only to return home after her roommates called her mom describing her self-destructive behavior. Barbra refused to answer any questions. Her therapist found it a challenge to figure out a creative means of connecting with her. Barbra loved to write, and through some of her journals and poetry, reluctantly shared after a year, it became clear that she was still in excruciating pain over the loss of her beloved father.

The anorexia and the bulimia distracted and cut her off from herself and her thoughts and feelings. The cutting became dependable and familiar, something that she could control, that would never abandon her, like her father once did.

Her rage and anger became self-directed. Barbra had started to binge drink and abuse amphetamines. She had two seizures, the last and final episode in her doctor's office. After two unsuccessful hospitalizations her therapist, physician, friends, and mother looked for a more dramatic intervention.

After a 2-month stay in a Christian-based residential treatment center, Barbra made remarkable progress, except for the cutting. She continued treatment for a few more months but remained silent, so her therapist did the talking for both of them. Her friends were often invited into the sessions. She was eventually able to resume work and attend a local college full time while still living at home, a major achievement.

But Barbra wanted to stop therapy. She'd often say "no one will care about me when I get better." Her therapist said she'd still be cared about, but in a less dramatic way. Her therapist knew she'd hear from Barbra again, as her recovery was incomplete. Under renewed stress Barbra would probably experience occasional slips that hopefully would not discourage her. The therapist assured her that she was loved and the door was always open for her.

Referral

Clients may be referred by several methods. Self-referral is common; or a relative, family member, friend, or peer may refer a client. In the school setting, a counselor or health educator could be the source. Work-site EAP may be another source, as well. Eating Disorder Organizations can provide a list of recommended eating disorder specialists as well.

Screening and Intervention

As a health educator, health counselor, family member, or friend, it is important to be as supportive as possible and make sure that an appropriate referral to a trained professional is made. Questions are not always the best approach. A compassionate observation from a friend or family member, such as, "You seem out of sorts today and anxious." "I know it's hard for you to talk, but I'm here if you want to." "I've noticed lately that you are not eating," or "I've noticed some cuts on your arm. I'm concerned" could be useful.

A health educator confronted with someone who is suspected or known to be a "cutter" as well

as a substance abuser, can interview him/her gently to get a history and general picture of his/her life. The educator should be prepared with appropriate resources for counseling and treatment.

Interview Questions. An interviewer should ask "What hurts you so badly that you have to resort to cutting or anorexia? What were you thinking and feeling before, during, and after you restricted food, binged, threw up, or cut? How long have you had these symptoms? What traumas or losses have you suffered in your life? Tell me about any substance-abuse or psychiatric history in your family" (Levenkron, 1999).

Screening Techniques. A helpful screening instrument, the Diagnostic Survey for Eating Disorders-Revised, can be utilized for an initial consultation for patients suspected of suffering from bulimia and anorexia (Johnson, 1985).

The Eating Disorders Inventory (EDI) is a scaled instrument that measures eating attitudes and behaviors of patients with anorexia and bulimia with a 64-item self-report questionnaire (Garner, Olmsted, & Polivy, 1983).

Another valid screening instrument is The Eating Attitudes Test, a 26-item self-rated scale covering attitudes and behaviors that could lead to the development of an eating disorder (Garner & Garfinkel, 1979).

The Danish Adoption Register for the Study of Obesity and Thinness, (Stukard, Sorensen, & Schulsinger, 1980) is a visual body-image survey used to see how men and women view their own body.

Treatment Approaches

The most commonly used treatment approaches are: Feminist Relational, Behavioral, Cognitive, Psychoanalytic Psychotherapy, Humanistic, Drug Therapy (Matlin,1993), Group, Family Therapy, Nutritional Counseling, Educative, Self and Body Acceptance/Anti-diet approach. Treatment can also include self-help groups such as Overeaters Anonymous.

Table 6.7
The Seven P's of Recovery—Getting It Together

A Lifetime Commitment

- **P**atience
- **P**ractice
- **P**ersistence
- **P**erseverance
- **P**ositive Outlook and Attitude
- **P**eace: Love, Trust, Hope, Faith for Self & Others
- **P**ro-Active: Give of yourself in collaboration with others

The focus of treatment is on the health and wellness of the whole person—mind, body, and spirit. With that in mind, moderate movement (exercise) which includes sports, dance, yoga, and nature walking as well as meditation, guided imagery, and stress management is strongly advised. In addition there are intensive outpatient treatment programs, day hospital programs, in-patient eating disorder hospitalizations, and residential and Christian-based treatment facilities.

Treatment and Management of Recovery

In her article, "The Body Speaks, the Body Weeps," Farber says the therapist should enable the patient to "develop the ability to move from the language of the body to expressive spoken and written language. Instead of saying 'I am fat' or 'I am ugly,' she might come to be able to say, 'I feel angry' or 'guilty' or 'sad' or 'ashamed' or 'frightened.'" (Farber, 1998).

In recovery, the therapist and patient establish a close trusting relationship where the therapist can be depended on to recreate a healthy, re-parenting-like attachment. This will include listening, coaching, advising, challenging the patient in an empathic, understanding, and insightful way, and behaving like a benevolent authority figure, when appropriate. Recovery is more insured when the patient reestablishes preexisting relationships and develops the capacity to have new relationships.

Recovery is a slippery, slow, arduous, and lengthy process. Under renewed stress of any kind a relapse, a temporary setback, a lapse, and a return to unhealthy coping can occur. Following is a list of the seven necessary elements of recovery.

Latest Research and Trends

Factors responsible for the proliferation of eating disorders have involved a nature/nurture understanding. Having first-degree relatives suffering from an eating disorder provide a model of disordered eating behaviors and attitudes. A multiple-gene configuration that interacts with environmental factors such as a mutation that affects the functioning of the hypothalamus, which plays a major role in hunger and satiety, might exist, which results in anorexia, bulimia, or another disordered eating (Bulik & Johnson, 2001).

Research on eating disorders and the athlete have proliferated since the late 1970s. Eating disorders occur more often in sports requiring weight control, such as wrestling, swimming, track, and running, as well as the "appearance sports" such as ballet, gymnastics, cheerleading, and tennis (Greenspan-Goldberg, 1991). The latest concern and research is based on the "Female Athlete Triad" Syndrome. Simply put, some athletes have gotten the notion that an extremely low body/fat ratio will make them more successful, that is, a "thin equals win" formula. Some coaches have unknowingly instilled, adopted, or encouraged this attitude.

Unfortunately, when a female loses too much body fat, she no longer has her menses. The syndrome resembles anorexia with one of its most insidious consequences, osteoporosis. Many of these athletes suffer from multiple bone breaks and the heartache of a shortened career.

Prevention of Addictions

Much has been written about the diet industry's financial interest in making weight loss a national obsession. The plastic surgery, pornography, and fashion industries are profiting off self and body insecurities, convincing us that we are not good enough as we are (Wolf, 1991). We need to be educated consumers and resist the cultural preoccupation with thinness. A man or a woman *can* be too thin! Culturally speaking, as long as we still have waiflike models put forth as seductresses, or bulked-up, big, "cut," V-shape, lean young men proliferating our magazines, print, and commercial advertisements, we'll be sending the wrong message to men and women of all ages and sizes.

Where to begin? It all starts at home. Appreciate parental impact on impressionable children and teens. Children observe dieting behavior and how parents treat themselves and their bodies. Parents are their role models; children identify with them. When an 8-year-old is preoccupied with what she's eating, with weight, thinness, bigness, with a critical self-appraisal based on appearance, parents must intervene.

Prevention is about education from an early age. Parents should be accessible and talk to their children about body image, good nutrition, eating disorders, and liking and loving themselves. A child must have stable and secure caretakers in caring relationships who are able to provide unconditional love in their primary years with limits, boundaries, and appropriate age expectations throughout their young adult years.

Primary prevention programs for addictions should be part of a school curriculum from kindergarten through college, including skills such as effective communication, conflict resolution, and empathy.

We are more than our bodies. We must focus on well-being, the health and wholeness of our mind, body, and spirit.

Internet Addiction

We have an interpersonal relationship with our computers. They are an extension of self, like an extended family. Our ease of interaction or frustration with our computer parallels how we interact with people in our lives. The Internet can be a marvelous global learning tool. The screen can be a canvas, the mouse a paintbrush, and our com-

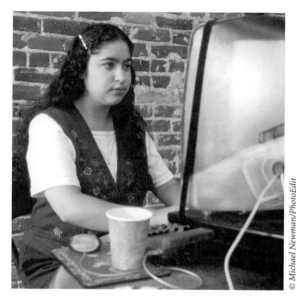

Internet addiction is one of the fastest growing forms of addiction in our times, particularly for young people.

puter, a companion. Children and teens can use the Internet to explore, to actively participate in a learning process involving gathering information for homework assignments and connecting to their friends through email and instant messages. So when does usage become *abusive* usage?

"While the typical student uses the Internet for 100 minutes per day, there is a small group of students that use the Internet to the degree that it interferes with other aspects of their lives. Approximately ten percent of Internet-using students have used the Internet to the degree that their usage meets criteria that are parallel to those of other forms of dependence." DSM-IV criteria for substance dependence was used as a screening tool for this exploratory study (Anderson, 2001).

As always, no matter what the presenting problem, health educators and counselors should be alert to other possibilities. Internet use is so common today that counselors should listen carefully for clues in this area.

Dr. K. Young, a psychologist, has paralleled Internet addiction with pathological gambling, using DSM-IV criteria as a guide. People are considered addicted when the answer is "yes" to five of the questions in Table 6.8.

Table 6.8
Screening for Internet Addiction

- Do you feel preoccupied with the Internet?

- Do you feel the need to use the Internet with increasing amount of time to achieve

- Have you tried repeatedly to cut back or stop using the Internet unsuccessfully?

- Have you lied to others, like family members, to conceal the extent of involvement with the Internet?

- Do you use the Internet to escape from problems or to relieve painful feelings?

- Do you stay online longer than intended?

- Is it interfering with any relationship in your life or work related commitments?

Source: From *Caught in the Net: How to Recognize the Signs of Internet Addiction and a Winning Strategy for Recovery* by K. Young, 1998. This material is used by permission of John Wiley & Sons, Inc.

The "ACE Model" which stands for anonymity, convenience, and escape, are three basic elements of cyberspace that serve to reward and reinforce addictive and pathological online behavior. Two evaluation forms to assess computer dependency are the Internet Dependency Intake Evaluation and the Internet Addiction Impairment Index (Young, 1998).

Case Study

Richard

Richard, an 18-year-old high-school graduate, decided to take a summer off before entering college. His parents were unhappy because they felt a job would provide structure and a connection with peers. They noticed he often spent hours on the Internet in his room.

That summer Richard grew edgy, moody, irritable, insecure, and self-critical, frightened about leaving home and starting college. Some days he didn't shower or change clothes. He would start and end his day online, eating most of his meals at his computer.

Richard's parents asked the high-school guidance counselor for a referral to a psychotherapist.

During the initial session with his therapist, Richard described himself as a "loner," saying the Internet and chat rooms offered him an opportunity to connect with people. He had few friends, and his one close friend was far away. They sent instant messages.

Through therapy, Richard realized that he appreciated a "real person" connection in his life, and that he had been avoiding the real world and growing up.

Dangers and Pitfalls in Cyberspace

Some people use the Internet to express what they would not say on the telephone or in person. Some people sometimes send angry, negative, and hurtful statements via email and instant messaging. There are thousands of hate Web sites, pornography sites, and off-color chat rooms where people speak and act out unusual and wild fantasies.

Some children, teens, and young adults post intimate profiles in cyberspace in an attempt to connect with others. Unfortunately, there are cyberspace predators too, seeking vulnerable prey such as children. These predators lure them through seductive language and promises, and coerce them to meet in person.

Health professionals and parents should emphasize the importance of keeping personal information personal. Remind young people to safeguard their telephone numbers and/or home addresses, and to keep their passwords secret. Meeting an online acquaintance in person can be dangerous, and should be strongly discouraged for safety reasons.

Prevention

Consumers, teens, young adults, parents, health educators and health counselors, and students should be aware of the potential for abusive usage of the Internet, as well as the dangers and pitfalls in cyberspace. Education must catch up with technology and the information age of the 21st century. No matter the age, computer usage needs to be time limited and self-monitored.

Parents need to actively monitor children's time on the Internet, and be aware of their children's purpose for being on the Internet. Educators and parents need to further research and discuss age-appropriate limits, boundaries, and guidelines for appropriate usage.

It can be wonderful to connect with a long-distance friend online. It makes you feel good, it's convenient and cost-effective, but it need not be a replacement for telephone or face-to-face contact. Like anything else in life, maintaining balance and moderation will prevent an overdependence or addiction to the Internet.

Gambling

Gambling has grown tremendously in the United States in the past two decades, becoming a major part of the nation's economy. Las Vegas and Atlantic City have been joined by riverboat casinos, Indian reservation casinos, online betting, off-track betting, and state lotteries. We are inundated with advertising for the lottery.

Though most people gamble recreationally and have some personal parameters (like knowing when to stop and how to gamble in moderation) approximately 3 to 5 percent of the population can be described as compulsive, pathological gamblers (Council on Compulsive Gambling of New Jersey [CCGNJ], 2002).

According to CCGNJ, "95 percent of teen gamblers are male; only 5 percent are female. Males tend to bet on sports, cards, dice, lottery, horses and casinos, while females bet on lotteries, casinos, play cards, racetracks and bingo."

A health educator or counselor in a classroom setting, community outreach program, or employee assistance program should check out the DSM-IV (see Table 6.9) which lists criteria as a screening guide in identifying people who could be suffering from a gambling problem. It is a challenge to assess those who may have crossed the line from recreational gambling to compulsive pathological gambling.

The Council on Compulsive Gambling of New Jersey (CCGNJ). has developed a guide for teachers/health educators to be alert to possible gam-

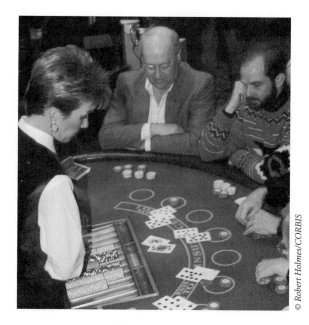

© Robert Holmes/CORBIS

Though recreational for many people, gambling can be a serious addiction with disastrous consequences for others.

bling problems in their students. Here are three of the 12 warning signs:

- Unexplained absences from school along with a sudden drop in grades

- Change in personality (such as irritability, impatience, criticism, or sarcasm).

- Gambling language in his/her conversation. (For example, exaggerated use of the words *bet, 5 timer, 10 timer, bookie, loan shark, point spread, underdog* or *favorite.*)

For a health counselor or educator, like any other addiction, an appropriate referral must be made after speaking to your student, client, friend, or colleague. Gamblers Anonymous is an organization that recommends abstinence from gambling. Consider a referral to a psychotherapist who can assess any underlying depression or anxiety disorder, provide a psychiatric evaluation, and, if indicated, prescribe medication. Many gamblers base their identity and self-esteem on whether they are a "winner" and get caught up in "catching up," or "making good on their losses." Family and friends

Table 6.9
DSM-IV Diagnostic Criteria for Pathological Gambling (312.31).

Persistent and recurrent maladaptive gambling behavior is indicated by five (or more) of the following:

- is preoccupied with gambling (e.g., preoccupied with reliving past gambling experiences, handicapping or planning the next venture, or think of ways to get money with which to gamble).

- needs to gamble with increasing amounts of money in order to achieve the desired excitement

- has repeated unsuccessful efforts to control, cut back or stop gambling

- is restless or irritable when attempting to cut down or stop gambling

- gambles as a way of escaping from problems or of relieving a dysphoric mood (e.g., felling of helplessness, guilt, anxiety, depression).

- after losing money gambling, often returns another day to get even ("chasing" ones losses).

- lies to family members, therapist or others to conceal the extent of involvement with gambling

- has committed illegal acts such as forgery, fraud, theft, or embezzlement to finance gambling

- has jeopardized or lost a significant relationship, job or educational career opportunity because of gambling

- relies on others to provide money to relieve a desperate financial situation caused by gambling

Source: From *Diagnostic and Statistical Manual of Mental Disorders,* Fourth Edition, Text Revision. Washington, D.C., American Psychiatric Association, 1994. Reprinted with permission from the *Diagnostic and Statistical Manual of Mental Disorders,* Fourth Edition. Copyright 1999 American Psychiatric Association.

need to be alerted not to "enable," or "bail out" the compulsive gambler but rather be supportive and make sure they get the appropriate help.

Early intervention is all about prevention. As with alcohol, drug, eating disorders, and Internet addictions, the negative influences of gambling must get the same attention at all levels. Children are very impressionable and parents can make the greatest impact in having conversations with children when they are young, at home and at school. Role models are important, too. Because young people watch adults carefully, we must be consistent in our words and deeds.

Summary

Because addictions and dependencies occur so often in American life, health educators and counselors should remain attuned to the spectrum of possibilities, and be prepared to address issues that may arise. Health educators and counselors can play a beneficial role in raising awareness of these issues. In the important areas of substance abuse, Internet addiction, and gambling, health educators and counselors must keep up to date on the latest information, data, and trends, and periodically review their files to keep current.

In the health field health educators and counselors contribute toward minimizing risks and negative consequences for individuals, families, and/or communities. They also provide accurate information, resources, and referral; help individuals begin the process of self-reflection and self-awareness; and provide support for those concerned about others. In some cases they facilitate and support change. Health educators and counselors play critical roles in maintaining wellness and regaining good health.

Key Terms

abstinence, 97
addiction, 101
assessment, 102
cessation, 101
dependence, 98

eating disorder, 106
intervention, 99
relapse, 100
withdrawal, 98

Questions for Discussion

1. Ryan is an 18-year-old freshman attending a local college who lives on campus and comes home on alternate weekends. His parents notice that he sometimes spends up to 5 consecutive hours on the Internet chatting with his friends and playing games. Ryan did not do well in his first semester and is now on academic probation. He gets angry with his parents when they suggest he limit his Internet usage.

2. Do you think Ryan is bordering on an Internet addiction? What counseling suggestions would you make to a parent to help manage Ryan's Internet usage? What suggestions would you make to Ryan if he consulted you?

3. Marta sees her friend Judy consistently throwing away her lunch at school and going to the bathroom after meals. What can you do as a friend if you suspect a potential eating disorder?

4. You teach a first-period class. One of your students, Tyrone, comes in late most Monday mornings. His eyes appear bloodshot, he looks tired and pale, and he even puts his head on the desk, on occasion. One day he stays after class to hand in an assignment, and as you are talking, you smell beer on his breath. You suspect he has been drinking on the weekends. How would you address this issue with Tyrone? What resources can you offer to him?

5. Larissa consults you with her concerns about her sister, Lena, who is 4 months pregnant. For several years, Lena has enjoyed a glass of wine or beer with her dinner, and has continued to drink alcohol even though she is pregnant. Larissa is worried about Fetal Alcohol Syndrome, and thinks Lena should stop drinking until she has her baby. What can you suggest?

Related Web Sites

http://www.cdc.gov
Centers for Disease Control and Prevention. Offers current news, Health Topics data, links to other sites, public health information, and other information.

http://www.edap.org
Eating Disorders Awareness and Prevention, Inc. Provides information on eating disorders, programs, links and resources, tips for helping a friend, prevention.

http://www.gamblersanonymous.org
Gamblers Anonymous. Offers questions and answers, history, current programs, resources, and links.

http://www.nida.nih.gov
National Institute on Drug Abuse. Contains information on trends, statistics, grants, research, prevention; specific information for parents, teachers, students, and young adults.

http://www.samhsa.gov
Substance Abuse and Mental Health Services Administration. Includes information about programs, conferences, legislative information, policy, statistics, workplace resources, mental-health services, treatment, and prevention.

Healthy Relationships

JOAN D. ATWOOD, PH.D.

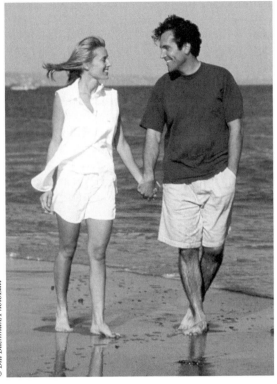

© Bill Bachman/PhotoEdit

OBJECTIVES

By the end of the chapter, the reader should be able to:

- Discuss psychological theoretical concepts underlying healthy relationships

- Present information on the developmental tasks associated with healthy relationships

- Examine and explore the role of love and intimacy in emotionally mature relationships

- Discuss the traps and pitfalls individuals encounter along the way to a healthy relationship

- Present information on contributing factors to healthy relationships

- Explore some skills necessary for building a healthy relationship

- Examine some communication pitfalls that can affect relationships

- Discuss research findings in the area of healthy relationships

- To present information on the traits of healthy relationships

Despite the importance of achieving constructive and satisfying relationships, and the enormous disappointments, hurts, and self-devaluation that failure in a relationship can entail, there is little research that has focused on the factors involved in what makes a **healthy relationship.** The U.S. Census Bureau (2001) reports that in 1997 there were 2,384,000 marriages in this country. Approximately 60 percent of them will end in divorce. Yet the literature mainly focuses on variables involved in unhealthy relationships and it is only recently that researchers are examining

Healthy relationships. Relationships in which positivity, growth, effective communication, and mature giving and receiving of love are standard.

117

factors that promote successful, healthy, and satisfying relationships (Julien, Markman, Leveille, Chartrand, 1994). It is interesting to note that while Americans value a healthy relationship and/or marriage above all else—ahead of money, satisfying work, and even health (Sollee, 1996), there is no training in the public school system or elsewhere as to how to accomplish this healthy relationship. Children learn early on that relationships and, ultimately for some, marriage, are socially and individually desirable states and that satisfying ones are the ideal goals; but children are not given any training or skill building for their most important relationship, which could possibly span 60 or 70 years. Because of their training, health educators, counselors, and marriage and family therapists are in a unique position to fill this gap.

It is the purpose of this chapter to explore the psychological factors and developmental tasks necessary for the formation of a healthy, stable, satisfying relationship. These tasks are examined pre-relationship and then in a relationship situation. Psychological factors hindering the completion of these tasks are presented, along with a discussion of the traps and pitfalls commonly encountered by couples who have not completed the tasks. There is then a discussion of the factors influencing healthy relationships, along with a presentation of many suggestions health educators and counselors can utilize with their students and/or clients. Throughout the chapter there are suggestions for educators and counselors as well as bibliographical references that direct the reader to more extensive materials. While most of the research presented focuses on marital relationships, the findings can be applied to any intimate relationship.

The Psychological Preparation for Healthy Relationships

Pre-Relationship Developmental Tasks

In order for a relationship to be successful and satisfying, relatively free from stress and turmoil, certain pre-relationship tasks should be accomplished. Partners in a healthy relationship are continuously changing and growing with respect to their personality development, interests, goals, and relationships with friends, relatives, and colleagues. In order for these changes to benefit the relationship, flexibility and sensitivity are required on each partner's part. This in turn necessitates the maturational skills necessary to cope with the partner's growth and define it as a benefit rather than as a threat. An intimate relationship often highlights and intensifies the emotional challenges necessary to achieve greater personal maturity, which, in turn contributes to greater relationship happiness. Personal maturity involves the successful negotiation of life tasks that each individual must face. Classical theorist Mahler (1975) believes that these tasks must include the following:

- The formation of a positive self-image which fosters spontaneity, curiosity, and more competent intellectual and social skills

- The separation and individuation of the person from their families of origin into a more self-reliant and confident individual

- The development of healthy self-esteem which allows for the capacity to love and give to others without feeling depleted or deprived

- The willingness to assume responsibilities and care-taking positions without feeling resentful or taken advantage of

- The capacity to achieve a balance in one's mental functioning between reasoning and emotions which allows one to develop the ability to empathize with another's feelings and position

An emotionally mature relationship requires mutual respectfulness of each partner's growth and changing needs and interests. More mature individuals can accommodate changing dimensions in their partners without feeling rejected, diminished, or threatened. They feel comfortable pursuing outside interests and bringing other important people into the relationship sphere. Although the capacity to function independently in an intimate relationship is most important, the ability to trust and rely on one's partner is an equally vital issue.

More secure individuals, who have come into an intimate relationship after completing the basic developmental tasks, are able to recognize and share fears, insecurities, and limitations, which allows for a reaching out in times of need, stress, or problems. In this way, both partners feel they are making important contributions to each other, which enhances the feeling of mutual dignity and respectfulness. While this issue of equality and mutual respectfulness may not be emphasized in other cultures, in American society where equality is a significant issue, it is a crucial factor in the smooth functioning of any intimate relationship, including marriage. For a detailed description of the psychological processes involved in finding a mate, see Atwood, 1993.

Relationship Developmental Tasks

Jim and Sara dated each other for about 6 months. They felt that they loved each other but they had so many arguments that they questioned whether their relationship could go the long haul. Jim wanted to go out with his friends; Sara wanted him to spend all of his spare time with her. She felt that at this point he should have outgrown the "hanging out with the guys" phase; he felt that she wanted to put him on a leash.

Once individuals have accomplished the earlier pre-relationship psychological tasks, it is helpful if they are able to apply their emotional maturity to certain developmental tasks in the relationship. A successful intimate relationship, marital or otherwise, involves accomplishing fundamental tasks, which are discussed throughout this paper.

Some of the more basic **developmental tasks** are:

> **Developmental tasks.** The maturational skills necessary for a healthy relationship including (1) positive self-image, (2) individuation, (3) expression of love without feeling depleted, (4) willingness to assume responsibility and care-taking and (5) a balance of emotions and reasoning.

- Continuing to grow as separate individuals in the relationship/marriage, while maintaining a working interdependence with themselves and society. This growth process is what is involved in one's maturing as a person and being respectful of the partner's individuality. It means working out differences in backgrounds, past experiences, and intellectual and personality styles with a spirit of cooperation rather than a power struggle;

- Bridging the transition from romantic love to the caring and nurturing involved in a longer term intimate relationship.

- Learning to compromise one's own needs with the needs of one's partner so that resentments and feelings of deprivations are held to a minimum.

- Mutually agreeing on the division of labor within the household so that the workload of relationship or marriage and raising a family (if there is one) are equally shared.

- If there is a marriage or a commitment ceremony, being able to make the transition from the initial romantic dyad or couple to the inclusion of children which brings about important changes in the relationship of the couple.

- Effectively managing conflict which is an inevitable accompaniment of a healthy relationship where both partners are expressive of their thoughts, feelings, and needs.

- Maintaining sexual interest so that the intimate relationship is the primary relationship in both its emotional and physical aspects.

The Role of Love and Intimacy in Emotionally Mature Relationships

This section discusses the role of love and intimacy in relationship/marriage. Again, this applies to any relationship or partnership where there is a basis of love, intimacy, and commitment. It would be unusual for a couple to maintain the intensity of romantic and erotic feelings that characterize the initial months of a relationship. Gradually, the excitement and passion of the early relationship is replaced by everyday concerns and tasks, which are important to the ongoing maintenance of the relationship. The newness of the sexual experience may diminish somewhat, and the conversations which previously revealed interesting information become more directed to practical matters. Hopefully, romantic love becomes supplemented by a deeper sense of caring and appreciation as the couple share life situations together, and the bonding becomes a source of friendship, love, and intimacy.

Love

Brian and Nicole thought they were in love. When they first met, they wanted to spend every waking hour with each other. Eight months later, although they still enjoyed each other's company and wanted to be together, they didn't feel the intensity of passion they felt in the beginning of their relationship. Now they were starting to question whether they were experiencing "true love" or whether they were simply infatuated with each other.

Most people, when asked why they are in a committed relationship or why they are together, reply that they are in love. Love involves acceptance. In fact, if there is any singular aspect to the feeling commonly described as mature love, it is acceptance. Loving, in its most developed form, involves the embracing of the loved person with a deeper appreciation and approval of that person just as they are. The bonding is cemented by the helpfulness and mutual maturing which each partner renders to the other, with a deepening of appreciation and respectfulness of the other's qualities and assets. It is an intuitive understanding and action of extending one's caring feelings to another, without expectations, judgment, or evaluation. This is not an easy task even for the most mature of couples, for socialization in American society involves being shaped by messages of what is prized and what is valued and what is less worthy of our attention and appreciation, and so on. Some individuals learn to be fearful of deeply accepting another because they feel that this might condone ways or qualities of being that are gener-

ally disapproved of by society. Furthermore, individuals mistakenly believe that the way to mature and improve themselves is to eliminate what they regard as their undesirable aspects and behaviors. They often are frightened of the process of opening up to, and accepting, aspects of themselves that they have judged unlovable. They fear that acceptance of these aspects will lead either to stagnation or to an unwanted redefinition of themselves. This creates tendencies to present "false selves" to their partners, which could lead to a lack of authenticity in the relationship.

Intimacy. Intimacy is crucial in any healthy relationship. The foundation of intimacy is basic trust and communication. Basic trust is the experience of positiveness toward oneself and those close to us. It allows individuals to feel accepting of themselves and to value their loving feelings. This self-acceptance promotes a more relaxed psychological state of mind, which makes for openness and allows couples to reach out toward each other with positive expectations of returned loving feelings. It diminishes unnecessary protectiveness and anticipation of hurts and rejections. This basic caring feeling toward oneself and others reduces the need to hide behind images, or to feel threatened that unacceptable aspects of ourselves will emerge (lost selves). Out of this positiveness, communication flows more readily and couples allow themselves to be more "real" or authentic. Where basic trust is present to a greater degree, partners are more mutually respectful of each other, and unrealistic expectations are minimized. As each partner more readily shares their feelings and difficulties, a better perspective of the needs and capabilities of each partner emerges.

As stated earlier, a sustained loving relationship requires the deeper appreciation and acceptance of one's partner as they truly are, not as we expect them to be. This does not mean that if there are significant difficulties that problems cannot be addressed and changes hoped for; rather, it means that one starts to work on these problems with patience and an understanding of this is how things are rather than an attitude of, "How can you be or act this way?"

Developmental Tasks and Emotional Maturity or Immaturity

The role of individual personality dynamics is important in that they are powerful factors that relate to the couple's mutual capacity for happiness. It is the degree of nurturance, acceptance, appreciation, and sense of emotional security which the individuals experienced through their childhood emotional development that will largely contribute to how they respond to their partner over time, and the level of intimacy that they will allow in the relationship. When we speak of levels of maturity, we are in fact, talking about the degree to which the person has been able or encouraged to develop their emotional and intellectual capabilities, along with a stabilized and positive sense of self. When there are blocks to this development, such as in childhood situations of abandonment, abuse, neglect, or overindulgence, the person might display troubled personality dynamics.

Personality dynamics means the patterned sets of feelings, emotional reactions, and behaviors human beings exhibit as a result of their interaction with their environment and significant others. These patterns serve important functions of helping individuals anticipate and manipulate the environment to serve their needs and to avoid pain, anxiety, or harm.

The human mind and brain functioning is established in such a way as to be able to shield from consciousness unwanted or painful aspects of feelings, thoughts, and experiences. This does not mean that these experiences are inactive. It simply means that individuals can consciously carry on activities without distraction, more or less, from these unconscious elements. This state of affairs carries with it both major advantages and disadvantages. The major advantage is that persons are often spared the immediate pain or discomfort of feeling states, which probably helps them to function more effectively in a current, immediate situation.

The major disadvantages are:

- People are under the illusion that their conscious mental activity is the major source of their decision-making functions, and that it represents the majority portion of what they would refer to as their mind or personality.

- They do not understand that there are major aspects of their decisions and behaviors that emanate out of this unconscious reservoir of feelings and rejected aspects of themselves.

- Feeling states which remain unconscious are free to play out in terms of substitutive behaviors which are not within awareness, or conscious choice. More importantly, however, the assumptions, which are contained within these feeling states, are beyond rational review. For example, if a young boy has a chronic experience of feeling unworthy because his mother is continuously unhappy, it would not be unusual for the child to blame himself for his mother's unhappiness. If he later goes on to repress this experience, the assumption which he made as a child that he must not have been lovable enough to make his mother happy remains in his unconscious unquestioned and accepted without reservation. He might therefore respond to the unhappiness in his spouse with discomfort and fear, unconsciously feeling that there must be something wrong with him because his wife is experiencing unhappiness.

- When feeling states are unconscious, they assume the form of nonlogical properties. Parts can stand for wholes, and rules of orderly logic and understanding may not be applicable. The best example of nonlogical or primary process thinking or feeling states is exemplified in dream states. Thus, if an aspect of our partner's behavior reminds us unconsciously of a parent's personality or behavior, it is not uncommon for the piece of behavior to become representative of that individual as a whole, evoking such reactions as "You're just like my mother!"

(For a detailed discussion on the effects of early experiences on later behavior, see Hendrix, 1988; Scharff & Scharff, 1991).

While each partner may have entered the relationship with a relatively stable personality, it is a recognized fact that longer-term exposure to a troubled personality of one partner can adversely affect the personality of the other partner in important ways. As long as each partner is catering to the needs of the other partner, no matter how maladaptive, the couple will manage to function together and feel that the relationship is viable. Pressure might then be brought to bear on the partner by the less-healthy individual to maintain the status quo. This situation is frequently encountered where one partner is an alcoholic. Despite the bitter complaints of the sober partner about his/her mate's drinking, she/he nevertheless maintains a control of the relationship, which endows him/her with esteem and power. When the alcoholic enters treatment and begins to make genuine changes in his/her personality and style of interaction, their mate may well sabotage treatment and subtly induce the spouse to resume drinking.

Relationship Traps and Pitfalls

There are many **traps and pitfalls** along the way in the developmental transitions. One would think that being in a "loving relationship" would diminish the anxieties, or conversely, increase the trust, that people experience with one another. This is often not the case, however, as witnessed by the number of partnerships which deteriorate once vows of marriage and/or commitment are exchanged. One of the main reasons for this is that the intimacy which marriage or a committed relationship brings increases the threat of exposure or rejection, which an individual may have feared through his/her life. The more important the partner becomes, the greater the trauma anticipated should she/he be disapproved of or rejected by their partner. It is important for health educa-

> **Traps and pitfalls of relationships.** Many mechanisms, conscious and subconscious, that can undermine and negatively impact a relationship. These can include defenses such as denial, projection, devaluation, and so on.

tors/counselors to be aware of the various defensive maneuvers that individuals employ in order to protect themselves.

Building up Protective Mechanisms.

Jane and Gerry knew each other for about 2 years. They were at the point where they were deciding if they should make more of a commitment to each other—perhaps get engaged. Jane believed she loved Gerry but felt he was very defensive. Every time she brought up an issue that she felt they should work on, Gerry would not address the issue, but instead focus on defending himself. No matter how much she tried to explain that she wasn't criticizing him, he continued to defend himself and the issue got lost in the argument. Gerry felt he just wanted to explain himself when Jane criticized him.

One of the most important underlying motivational drives is the need for individuals to maintain a sense of security, diminished anxiety, and intact sense of self. This motivational system gives rise to the emphasis on individuals' need for self-protection, which easily outweighs conscious considerations of love and romance when individuals feel themselves to be in any way threatened. It is important to note, as Sager (1975) points out, that defense or protective mechanisms are not necessarily pathological. If they do not become permanent ways of avoiding reality, they can have adaptive value. If, however, they cause distancing and/or excluding, they can lead to problems in a relationship.

Individuals' intellectual capacity to reason, anticipate, project, and analyze provides them with powerful tools to adapt and protect themselves. If they are accurate in their appraisal of the current situation and its potential problems or harms, then these processes serve them well. If, however, past wounds and sensitivities cause them to misinterpret present circumstances, then what was a positive asset now becomes a significant limitation, and they are likely to become defensive and emotionally restricted in the face of an anticipated unpleasantness, harm, or rejection. The significant reasons for how these processes of misinterpretation develop are discussed in a later section. The main point is that these personality dynamics are instrumental in whether the relationship will contain greater harmony or greater discord.

Protective measures are built up over a lifetime of experience and become incorporated into an individual's personality makeup. They are experienced by the people as a natural part of themselves, and more importantly, are felt to be a necessary part of their secure functioning. Because these protective mechanisms are experienced by the individual as part of him/herself and necessary for survival, they are clung to with the belief that greater harm or threat will come if they are questioned or let go of. Because most of what individuals dislike about themselves, and are rejected for by others, is in reality their defensive maladaptive maneuvers. They are often in the paradoxical situation of suffering from the very same processes from which they are convinced they need to protect themselves. Generally, individuals will not change despite their complaints of suffering or rejection until they can experientially understand that the way they are trying to defend against hurt and rejection is their major problem.

Painful or emotionally depriving experiences in childhood create a need to compensate for the effects they have had on self-esteem and feelings of self-worth. Individuals then develop expectations of self and others to offset these deprivations and handicaps to self-esteem and set about to fashion a self-image that excludes what is judged to be undesirable personality features. They long for the acceptance and unconditional love that would have been helpful in the past, and transfer these expectations onto the people who become most important in their life. They think, "Surely if I am loved, those who love me will be willing and able to fulfill all my needs and expectations (Hendrix, 1988). In this way, they endow their partners with qualities and capabilities to help them accomplish this task only to later become disappointed and angry when their partner falls short of their expectations. Often, as a result of this process, which may be acted out quite unconsciously, they become angry and demand the most from those who are closest and most caring.

The need to protect oneself at all costs is most difficult for couples to understand because, for the most part, they are unaware of their underlying feelings. There can be many types and degrees of protective measures invoked, as well as different vulnerabilities, which are triggered by an intimate committed and/or marital relationship. People who have been living together for one to several years and then marry or have a commitment ceremony may find an escalation of conflict in their relationship which did not exist while they were living together.

These patterns of behavior, with their attendant needs, expectations, frustrations, disappointments, and disillusionments, are powerful processes because they represent attempts by the person to repair hurts and wounds from the past. These hurts do not necessarily have to be traumatic events or devastating occurrences. They can be the day-to-day insensitivities and subtle lack of parental responsiveness which accumulate over time to undercut a child's confidence and positive feelings for life and appreciation of themselves. While these reparative processes can become maladaptive when they are transferred intact onto partners, they nevertheless are attempts by persons to repair themselves and bring solace to their inner discomfort. If that positive energy can be harnessed and redirected, that individual then has the opportunity to attempt the healing process with different tools.

In evolving defensive mechanisms to protect themselves, as occurs in the process of worrying, individuals are attempting to anticipate, predict, and thus control a potentially threatening situation. Capacities for anticipation and prediction are dependent on memories of past experiences. When individuals recall past events and project them into the future in anticipation of trying to cope with what they feel is about to happen, they have a sense of power and control. They gear their forces up and feel a certain strength even if it means stirring up and holding onto negative feelings of anger or hurt. If their estimation of the current situation and its similarity to past experiences is accurate, then the behavior is adaptive. If there are significant inaccuracies or misperceptions either about the present situation or the way things happened in the past, then they are susceptible to maladaptive behaviors.

One of the difficulties in this whole process of adaptation through anticipation and comparison with the past is that the individual is dealing not only with factual events, but constellations of feelings, some or all of which may be unconscious, which alter the memory or understanding of these events. Therefore, not only is the actual recall of events open to error, but the understanding of the dynamics involved in these events may even be faulty. As in the example given earlier, a mother's chronic unhappiness stemming from an unhappy marriage and personal conflicts can easily be erroneously experienced by a child as resulting from some fault of his in being able to make his mother happy. This set of experiences is then laid down in the child's memory and reproduced in his current feelings as they may apply to experiencing his partner's unhappiness. Her distress may evoke anticipatory defensiveness in dealing with her unhappiness, which may have little to do with him. This then might lead to his withdrawal of empathy, intensifying his partner's unhappiness.

If past hurts have been prominent, then the activation of these anticipatory defenses is most often involuntary. This set of circumstances leads to a situation where the individual repeatedly experiences negative outcomes of his/her behavior and is puzzled as to how this comes about. Because the defensive maneuvers are not within his/her consciousness, the person is unaware how the defensiveness may contribute to, or bring about the very results that they are trying to avoid. A common example is of a shy and insecure young man who attributes a considerable amount of the insecurity to the fact that women do not respond to him, when the more complete picture is that he will attend a party and relate only minimally, if at all, to the women at the party. His fear of anticipated rejection almost automatically evokes behaviors that cause him to remain on the periphery of activities, or to only have brief and awkward conversations with women he is introduced to.

Another significant difficulty with the anticipatory system of defense is the fact that partial similarities in the current situation are likely to trigger stronger defensive reactions, which were geared to more comprehensive dangers in the past. For example, a wife might have some similar characteristics to her husband's rejecting or controlling mother. This could cause an unconscious major distancing maneuver on the husband's part because the part-identification triggered a global defensive reaction to an unconsciously perceived mother figure.

Defense Mechanisms. As individuals experience many aspects of life, there are always potentially conflicting or opposite aspects of situations. While people need a degree of protection in their lives through predictability based on the projection of past experiences onto current situations, this process is also responsible for holding onto negative and painful experiences which not only continue the pain, but also reinforce negative notions about themselves, and of the world as a dangerous or threatening environment. Protective mechanisms that are typically used by couples are (1) denial, (2) projection, (3) externalization and devaluation. These defense mechanisms are employed by individuals in an intimate, committed relationship in order to avoid anticipated hurt or rejection. The first three major defenses are listed below

Denial. Chief among these defenses is denial, which allows persons not to attend to, and be actively aware of, their behavior, expressions, or verbal communication, which reveals the truer underlying aspects of their thoughts and feelings. They will disavow evidence, which disputes their own consolidated view of themselves, fearing that any contradiction to their self-image will render them vulnerable to hurt, humiliation, or criticism. Denial allows for the addition of other mechanisms of defense such as projection or externalization.

Projection. Projection is a fundamental process occurring out of a need for stability and protection which involves the transfer of inner states of mind or qualities onto the environment. The recipient of the transfer may either be a spouse or significant other, or the environment itself in the form of negative vibrations attached to a situation. Because repressed aspects of our life remain active and influential, even though they remain beyond everyday awareness, projection is one mechanism to discharge the inner emotional tension that these unconscious aspects generate. In projection, the individual finds in others what he/she has been unable to accept in him/herself and can direct his/her energies to disparaging or criticizing others for these attributes. Other common means of discharging inner tension is through the pursuit of pleasure, sexuality, or mood-altering substances such as drugs or alcohol.

Devaluation.

> Tim and Carolyn dated about a year and a half before they married. For the first 6 months of their marriage, they both agreed they were happy. Then Carolyn said Tim started saying "mean" things to her. He used to like the softness of her body. Now he teased her and said she could lose a few pounds. He used to think she was very intelligent. Now he frequently asked her if "she got it yet," and on occasion would even say, "Duh!" to her, indicating that she was being stupid. Carolyn felt he was chipping away at her self-esteem and wished he would stop. She also questioned whether his feelings for her had changed.

Projection is often coupled with devaluation, which is the process of lowering the esteem or worth of the significant other by the projector, so as to avoid anticipated devaluation of oneself. By making the other person less meaningful and valuable, any potential loss of that person is more easily borne, minimizing the risk of feeling loss, hurt, and rejection.

A detailed exploration of the varied defense mechanisms and their role in intimate relationships is beyond the scope of this chapter. However, it is helpful to address their main attributes:

- Defenses frequently make their appearance in a more intensified way when intimacy deepens, with its concomitant threat of rejection or abandonment in those individuals with underlying and significant emotional insecurities.

- Defense mechanisms are necessary for normal adjustment but may become intensified, leading to restricted and maladaptive behaviors and inner emotional suffering. Intensifications of defensive operations because of current precipitators may reactivate past vulnerabilities to the point where there is significant misinterpretation of present events.

- Because defenses are replays of the past (anticipation and prediction foster reenactment of past emotional experiences) there are unconscious, accompanying belief systems which are themselves repressed and not accessible to rational processes. The individual is usually convinced he/she is operating under adult, rational processes and these processes are what make him/her who they are. Direct challenges to these beliefs, behaviors, or attitudes are frequently met with frustration, anger, or a feeling of being criticized.

- These defenses create, for better or for worse, a stabilized sense of self which may be more or less realistic than the individual appreciates. This may be a serious problem in intimate relationships where there is significant discrepancy between the actual and idealized self.

- As the individual feels increasingly threatened, she/he tends to cling more to the defensive operations, creating a vicious cycle of attack and defense with the spouse. This conflict leads to a confusion of what the truer nature of the actual here-and-now problem between the couple actually is, as opposed to reactivation of premarital emotional problems.

- When defensive operations are more intensely mobilized, persons become hyperfocused on the current triggers of their sense of being threatened or hurt by their spouse, and so have a much diminished awareness that the hurt and threat they are currently experiencing derives from a more fundamental and relevant set of past experiences. Indeed, the current interaction or trigger may only represent a smaller part of their underlying vulnerability with its accompanying hurt and pain.

- Because defenses are ubiquitous in personality makeup, it is easy for each spouse to cite the defenses of their partner as being responsible for the conflict, and avoid appreciating how each partner is contributing to the conflict.

There are many strategies for engaging and assisting relationship conflict brought about in some measure by defensive operations triggered by the underlying emotional vulnerabilities of one or both of the partners. Given the aforementioned factors in defensive maneuvers, it is helpful to bring the couple together in an atmosphere of patience, acceptance, and noncritical observation of what is transpiring at the individual and couple level. This exploration fosters a mutual search of themselves as individuals as well as a couple, so as to reduce the fear of being criticized and rejected. When people come to understand that their misperceptions, maladaptive behaviors, and objectionable aspects of their personalities are understandable past attempts to cope and adapt, they are able to accept emotional correction more easily, and bring a compassion and empathy to the arena, which is healing to both themselves and their spouse. When couples can realized that they are reliving past hurts and vulnerabilities, rather than being labeled as "crazy" or "unreasonable," they now understand how their past needs to protect themselves account for what appears to be unreasonable behavior.

Relationships that have a foundation of health will be able to withstand these revelations of the truer nature of their spouses and will grow from the experience of openness and realness in the relationship. The defensive operations account for the problems more than the feelings themselves.

A frequent experience in couple's arguments is to have a spouse whom has been just accused of various types of behavior answer with an unbelievable "but that's just the way *you* are!" The process of projection blinds couples to those qualities within themselves that they find objectionable. They are then less able to identify these qualities and accept them as parts of themselves so as to bring meaningful help to themselves rather than to become condemnatory. For a detailed description of therapy with couples, see Atwood, 1992; Atwood & Maltin, 1992; Atwood, 1993).

Healthy Relationships

The prior discussion examined the individual personality factors, the pre-relationship tasks, and the relationship tasks necessary for the foundation of a healthy relationship. The following sections explore healthy relationship functioning. In distinguishing between superficial and intimate relationships there are certain changes that take place in a relationship (http://www.the.net/wise/relationships/healthy_relationship.htm).

- Interaction between the two individuals occurs more often for longer periods of time and in a wider range of settings.

- When separated, the two individuals attempt to resolve the proximity and when it is regained, they feel more comfortable.

- The two individuals disclose secrets and are more open in criticizing and praising one another.

- The two individuals develop their own method of communicating and become increasingly more efficient in communicating with each other.

- They develop agreed-upon goals and stable interaction patterns

- Investment in the relationship increases, enhancing its importance in the two individuals' lives.

Learning Good Relationships Skills

Sollee (1997) speaks of healthy marital relationships but her principles can easily be applied to committed relationships of all kind. She theorizes that love and committed relationships are actually skill-based propositions and that what makes the difference between relationships that work and relationships that do not are learned behaviors and skills. She believes that important skills are conflict management and resolution. The problem is not that individuals have differences of opinion, it is rather how they handle those differences. She believes that potential intimate partners should take pre-committment preparation courses. This author wholeheartedly agrees.

Some Relationships Skills

Mutual Self Disclosure. The building of intimate relationships depends not only on effective communication and learning skill enhancement techniques, but also on mutual self-disclosure. Self-disclosure refers to each partner revealing personal information to the other. As a relationship progresses, the amount and intimacy of self-disclosure usually increases in a stepwise progression as one person's self-disclosure is responded to in kind by the other. Thus, when one partner reveals something about himself or herself, the other is expected to reply with an equally personal revelation—a process referred to as reciprocity.

Self-disclosures usually entail some form of risk and vulnerability. Usually, the more information that is disclosed, the greater the risk and generally the more vulnerable the person feels. A person who reveals something of his or her real self may fear rejection, especially if the revelation is highly negative. Revealing such information may enable the partner to put the other person in an inferior position, to make excessive demands, or to continually confront their partner with the past. Generally speaking, the greatest obstacle to self-disclosure is fear of being judged and being found lacking in some trait.

Intimacy involves the dropping of masks (or the false selves) and the lowering of defenses by each partner, together with the sharing of beliefs, hopes, feelings, values, achievements, and disappointments. This does not mean that partners must "tell all," but it does mean that building a relationship based on trust and intimacy is being more open and coming to know each other more fully—being more "real" and authentic.

To facilitate self-disclosure, it is suggested that partners try not to judge each other's behavior. They should try to refrain from giving advice to each other. This only serves to put one in a superior position. They should try not to interrogate their partners in order to get all the details. In other words, they should try to get involved, but they should also try not to intrude. It is helpful for partners to try to refrain from issuing commands, orders, or threats in order to get the upper hand. It would be helpful if partners tried to listen and understand each other's feelings and needs.

In sum, the building of intimacy requires the lowering of defenses and the dropping of masks by each partner, together with the willingness to share beliefs, hopes, feelings, values, achievements, and disappointments.

Establishing Ground Rules. Ground rules, or the structuring of relationships, usually apply to three areas: (1) goals—what the couple want from the relationship, (2) roles and responsibilities—the behavior each partner will enact in order to achieve the goals, and (3) norms—acceptable and expected patterns of behavior considered right or appropriate for their situation. People try to meet various personal needs—for love and affection, self-esteem and worth, emotional support and security, the sharing of common interests and activities. It is important that the relationship goals meet both partners' needs, and that there is an agreement of common goals that are satisfying to each.

Once the goals are agreed upon, the question becomes what will each do to accomplish those goals? This refers to roles and responsibilities. The words and actions of the role are borrowed from the script—the set of directions the actors follow in order to convey the story. The script tells the partners how, when, and where to behave (Atwood, 1997). Each role has certain role expectations that carry with it certain individual interpretations but there are also social expectations that define the role. Problems can arise at any juncture. If the goals are not specified, individuals can have discrepant definitions of what the common goals are. This could also cause one person's goals not to be met. If the roles are not spelled out, conflict can arise. One person may see the role in one way; the other in another way. Or there may be role overload and/or role conflicts. This is easily demonstrated by the "super mom," a mom who feels responsible for 'every' thing in the relationship.

It is helpful for individuals to establish ground rules. In order to maximize their effectiveness, such rules are more likely to be effective when (1) the couple has similar backgrounds, goals, beliefs, and values; (2) the rules have been discussed, understood, and agreed upon by both partners; (3) the rules are realistic and comfortable for both; and (4) the rules are periodically reviewed and updated.

Establishing Boundaries

Boundaries describe the limits individuals keep in regard to how much they will bend for other people. For example, Vera, a massage therapist, finds herself continually asked by her friends for small, free massages. She clarifies what she is willing to do and what she is not willing to do (draws a boundary) when she says, "As a friend, I can rub your shoulders for a minute or two, but if you want a full professional massage, I'd be happy to discuss my fees with you." This lets her friends know that she cares about them, but that she does not offer her services for free. (Someone with looser boundaries may find herself giving free massages, and then resenting it.)

The term *boundary* is also used to clarify differences among people; in fact, some people's definition of " 'boundary' is 'the place where you end and I begin.' " An example of this type of boundary is when we respect others' views of the world and opinions without necessarily taking them on as our own.

Boundaries vs. Barriers

Some people confuse boundaries with barriers between people, but the two are actually quite different in a few ways:

- Barriers promote extreme separateness and lack of communication and intimacy. Barriers are built to protect ourselves by keeping others out. For example, Alison battled her mother's controlling tendencies all her life. As an adult, she found no other way to handle her overbearing mother than to move far away and see her mother very little, thus creating a barrier between the two.

- Boundaries promote distinction, but they also can foster closeness between people. Boundaries allow individuals to remain close to others and still be separate; they allow people to be themselves. If Alison created boundaries with her mother by gently but firmly establishing that she would not change who she is to please her mother, there's a great chance that she could see more of her mother and the two could have a better relationship, with both being comfortable in who they are.

- A lack of boundaries often leads to the addition of barriers. The barriers come in the form of withdrawing from the relationship physically (as in the above example), or emotionally (as in not sharing one's thoughts and feelings, feeling victimized, not feeling comfortable and close, the addition of passive-aggressive behaviors, or a host of other relationship difficulties).

Resolving Conflicts

It is inevitable that conflicts and disagreements will occur in any given relationship. It is not a problem that these disagreements occur, but it is important how the individuals resolve the disagreements. Conflict can arise from many issues and at many different levels. Some of the more common conflicts are: money, sex, power struggles, decision-making, gender roles (traditional vs. egalitarian), jealousy and possessiveness, and unmet needs and expectations. Conflicts tend to have negative effects on relationships unless the frequency and intensity of the conflicts are low, there is background of positive interaction between the partners, and the couple is skilled in conflict-coping capabilities.

Conflict can be constructive in a relationship if it assists the couple in developing conflict-resolving skills. It can also help the individuals better understand each other so that they can avoid future conflicts.

Helping Relationships Grow

Acceptance is crucial in a relationship. It means that neither person takes a judgmental attitude toward the other. It does not mean that there is total agreement; rather it means that each frame of reference is respected and that if disagreements arise, there is not rejection of the person. Acceptance allows the person to feel free to share his or her feelings and beliefs with their partner.

Caring is also a healthy relationship ingredient. It may be expressed in words or actions. It could be behavioral or emotional in terms of support. Caring involves respecting the rights and ideas of the other person. It also means maintaining a balance between separateness and togetherness—building mutuality togetherness while giving each other the freedom to grow as persons.

Friendship is vitally important in healthy relationships. Friendship is being concerned about meeting one's partner's needs as well as one's own. When there is trust between partners, each can then be sincerely concerned about and attentive to his or her own needs, and freer to relax and be concerned about meeting his or her partner's needs. In this way a positive loop is established in the relationship.

Commitment

Commitment refers to the avowed intent of each partner to maintain the relationship. It serves as a stabilizing influence in the relationship and tends to restrain the types of behaviors the partners engage in. Commitment can be measured by duration, intensity, and priority. *Duration* refers to how long a person is willing to give unre-

served love and support to another. However, time span may have little to do with the quality of a relationship. Many marriages or relationships endure but the quality of the relationship is poor and the satisfaction of the individuals is low. *Intensity* refers to the strength of feeling and depth of concern for one's partner. *Priority* is the extent to which concern takes precedence over other matters, such as work, hobbies, family, and other relationships. *Commitment* can be measured by the value placed on the relationship and the willingness to take the responsibility for maintaining it.

Problems arise when the partners in a relationship are not equally committed. This is commonly known as the "principal of least interest." The person with the least interest in the relationship is more likely to exploit the other. The person with the least commitment may dictate and manipulate the development of the relationship since she/he will not be as badly hurt if the relationship ends. It is important to point out that relationships do not simply need an equal level of commitment in order to endure in a satisfying manner over a long period of time. It is rather that relationships require a high degree of commitment from each partner. Otherwise neither partner is likely to devote the time and effort needed to maintain the relationship.

A Realistic View of Oneself

Understanding oneself is key to participating in a healthy relationship. In order for a relationship of any kind to survive, individuals must have a realistic view of themselves. They should understand their assets, their liabilities, their motives and goals, beliefs and values, their aspirations for personal growth and achievement. Thus, t is helpful to examine one's self-identity. It is also important to explore one's life plans, the skills one needs to achieve the goals she/he has set. It would be also helpful for the couple to explore values they consider important. How would they define a fulfilled and meaningful life?

A Realistic View of One's Partner

Being realistic about one's partner means that one has an accurate picture of their partner, their assets, and their liabilities. Here it is also important to explore your partner's values and beliefs, their picture of a fulfilled and meaningful life.

A Realistic View of the Relationship

Partners should develop an accurate view of the relationship. What do they each want in the relationship? For themselves? For their partners? Do both agree on what they want out of the relationship? Do both have similar and realistic views about their goals, roles and responsibilities, ways of communicating, resolving conflict, levels of satisfaction, and degree of commitment?

Intentional Rituals

At a Smart Marriage conference (*http:www.smart-marriages.com*), Doherty (2000) proposed that healthy relationships are where the two individuals are conscious, deliberate, and planning about building and maintaining a sense of connection over the years. He compares this to people who are on autopilot, individuals who allow their lives to control them instead of them controlling their lives. He suggests that couples incorporate rituals into their relationship. Rituals are repeated, consistent, significant interactions that have positive meaning for the two individuals. Rituals are what distinguish routine relationships from ones that have emotional meaning. He suggests three types of rituals that create intentionality in relationships: (1) intimacy rituals, (2) community rituals, and (3) talk rituals. *Intimacy rituals* refer to shared special times. *Community rituals* are where the two people give and receive community support such as joint involvement in their religious community, neighborhood activities, friendship activities, or volunteer activities. *Talk rituals* are when couples spend at least 15 minutes of uninterrupted, nonlogical, nonproblem-solving talk every

day. Gottman (1994) agrees when he discusses emotionally intelligent marriages where couples or individuals can learn to become emotionally intelligent. His findings are applicable to any committed, intimate relationship. Thus, the emphasis in this section is on skill building and creating intentional, conscious relationships. Crucially important also in building healthy relationships is effective communication.

Effective Communication

In order for healthy relationships to develop, it is essential that the partners learn to communicate effectively with each other. There are two types of **effective communication** that are important for purposes of this chapter: (1) cognitive communication which involves facts and information about the surrounding world, and (2) affective communication which is how two people feel about each other, their experiences, and the world around them.

Generally, verbalizations are used to communicate cognitive information. Nonverbal messages also communicate information. These are conveyed by facial expression, gestures, eye contact, voice inflection, pauses, odors, dress, touch, body movements, body postures, and other types of body language. Problems arise when verbal and nonverbal messages conflict. In healthy relationships there is a congruence between verbal and nonverbal messages. For example, if one individual asks the other to a football game and the other replies, "Yes, I'd love to go" but says so in a very dull uninterested voice, there is a discrepancy between the verbal and nonverbal message.

In order to foster good **communication skills** in couples, health educators or health counselors

Effective communication. Communication characterized by listening, receptivity, specificity, honesty, respect, and nonjudgment.

Communication skills. Methods of effective communication, practiced as sender and receiver, using verbalization and nonverbal messages.

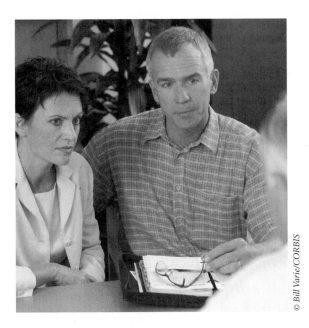

Healthy relationship skills are essential in maintaining loving, committed relationships.

can make certain helpful suggestions to their students or clients. They are:

For the Sender

- **Be specific:** Get to the point. Beating around the bush is frustrating for the other person and often the main point gets lost.

- **Express feelings and perceptions,** not facts. This keeps discussions from escalating because it is difficult for the other person to become annoyed if a person is describing how she/he feels.

- **Examine body language.** Body language should help to get messages across, not be detrimental to communication. Some examples are: speaking in a bored or monotone voice, avoiding eye contact, or yawning as compared with consistent eye contact, leaning toward the person, and so on.

- **Allow for the other person's perspective.** Each person has his or her own frame of reference and it is important for him or her to express

that perspective and be heard by the other person.

- **Use feedback.** Giving the other person feedback helps them to feel heard.

For the Receiver

- **Pay Attention.** Maintain eye contact and avoid external distractions.

- **Read body language.** Pay attention to the other person's body language.

- **Uncover hidden meanings.** There are times when words can obscure true feelings. For example, asking the question, "Do you love me?" may mean, "I'm feeling insecure right now." Make the covert, overt. If the message is to be interpreted correctly, then the hidden meaning must be made clear.

- **Ask for clarification.** If there is a statement or feeling made by a partner that is not understood, they should ask for clarification.

- **Maintain an accepting attitude.** Encourage the sender to communicate his or her thoughts openly, without fear of ridicule or rejection.

Analyze Meta-Communication

Meta-communication is the communication about the communication. It involves such factors as: (1) the amount of relevant communication given vs. extraneous, irrelevant communication; (2) the emotional climate created by talking about problems; (3) whether one person does most of the talking and one does most of the listening; (4) whether certain topics or problems create difficulties in understanding and reaching agreements; and (5) whether the communications are generally rewarding or aversive.

Effective and positive communications are important to relationships at every stage. Even in intimate relationships that have endured for some time, communication patterns can deteriorate. One indication of a failing relationship is the inability of the partners to talk about their problems. At the extreme end of the continuum is when two people exist in total silence—each has given up trying to get through to the other.

Common Communication Pitfalls

- Bringing up the past.

- Talking too much about one subject.

- Instead of listening, thinking about what to say next.

- Focusing excessively on problems.

- Being critical about something that cannot be undone.

- Losing one's temper or becoming too emotional.

- Sending discrepant or conflicting messages.

- Choosing the wrong time to discuss a toxic issue.

- Not considering the other person's frame of reference.

- Disqualifying or distorting the other person's message.

- Not being honest with the other person.

- Mindreading—telling your partner what she/he is thinking, feeling, or meaning.

- Not paying attention to your partner's feedback.

- Being insensitive to the feelings behind the words.

- Being irritable, impatient, or hostile to your partner.

- Exaggerating or overestimating your partner's statement so that they fit in with your frame of reference rather than hearing them for what they were intended.

Gottman & Silver (1999) researches communication patterns in couples. First he asks the couple to discuss a problem. He believes that in 5 minutes he is able to predict if they will divorce and he reports that he does this with 82 percent accuracy.

He has summarized the indicators. They are outlined as follows:

1. **Harsh Setup:** The most obvious indicator that the discussion and the relationship are not going well is when it begins negative and accusatory—with criticism and/or sarcasm, a form of contempt.

2. **The Four Horsemen:** One or more of the Four Horsemen is present. They are: criticism, contempt, defensiveness, and stonewalling.

   Criticism: This is different from a simple complaint. A complaint focuses on a specific behavior but a criticism throws in blame and general character assassination.

   Contempt: Sarcasm and cynicism are types of contempt as well as name-calling, eye rolling, sneering, mockery, and hostile humor. This form of communication conveys disgust to the other person and leads to more conflict. This is fueled by long-simmering negative thoughts about the partner.

   Defensiveness: The reaction to the criticism and contempt is being defensive. This is actually a form of blaming your partner and escalates the argument.

   Stonewalling: This is when a partner (it is usually the male) avoids a conflict, and the relationship altogether, rather than confronting his wife. He tends to look away or down without uttering a sound. He sits like an impassive stone wall and acts as though he does not care what his partner is saying.

3. **Flooding:** Flooding means that a partner's negativity is so overwhelming, and so sudden, it leaves the other partner shell-shocked. Gottman (1994) predicts a relationship/marriage will end in divorce when habitual harsh startups and frequent flooding occur, brought on by the relentless presence of the Four Horsemen during conflicts.

Gottman (1994) has also monitored couple physiological readings and describes the physical reactions during flooding to be increased heart rate, sweating, and so on. When this occurs, an individual's abilities to process information are reduced, meaning it is harder to pay attention to what others are saying. In these situations, creative problem solving does not stand a chance.

4. **Failed Repair Attempts:** Gottman (1994) places great importance on failed repair attempts. They refer to efforts couples make to de-escalate the tension during touchy discussions so they do not get out of hand. In this manner flooding is prevented. He believes that whether they succeed or fail is a crucial part of the pattern.

5. **Bad Memories:** Couples who are deeply entrenched in a negative view of their partner and relationship (memories of their commitment/wedding day, first date, old favorite hangouts, and so on) often rewrite their relationship/marriage, for the worse. Gottman presents factors that contribute to making a marriage or relationship work. They are listed below.

Gottman's Seven Principles for Making Marriage Work (1999)

Principle 1: Enhance Love Maps

Love maps are where individuals store all of the relevant information about their partners. Emotionally intelligent couples are intimately familiar with each other's worlds—they are best friends. They have made plenty of cognitive room for each other in their relationship/marriage. They remember the major events in each other's history, and they keep updating each other as their world changes. (When she orders his salad, she knows he likes the dressing on the side. When she works late, he tapes her favorite show). Gottman claims that without a love map, one cannot really know his or her partner and if one does not really know someone, how can one love him or her?

Principle 2: Nurture Your Fondness and Admiration

Emotionally Intelligent Couples do not just know each other; they build on and enhance this knowl-

edge in many important ways. They use their "love maps" to express not only their understanding of each other, but their fondness and admiration as well. Fondness and admiration are two of the most crucial elements in a rewarding and long-lasting romance. Even though they may be annoyed at times by their partner's personality flaws, they still feel that the person they married or are in a relationship with is worthy of honor and respect. Gottman says that when this sense is completely missing from a relationship, it cannot be revived.

Principle 3: Turn Toward Each Other Instead of Away

Gottman states that romance is kept alive each time one of the partners values the other during the course of the day. He believes that this stabilizes the relationship and its ongoing sense of romance. Partners who do this put money in the bank.

They build up emotional savings that can serve as a cushion when times get tough, that is, when they are faced with a major life stress or conflict. When conflict arises they will better be able to make allowances for each other and maintain a positive sense of each other and their relationship/marriage.

Principle 4: Let Your Partner Influence You

According to Gottman the happiest, most stable relationships/marriages in the long run are when husbands treat their wives with respect and do not resist power sharing and decision making with them. When they do disagree, these husbands actively search for common ground rather than insist on getting their way. This open attitude heightens the positive in the relationship and serves to strengthen the couple's friendship.

Principle 5: Solve Your Solvable Problems

Gottman suggests that couples should attempt to put themselves in their partner's shoes while listening intently to what they are saying. They then should communicate empathetically that they see the dilemma from the other's perspective. Couples can do this by (1) softening their startup,

(2) learning to make and receive repair attempts, (3) soothing themselves, (4) compromising, and (5) being tolerant of each other's faults.

Principle 6: Overcome Gridlock

The goal here is not necessarily to solve the problem, but rather to move from gridlock to dialogue. The goal is for the couple to be able to talk about the problem without hurting each other. Each relationship has differences that will remain unresolved, but it is the degree and quality of dialogue around these differences that makes the difference as to the satisfaction in the relationship. A gridlock is usually caused by a problem in the relationship that the person believes is not being addressed or respected by his or her partner.

Principle 7: Create Shared Meaning

A committed relationship is not just about the tasks of creating a home, raising kids, splitting chores, and so on. It is also about creating an inner life together—a culture rich with symbols and rituals, and an appreciation for the roles and goals that create linkages, leading to an understanding of what it means to be part of the family.

Successful couples are those who know how to discuss their differences in ways that actually strengthen and improve the intimacy in their relationship rather than break it apart. If a couple does not know how to successfully handle their arguments, they will not learn how to deal with other things that come up in the course of the relationship. Sollee (1996) believes that every happy and successful couple has about ten areas of disagreement that they will never resolve. These couples learn to "dance" in spite of the differences with behaviors and skills necessary to successfully resolve conflicts. Other theorists such as Robinson (1997) also have contributed to the thinking in this area.

Robinson's Three-Step Approach

Robinson (1997) promises to help couples in three sessions or less, to improve their relationships by changing the way they communicate. He explains his three-step approach consisting of (1) creating intimacy, (2) avoiding fights, and (3) solving problems without bruising egos. He claims that he has found the right theory about what makes "humans tick" and says his technique can apply not just to create more intimacy in already successful couples, but even in the most conflicted of relationships.

He believes that the key to getting partners to listen to each other is to give them plenty of the three As; Acknowledgment, Appreciation, Acceptance. When a discussion begins to get a little heated, the first thing individuals should do is to *acknowledge* their partners' experience by validating it and conveying understanding. This creates trust and a willingness to listen and understand their point of view. *Appreciation* is the art of telling one's partner what you like about him/her. Through this expression, the partner is assisted with letting go blaming or becoming defensive. *Acceptance* consists of loving one's partner unconditionally, "warts and all." This is not simply a behavior, it is a perception change. When individuals feel accepted, they do their best to make their partners happy and this, he believes, contributes to true intimacy.

Creating Intimacy

Robinson goes on to say that intimate couples push each other's "love buttons." Just as we are all familiar with someone "pushing our buttons"— referring to the negative ones, we can probably list them in 10 seconds—it is helpful if couples push each others "love buttons" by doing something for the other that is simply loving. Successful couples do this naturally but any couple can begin this process. Successful couples create love without words. They learn how to charm each other's hearts without uttering a single word. They do this by nonverbally communicating their appreciation. Four methods Robinson describes are (1) mirroring, where the couple mimics each other's body position as a form of connection; (2) touching, where each partner touches each other in caring, nonsexual ways; (3) simply smiling; and (4) "electric sex," where the couple simply sits facing each other and breathes rhythmically together for at least 5 minutes. Robinson (1997) believes that each of these techniques foster and contribute to a healthy relationship.

Avoiding Fights

Avoiding fights is the second technique Robinson emphasizes. To do this, he believes couples must give up their insistence to be right. Successful couples communicate without blame. Robinson stresses not arguing by using a technique called spooning where the couple lies next to each other, one holding the other from behind, and breathing rhythmically together. Robinson claims that when couples share this form of energy, the need for arguing subsides. Once the need for argument leaves, the individuals are able to communicate their needs by using feelings and expressing their vulnerabilities. The partner's "blame detector" will not be triggered and a fight will have been successfully avoided.

Solving Problems without Bruising Egos

The third step Robinson uses is solving problems without bruising egos. Successful couples speak to each other in ways that enable them to understand each other. Nonsuccessful couples claim that the other is not listening to them. Robinson uses metaphors to describe the communication and to teach couples how to speak to each other. He stresses that all of these considerations should be taken into account when asking your partner for a behavior change. The request needs to follow acknowledgement, appreciation, and acceptance, and have correct timing. Vulnerabilities and feelings need to be shared for the other partner to understand why the behavior change is warranted and for them to follow through with the request.

Once all of these steps are accomplished, a few other things are needed to keep love alive. Robinson instructs couples to do special things for each other each week, communicate in a loving and effective manner, and do a weekly housecleaning. This means to sit down once a week and review what happened throughout the week. Any resentment, feelings of anger or frustration, and so on need to be aired and cleaned out so the buildup of emotions most couples face will not occur.

Thus far, we have explored the psychological conditions necessary for the formation of healthy relationships; we have explored the developmental tasks necessary for healthy relationships; we have presented a discussion on the skills necessary for maintaining a healthy relationship, along with a discussion of research findings regarding the factors contributing to healthy relationships. The next section presents what a healthy relationship "looks like." Often in counseling situations, clients want a description of what the desired behavior "looks like." They appear to be looking for a template of how to behave. Although there is no one template that can be presented, there are certain characteristics common to healthy relationships. They are listed below.

What Is a Healthy Relationship?

Partners in healthy relationships share these characteristics:

- The individuals feel comfortable with themselves and their lives.

- Relationships/friendships come naturally into their lives.

- They are open to allow their relationship to unfold before making judgments about the type of persons that would be appropriate for them.

- They allow relationships to grow at their own speed. As the old saying goes, "They would rather have them smolder like embers than flame high and burn out quickly."

- They feel that they and their partner have different strengths and weaknesses in different areas. Ideally, they compliment each other.

- The relationship feels safe, gentle, and comfortable. The individuals do not hurl angry statements. There are no intense dramas in the relationship.

- It gets easier to be together and share their lives the more they get to know each other. They find out new things about each other as they both grow and mature.

- Partners want each other to realize their individual dreams and will help them to achieve them.

- Each individual is a self-sufficient and complete human being.

- Each person takes responsibility for his or her own happiness. It is not the partner's job to make him or her happy.

- They do not use negative tactics for getting their own way or dominating. Criticism, put-downs, guilt, shame, intolerance, neglect, combativeness, aggression, silence, and threats are not common.

- When they speak to each other, it is mainly with love, acceptance, and approval.

- They respect and support each other's ideas, beliefs, and wishes, no matter how different from their own.

- Their self-esteem improves when they are together.

- Their circle of friends grows.

- They do little things to please each other.

- When something bothers one or the other, the partner is truly concerned.

- They help each other to resolve problems.

- They assist each other to find time for their own individual interests.

- They share in responsibilities, even with things that are unpleasant or mundane.

- They feel that their time is equally valuable.

- They encourage each other to freely try new things, take chances, and to make mistakes (within the relationship contract).

- They develop a common spirituality that provides them peace and enables them to evolve into consciously aware human beings.

In short, they provide the security, love and nurturing for each other that enables them to evolve into consciously aware, cosmically or higher-power-connected, socially productive, community-involved human beings.

Summary

The divorce rate in this country is approaching 60 percent. There is a wealth of research on why people divorce, factors that predict divorce, emotional responses to divorce, and so on. Until recently there has been very little research on healthy relationships. It is startling to learn that in this country, people rate a happy relationship/marriage as most important to them. We are trained from childhood that an intimate, committed relationship and/or marriage is a desirable adult state to which we should all aspire. Yet, we have no school-based educational programs to teach us the skills necessary to be in a successful relationship. There are no courses that assist us with conflict resolution or negotiation and compromise. Even at the college and university level, there are no practically based courses focused on relationship skill enhancement. We are basically told that a partnership/marriage will be the most important relationship we will be in, that it is one we will spend the great majority of our lives in, but we are not given any idea as to how to accomplish it successfully!

Although some religious institutions do provide marriage preparation courses or offer premarital counseling workshops, and have adjusted lately to be more skill-based and contain practical information, in general, our society is still a very long way from providing our children with the skills necessary to embark on the most important relationship of their lives. Health educators, health counselors, and marriage and family therapists are in a perfect position to institute some of these courses in the schools. This chapter is a first step in initiating such a program. Its purpose is to provide health educators and counselors with a foundation of the factors involved in healthy relationships.

Key Terms

communication skills, 130
developmental tasks, 119
effective
   communication, 130

healthy
   relationships, 117
traps and pitfalls of
   relationships, 122

Questions for Discussion

1. What makes a healthy relationship? Are there any aspects that weren't mentioned in the chapter that are personally important to you?

2. Describe some communication pitfalls in relationships and specific strategies to promote good communication.

3. What suggestions could you give to a client to enhance his or her communication as a sender? As a receiver?

4. Describe the importance of the following in a relationship: a) boundaries, b) commitment, and c) ground rules.

5. How does realism factor into a healthy relationship? What must a person be realistic about? Why?

Related Web Sites

http://www.smartmarriages.com
Coalition for Marriage, Family and Couples Education, L.L.C. Offers discussion of topics ranging from the future of marriage, marriage rituals, marital therapy, and so on. Includes a directory of programs and resources, legislation, and marriage reports.

http://www.aamft.org
American Association for Marriage and Family Therapy. Offers information to the public on locating a family therapist, books and articles, information on family problems, FAQs. Also offers resources for family therapists and mental health practitioners, including legislation and policy and legal/ethical information.

http://www.relationship-talk.com
Offers relationship advice, how-to guides, forums, personal stories, relationship counseling info, recommended reading, and relationship links.

http://helping.apa.org/family/
American Psychological Association Help Center. Provides articles on family relationships, mind/body connection, therapy, psychology in daily life, and more.

http://www.isspr.org
International Society for the Study of Personal Relationship. Dedicated to all aspects of personal relationship, including discussion, conferences, publications, links to professional organizations, journals, social science resources, and relationships in the popular media.

Counseling in Human Sexuality

EVA S. GOLDFARB, PH.D.

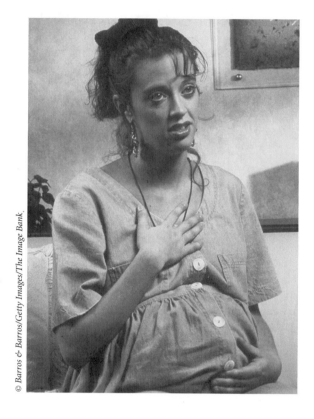

© Barros & Barros/Getty Images/The Image Bank.

OBJECTIVES

By the end of the chapter, the reader should be able to:

- Differentiate between sexuality education and sexuality counseling

- Know the characteristics of an effective sexuality counselor

- Know the three main root causes for someone to seek sexuality counseling

- Understand the components of the PLISSIT model for sexual counseling

- Understand the major counseling issues related to sexual orientation

- Understand the major counseling issues related to unintended pregnancy and prevention

- Understand the major counseling issues related to sexually transmitted infections

- Understand the major counseling issues related to sexual dysfunctions

- Understand the major counseling issues related to sexual assault/abuse

Sexuality Educator as Counselor

One of the most essential skills a sexuality educator must have is the ability to recognize his/her role and professional boundaries. The health educator's job is largely that of primary prevention, helping people to make appropriate decisions about their health-related behaviors and to avoid problems while achieving for themselves maximum health. A counselor, by contrast, could be considered to be secondary prevention, helping people to deal with problems that have already arisen. The line between the two, of course, is not always so obvious. Often, education itself can help people to resolve problems, conflicts, or questions they have about a topic while counseling can often be quite successful through giving information. In the area of sexuality education, this line can become particularly blurred. It is important for the educator who does not have professional training as a counselor to respect the limitations of her/his professional expertise.

Having said that, of course, in reality it is not an easy thing to do. When someone has a problem and needs help or advice, often she or he will seek out a trusted person, someone in whom they feel they can confide. When it comes to the topic of sexuality, this becomes a particularly delicate task given the likelihood that the problem will be of a personal nature. Many people may be either too embarrassed or too afraid to seek out a professional counselor. If, however, they know a sexuality educator who is comfortable discussing sensitive issues, who establishes ground rules with all clients and students that include confidentiality and respect for individuals and diversity, and is approachable, the person with a particular problem or concern may very well seek out that educator. Although trusting educators can come from any discipline, sexuality education, due to the inherently personal nature of the topic, is more likely to raise issues for students and thus, the sexuality educator can expect to find her/himself in the role of counselor with relative frequency. Knowing how to handle that role effectively and professionally will be critical.

Characteristics of a Successful Sexuality Counselor

It is extremely important that anyone offering counseling in the area of sexuality is comfortable and not embarrassed talking with someone about sexual issues. Discomfort on the part of the counselor will limit any discussion a person may have on sexuality-related concerns. Comfort discussing sexuality does not come naturally or easily to most people. Knowledge of the topic and practice talking about it with others is the best way to gain comfort and confidence. Being aware of one's own particular biases, beliefs, and values and how these might affect the counseling one provides is always

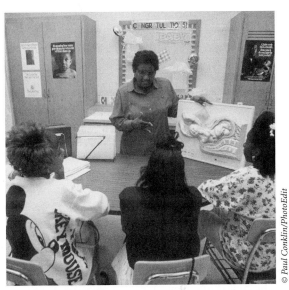

© *Paul Conklin/PhotoEdit*

A sexuality educator/counselor must be comfortable discussing a range of highly personal subjects with honesty and openness which inspires the same in the client.

a central concern. With every question or problem that comes before the counselor, he/she should ask him/herself, "In what ways will my own values, prejudices, or discomfort with the issue affect my ability to provide good counseling to this person?"

Someone who provides counseling should be able to recognize a sexual concern or problem presented by the person seeking counseling, and allow him/her to express this concern in his or her own way. The counselor must also be able to discuss the person's sexual concern in an appropriate manner, giving both the counselor and the client permission to be a sexual human being.

The characteristics of a professional who is comfortable providing education/counseling in sexuality include:

- An awareness of and comfort with her or his own sexual attitudes and values, and a sensitivity to the fact that they may differ from those of the person seeking counseling.

- Knowledge of the range of sexual behaviors, questions, and concerns about which a person is likely to seek counseling.

- The skill to recognize sexual concerns and the ability to handle them appropriately, including referral to a trained professional where necessary. (Weerakoon, 2001)

Within the field of sexuality, there are certain problems, conditions, and concerns that really require the expertise of a professional counselor or therapist. Often, however, some information, understanding, and permission giving are all that are needed. A good educator or other health professional can often fulfill that role.

Three Root Causes for Sexuality Counseling

The first thing, then, that an educator/health professional must do is to determine if he or she is the appropriate person to provide counseling. To do this, she or he must know the reason counseling is being sought. In the realm of sexuality, there are really only a few possibilities. Having this information can help the educator/counselor determine the appropriate course of action. Regardless of the actual issue at hand, the three root causes—the question behind the question—for someone seeking sexuality counseling are (1) information-seeking, (2) the question "Am I normal?," (3) the need to deal with a problem.

Information-Seeking

At the root of many questions or concerns people have related to sexuality is the need for information. "I'm afraid I may have been infected with HIV last night," can be a statement from someone needing to know how a person can contract the virus, and what she or he should do about it. In this instance, providing information about how HIV is and is not transmitted can help the person to assess his/her risk of infection. Further information about testing options, safer sex, and communication with sexual partners may be exactly what the person needs. Providing information is a central component to sexuality counseling and in most cases, a good knowledgeable educator is perfect for that role. Of course, no matter how knowl-

edgeable one is, no one is an expert on every topic. Knowing one's limitations again is key. If the educator does not know the answer, he/she can promise to help find the answer, or refer the person to someone with the appropriate information.

Am I Normal?

This type of question is especially typical of adolescents and young adults. However, people young and old ask themselves this question about an array of topics throughout their lives. "What if one breast is bigger (fatter, longer) than the other?" "One of my testicles hangs lower than the other." "Sometimes I get so angry at my girlfriend that I want to hit her." "I think about sex all day and all night." "I masturbate every day, is this okay?" All of these questions or concerns may have at their core the question "Am I normal or is something wrong with me?" One reason this kind of concern is so common is that we have very little accurate information about what *most people* are like, what they do or think when it comes to sexuality. The media tends to portray a very skewed picture of sexual behavior and relationships. While friends talk about sex, the information exchanged is rarely open, direct, or accurate, leaving false impressions and many questions about what is and is not acceptable. In this situation, accurate information, along with assurance and support, may be sufficient to ease a person's concerns.

It is extremely important for the educator/counselor to remember to keep their own values and biases in check when providing counseling to someone. Daily masturbation may seem excessive (or too infrequent) to the counselor, but that does not mean it is, or that it is abnormal. There are some good studies that have been conducted on people's sexual behavior that can provide the counselor with a better understanding of what is truly in the norm from a statistical standpoint (e.g. Lauman et al., 1994). Of course, being outside of the norm does not mean someone is not normal. While *most* people may not watch pornography on a regular basis, for example, that does not mean that a person who does is strange or bizarre in some way. For the person concerned about how often she or he masturbates, as long as masturbation does not become such a preoccupation that it interferes with the person's ability to get on with her or his day to day life, then it really is not a problem.

If someone asks a question or offers information that leads the educator to suspect that there may indeed be a serious problem (the person who is concerned about hitting his/her girlfriend, for example), appropriate referrals need to be made to a trained counselor, medical professional, or therapist. It is important to offer understanding and support to the person for having sought help. But the educator must make it clear that providing the person with the help he or she needs requires skills and training that are beyond the counseling scope of the educator.

Dealing with a Crisis

A traumatic event, either recent, in the past, or on-going, can (and hopefully will) cause a person to reach out for help. In most crisis situations, the primary role of an educator is to offer support, empathy, and understanding, and most of all to help the person receive services from an appropriately trained therapist, counselor, medical professional, or other service provider. Knowing who to contact and how to help a person to make and keep an appointment, as well as following up with the person, are knowledge and skills that are necessary to get that individual the help he or she needs. It is critically important in these cases for the educator to know her/his limits.

Finally, while confidentiality is always a golden rule in providing any kind of counseling, it is important for the person providing the counseling to know the instances in which the law requires that confidentiality must be broken. It is also important, if the counselor suspects that reportable information is forthcoming, that he/she warn the person that certain information must be reported. In most states, this includes information that would lead the professional to suspect that a person is about to cause harm to him or herself or to someone else. In some cases, crimes or assaults that have already been committed, if perpetrated against a minor, are also required to be reported.

Healthy Sexuality

Sexuality education should focus on promoting healthy sexuality rather than only on disease and problem prevention. Just as health is much more than merely the absence of disease, sexual health is much more than the absence of sexual problems or disease. The World Health Organization (WHO) has defined sexual health as "the integration of the somatic, emotional, intellectual, and social aspects of sexual being, in ways that are positively enriching and that enhance personality, communication, and love," and has added that "Fundamental to this concept are the right to sexual information and the right to pleasure." (World Health Organization, 1975, section 4.1) For most people, maintaining sexual health includes successfully resolving occasional or ongoing problems or concerns that arise throughout the person's lifespan. Many of these concerns are not really problems themselves, but are cause for concern or alarm for the person. Helping people to deal with those concerns and to integrate the information into their lives in a way that will help them to feel good about themselves, their bodies, their relationships, their interactions, and their futures, is an important goal of sexuality education. Much of this can be accomplished through education. Sometimes, however, additional one-on-one educational counseling is required.

PLISSIT—A Model for Sexual Counseling

The **PLISSIT** model for sexual counseling (**P**ermission, **L**imited **I**nformation, **S**pecific **S**uggestions, **I**ntensive **T**herapy), developed by Annon (1976; Green, 1994) is an effective tool for counselors to determine the level of information that is needed for a particular situation as well as to evaluate their own comfort level regarding sexuality

PLISSIT. A model for sexual counseling, meaning Permission, Limited Information, Specific Suggestions and Intensive Therapy.

counseling. It may also be a useful tool in identifying areas where an educator/counselor might need further training or information. The model involves four levels of counseling that are increasingly involved and require higher levels of comfort and counseling skills. The discussion here will focus on the first three levels as they might pertain to the sexuality counselor. The last level usually requires the skills of a trained therapist. The model is as follows:

Permission. A person who seeks out counseling will look for "permission" to feel the way they are feeling about a problem. It is up to the counselor to grant that permission. The person may start out with a comment or question that is very innocent or subtle. By doing that, he or she is often looking to the counselor for acceptance and permission that it is okay to talk about sexuality issues or concerns. Because a sexuality educator is not a trained counselor, the person may be testing to see if it is safe to talk with him/her about a sexual concern. It is important for the educator/counselor to let the person know that it is perfectly fine to think about, explore, and talk about how they are feeling. The first level for dealing with sexual difficulties often is being given permission to engage or not to engage in certain sexual expressions. It is important for people to hear that their thoughts, feelings, desires, fantasies, and behaviors are natural and acceptable as long as they do not bring harm to themselves or others. It may also be important for them to hear that they are not the only ones with those thoughts, feelings, or experiences. (Koch, 1995, p. 308) Good listening is a critical skill at this point. When a counselor listens to someone discuss their sexual concerns, that counselor gives the message that she or he cares and that the counselor sees the person as a sexual being. It is important for the person to have her or his feelings validated and to be reassured that his or her concerns are normal (Rodecker & Bullard, 1981). Sometimes, helping people to give themselves permission to be sexual may be enough to overcome some sexual concerns or difficulties.

Limited Information. This level of counseling requires the counselor to provide the basic informa-

tion a person has requested. People need to have their questions answered. Sometimes this simply means giving an answer to a question someone asks. Other times, it may mean anticipating a question that seems likely, and answering it. People have received much misinformation about sexuality. Often, just becoming more knowledgeable about a topic can help to solve a problem or overcome a sexual difficulty. Becoming more sexually educated about topics such as those discussed in this chapter can help people to re-examine their beliefs, attitudes, and behaviors and potentially decrease the problem they are experiencing. This is also a time to listen to the person's concerns and to reaffirm how they are feeling or help him or her to further explore those feelings. It is important to remember that the responses the counselor gives must not minimize the person's feelings ("Oh it's silly to be worried about that"), nor be what the counselor thinks the person wants to hear. Honest answers with a caring, empathetic approach are needed.

Specific Suggestions. There are specific techniques and strategies people can employ to help them diminish problems or concerns they are experiencing. Depending on the situation, some suggestions might include: increasing self-awareness, working on improving the quality of their overall relationship; learning and using effective communication skills; leaving a relationship; masturbating; practicing sensate focus and a variety of other sex therapy techniques; getting a medical examination; joining a support group or activist organization, and so on. This level of counseling is often better left to a trained sexuality therapist or counselor. Some specific suggestions for action, however, can appropriately be made by an educator/counselor depending on the issue and the level of comfort and expertise of the counselor.

Intensive Therapy. Although the vast majority of people experiencing a sexuality-related concern or problem can be helped through receiving permission, limited information, and specific suggestions (Annon, 1976), some people will require intensive therapy or other intervention by a trained professional to overcome their difficulty. It is important for an educator/counselor to recognize when a problem is beyond the scope of their abilities and be able to refer a person to an appropriate source for help.

When presented with a person seeking sexuality counseling, the educator should ask him/herself, What is being required of me? What level of counseling intervention is needed according to the PLISSIT model? What are my knowledge, skills, and comfort levels relative to this issue? Am I the best person to handle this? When these questions are answered honestly and satisfactorily, the educator/counselor can take appropriate action to provide the best possible counseling for an individual.

We are all sexual beings with our own histories, beliefs, and experiences that affect how we see the world and how we react to various issues related to sexuality. Every counselor has biases and values that will influence the counseling process. Giving oneself permission to feel sad, angry, or uncomfortable is an important part of being an effective counselor. Even more important, though, is keeping those feelings and beliefs from interfering with providing appropriate guidance to someone else. The first step to accomplishing this is to recognize and acknowledge one's own biases. While they cannot be ignored or locked away, if they are dealt with openly and honestly they are less likely to threaten the integrity of the counseling process. Sometimes, however, a counselor may have feelings on a topic that are so strong that it is impossible to divorce him/herself from them sufficiently to providing nonjudgmental counseling on that issue. In those cases, it is important to recognize that he/she is not the appropriate person to provide counseling.

Case Study

A Difficult Decision

Amy teaches 10th-grade health. One day, after a unit on sexual decision making, one of her students, Debbie, comes to see her. Debbie tells Amy that she always thought that she would wait until she was much older before having sexual intercourse. Now, though, her boyfriend of 6 months, who she really loves, wants to have sex with her. While he said he is willing to wait, she thinks his patience will not last forever and she is afraid she is going to lose him. On top of that both of her closest friends have already had sex and her one friend, Claire, has told her that practically everyone in the 10th grade is already doing it. Frankly, Debbie confides, she is actually quite curious about it and doesn't want to be the only inexperienced one in her class.

Amy's personal belief is that 16 is far too young to be having sex and that, in fact, people should wait for marriage or at least engagement before having sexual intercourse. She stops for a moment and thinks about her beliefs and whether expressing this idea will help Debbie to make the right decision. As she thinks about what Debbie has said, Amy decides that Debbie may be asking whether she is "normal" for wanting to wait longer. She also considers the PLISSIT model and decides that both permission-giving and limited information would be most helpful in this case. So, Amy decides first to validate Debbie's concern and to acknowledge that she must really be under a lot of pressure. Then, Amy provides Debbie with important information and statistics about how many 16-year-olds are actually having sex, to show her that in fact, not everyone is sexually active. Amy explains to Debbie that it is quite normal not to be ready for sex. They also talk about peer pressure and the desire to fit in. And they discuss Debbie's fear that she might lose her boyfriend and what that would mean.

Finally, Amy decides that she must put her own bias aside in order to provide Debbie with important information she needs. She asks Debbie if she has thought about contraception and talks to her about the importance of being prepared and safe if and when she does decide to be sexually active. They talk about the various options that are available for pregnancy and STD protection, and then Amy gives Debbie some additional resources where she can get more information and services.

Debbie now is armed with a lot of information and food for thought. She thanks Amy for her help and says she feels better about not being ready for sex and feels relieved after having this conversation. She also thanks Amy for the information about contraception because she knows it will come in handy some day.

Issues for Sexual Counseling

The educator will greatly enhance his/her effectiveness as a counselor by being knowledgeable about those sexuality-related issues that most often cause people to seek guidance or advice. Following is information on some topics related to sexuality that are the basis of the most common problems or concerns for which people may seek some help or guidance. Having accurate information in these areas as well as knowledge of appropriate resources is essential for the educator who seeks to offer some counseling.

Sexual Orientation

What if I'm gay? How does someone become gay or lesbian? Can a person change his/her sexual orientation? How do I tell my friends/co-workers/family that I am gay? I am afraid that if people find out I am gay I will get harassed. Am I normal?

All of these are common questions associated with sexual orientation. Some issues surrounding sexual orientation may require professional counseling. Most people, however, can gain a lot from a combination of information, reassurance, trust, and support.

Sexual orientation is one of the four components of a person's sexual identity. It refers to the erotic or romantic attractions one has to individuals of a particular gender. The other components are *biological sex* which is our physiological makeup as either males or females; *gender identity,* which is our own perceptions or feelings of being a man or a woman, boy or girl; and *gender role,* a society's expected traits and behaviors of people based on their gender, that is, masculine and feminine traits and behaviors.

Sexual orientation. One of the four components of a person's sexual identity, which describes a person's attraction to and behavior with their own or opposite gender.

In American culture, typically three sexual orientations are recognized: heterosexuality, attraction to people of other genders; homosexuality, attraction to people of one's own gender; and bisexuality, attraction to people of both genders. People with homosexual orientations are sometimes referred to as gay (both men and women) or as lesbian (women only). In reality, a person's sexual orientation can be viewed as falling along a continuum with more than just three orientations. Alfred Kinsey first suggested that sexual orientation was more fluid by introducing a seven-point scale that has come to be known as the Kinsey scale (Kinsey, Pomeroy & Martin 1948, 1953). Based on interviews with more than 10,000 people, Kinsey identified seven sexual orientations ranging from "0" to "6" which represent "exclusively heterosexual" to "exclusively homosexual." If a person's behavior was exclusively with people of the other gender, she/he was categorized as a "Kinsey 0." A person whose sexual behavior was exclusively with people of his/her own gender was identified as a "Kinsey 6." Those people falling within categories 1 through 5 had various degrees and combinations of same and other gender sexual experiences, with a "Kinsey 3" being considered bisexual.

While Kinsey's work was ground breaking, in that it changed the way we look at sexual orientation from just three discreet categories to a continuum, later researchers and theorists expressed two major criticisms of his work. First, some believed that it didn't make sense to categorize people based solely on their behaviors. While behavior may seem like the obvious way to tell someone's sexual orientation, and, in fact is the way that our culture tends to categorize people, consider the person who has not yet become sexually active with other people. Should we assume that this person does not have a sexual orientation yet? Most people can remember having sexual and romantic attractions to other people long before they chose to engage in sexual behaviors with others. Just as heterosexual adults can remember being "straight" from the time they were young, homosexual adults can remember being gay or lesbian from the time they were young as well. One study of approximately 1,000 gay people found that gay men remembered having erotic same-gender feelings beginning around age 14 while lesbian women remembered such feelings beginning closer to age 16 (Bell, Weinberg, & Hammersmith, 1981)

Nonetheless, in adolescence, a period during which young people experience an increase in the production of the sex hormones estrogen and testosterone, sexual experimentation is common and questions about one's sexual identity and orientation commonly surface. A teenage boy who considers himself to be heterosexual may all of a sudden find himself experiencing an erection while looking at a picture of a man in an underwear ad. A 16-year-old girl may feel sexually aroused sleeping next to her female best friend at a slumber party, after years of having done so without that reaction. One of the first questions they may ask themselves is: Am I gay? The answer, of course, is that they may be gay or straight, but that one experience is not the determining factor. As they grow, most people begin to see a pattern of arousal that will indicate to them—if they are open to seeing it and accepting it—what their sexual orientation is. So while orientation is often established at a young age, a person may not recognize a personal identity as either straight or gay until adulthood. Sexual orientation develops across a person's lifetime—different people realize at different points in their lives that they are heterosexual, gay, lesbian, bisexual, or somewhere else along the continuum. In a large-scale study of junior and senior high school students in Minnesota, 88.2 percent described themselves as predominantly heterosexual, and 10.7 percent were unsure of their sexual orientation. Uncertainty about sexual orientation declined with age, from 25.9 percent among 12-year-olds to 5 percent of 17-year-old students. This suggests that, especially in younger teens, uncertainty about sexual orientation is a normal part of development. It also suggests that in most cases, those who are unsure ultimately end up identifying as heterosexual (Remafedi et al., 1992).

Consider another problem with identifying sexual orientation based only on behavior. What about the woman who has only had sexual experiences with men, in other words what would be categorized as strictly heterosexual experiences, but who is attracted almost exclusively to other women? What would be her sexual orientation? Based on a strict behavioral model, we would have to identify her as being heterosexual. Yet, if her attractions are really geared to women but either women are unavailable to her, or she is afraid to express her sexual attractions to women for fear of being ostracized by her family and friends, she might be more appropriately categorized as homosexual or lesbian. Others would argue that neither category fits exactly right. What about the man who has had penile-vaginal intercourse several times with different women but has experienced same-gender oral sex twice?

This brings us to the second major objection to work by Kinsey and others who have tried to categorize sexual orientation. Many critics object to the need to categorize or label people at all. Consider these objections for a moment. Why do we, as a culture, insist on labeling people based on sexual orientation? How is the information useful? What do we do with it? Also, consider to whom we tend to apply it. How often do we hear rumors that a famous celebrity, often a sex symbol, is *really gay?* In contrast, when was the last time there was a rumor floating around about someone *really being straight?* Because we assume that heterosexuality is the norm, anyone who is other than heterosexual is at risk for being considered different, or odd, which can lead to discrimination or worse.

What causes our sexual orientations? The research thus far has been inconclusive. In attempting to explain sexual orientation, however, researchers and theorists have typically focused on the question of why some people are homosexual or bisexual. There has been no consideration of the topic from the perspective of why some people might be heterosexual. Because heterosexuality is considered "normal" it has not seemed important to investigate its origins. One must ask the question, then, why do we want to know the origins of homosexuality? What would we do with the information that we find? These issues are important to consider when we look at characteristics that are associated with a person's developing sexual orientation.

Although research into the origins of sexual orientation has been plentiful, how a particular sexual orientation develops in any individual is not well understood by scientists. Various theories have proposed differing sources for sexual orientation, including genetic or inborn hormonal factors and life experiences during early childhood. Most scientists share the view, however, that sexual orientation is shaped for most people at an early age through complex interactions of biological, psychological, and social factors. What is pretty evident, however, is that once a person's sexual orientation is established it is not subject to change.

Sexual Orientation Issues and Counseling

Because heterosexuality is considered to be normal and natural by our culture, a heterosexual identity is not likely to be seen as problematic by an individual and not likely to be a reason for someone to seek counseling. The most common concerns or questions related to sexual orientation are How do I know if I'm gay? Or I think I might be gay, what can I do about it? Other concerns will come from people who know they are gay or lesbian and are dealing with questions about **coming out,** which is the process of acknowledging one's gay, lesbian, or bisexual attractions and identity to oneself and disclosing them to others. Such questions may include to whom a person should come out, or whether to come out in a particular setting or at all. The third main area in which one may seek out help or advice is related to the well-justified fear or concern about anti-gay discrimination or violence.

Coming out. The process of acknowledging one's gay, lesbian, or bisexual attractions and attractions and identity to oneself and disclosing them to others.

Homosexuality and Mental Health

Psychologists, psychiatrists, and other mental-health professionals agree that homosexuality is not an illness, mental disorder, or emotional problem. Much objective scientific research over the past 35 years shows us that homosexual orientation, in and of itself, is not associated with emotional or social problems. At one time, homosexuality was thought to be a mental illness largely because mental-health professionals, like the rest of society, had biased information about homosexuality since most studies on gay men and lesbians were conducted only with people in therapy. When researchers examined data about gay people who were *not* in therapy, the idea that homosexuality was a mental illness was found to be untrue (American Psychological Association, 2001).

Harassment and Violence toward Gay, Lesbian, and Bisexual Youth

Gay, lesbian, and bisexual adolescents, however, do experience more physical and mental-health problems due to prejudice, discrimination, and violent messages and behaviors directed at them by their families, schools, communities, and the culture at large. Gay, lesbian, and bisexual youth are more likely than heterosexual young people to miss school due to fear, to be threatened by other students, and to have their property damaged at school (Garofalo et al., 1998). Research on gay, lesbian, and bisexual youth have also found that they were more than four times as likely to report being threatened with a weapon on school property than heterosexual students (Garafolo et al., 1998), and that they are more likely to report physical abuse than heterosexual adolescents (Saewyc et al., 1999).

Coming Out

Why would a gay, lesbian, or bisexual (GLB) person be concerned about coming out? Because of false stereotypes and unwarranted prejudice toward them, the process of coming out for lesbians and gay men can be a very challenging process, which may cause emotional pain. Lesbian and gay people often feel different and alone when they first become aware of same-gender attractions. They may also fear being rejected by family, friends, coworkers, and religious institutions if they do come out.

In addition, gay, lesbian, and bisexual people are frequently the targets of discrimination and violence. This threat of violence and discrimination is an obstacle to lesbian and gay people's development. In a 1989 national survey, 5 percent of gay men and 10 percent of lesbians reported physical abuse or assault related to being lesbian or gay in the past year; 47 percent reported some form of discrimination over their lifetime. Other research has shown similarly high rates of discrimination and violence (American Psychological Association, 2001).

So, why do people come out? Coming out is a way for gay, lesbian, and bisexual people to live their lives openly and honestly. Gay, lesbian, and bisexual people come out because staying "in the closet" keeps the important people in their lives from knowing about a big part of their identity. Hiding one's sexual orientation can be very stressful, lonely, and isolating. While many GLB people are concerned about coming out for fear of rejection, in most cases, the stress of keeping a secret from the people they are close to ultimately outweighs the fear of losing acceptance and love. Coming out is an important decision that people should be able to make on their own terms—when they want to, to whom they want to. Fear, misinformation, stereotypes, and societal prejudice can make coming out a very difficult process for both GLB people and for the friends and family they come out to. There are a number of organizations that can provide support for gay, lesbian, and bisexual people who want to come out to their families and friends and also support the people in their lives to whom they come out. Parents and Friends of Lesbians and Gays (PFLAG), is an organization that provides help and support to gays and lesbians and the people they love and who love them. PFLAG has chapters throughout the country.

Messages for Gay, Lesbian, Bisexual, Questioning Youth, and Others

People of all sexual orientations must be given support to respect and like themselves for who they are, and reassurance that no matter what gender or genders they find themselves attracted to, those attractions can be normal and healthy. While no one but the person him/herself can know for sure what their sexual orientation is or will be, they should be given affirmation for who they are and support to lead sexually pleasurable and healthy lives.

Pregnancy and Contraception

The decision about whether or not to have children is one that most people will face in their lifetime. The term **family planning** refers to the conscious decision one makes about having a family, including when to have children, how many, and how far apart. Although at one time there was an assumption that all people would eventually choose to become parents if they could, it is becoming more and more acceptable for people to make the conscious choice *not* to become parents. The stigma that was once associated with "childless" couples, has now given way to an accepting view of "child-free" couples. Not everyone wants to be a parent, not everyone is able to be one, and not every person would make a good parent. The choice of whether or not to have children is an important one that should not be taken lightly. Planning parenthood, rather than just "letting it happen" has some very clear advantages.

In today's world, people have many options for engaging in vaginal-penile intercourse without getting pregnant. Before choosing a particular contraceptive method, it is important for a person or couple to ask such questions as: Is it safe? How

Family planning. The conscious decision one makes about having a family, including when to have children, how many, and how far apart.

Table 8.1

Comparison of Contraception Effectiveness, Number of Pregnancies per 100 Women During First Year of Use

Method	Typical Use	Perfect Use	Protection Against Sexually Transmitted Diseases	Cost
Continuous abstinence	0.00	0.00	complete	none
Outercourse	N/A	N/A	good	none
Norplant®	0.05	0.05	none	$500–$600 for exam, implants, and insertion $100–$200 for removal
Sterilization				
Men (vasectomy)	0.15	0.1	none	$240–$520 for vasectomy
Women (tubal)	0.5	0.5	none	$1,000–$2,500 for tubal sterilization (Vasectomy costs less because it is a simpler operation that can be done in the clinician's office)
Depra-Provera®	0.3	0.3	none	$30–$75 per injection. May be less at clinics. $35–$125 for exam. Some family planning clinics charge according to income. $20–$40 for subsequent visits plus medication.
IUD				
ParaGard® (copper T 380A)	0.8	0.6	none	$150–$300: exam, insertion, and follow-up visit
Progestasert®	2.0	1.5	none	Some family planning clinics charge according to income.
The pill				
Combination	5.0	0.1	none	$15–$25 per monthly pill-pack at drugstores. Often less at clinics.
Progestin-only	5.0	0.5	none	$35–$125 for exam. Some family planning clinics charge according to income.
Male condom	14.0	3.0	good	25 cents and up: dry 50 cents and up: lubricated $2.50 and up: plastic, animal tissue, or textured Some family planning centers give them away or charge very little.
Withdrawal	19.0	4.0	none	none
Diaphragm	20.0	6.0	some	$13–$25 $50–$125 for exam. Often less at family planning clinics $4–$8 for supplies of spermicide jelly or cream.
Cervical cap				$13–$25
Women who have not given birth	20.0	9.0	some	$50$125 for exam. Often less at family planning clinics.
Women who have given birth	40.0	30.0	some	$4–$8 for supplies of spermicide jelly or cream
Female condom	21.0	5.0	good	$2.50
Predicting fertility				
Periodic abstinence	20.0		none	$5–$8 and up for temperature kits (drugstore)
Post-ovulation method		1.0	none	Free classes often available in health and church centers
Symptothermal method		2.0	none	
Cervical mucus (ovulation) (method)		3.0	none	
Calendar Method		9.0	none	

Table 8.1 *(continued)*

Method	Typical Use	Perfect Use	Protection Against Sexually Transmitted Diseases	Cost
Fertility awareness methods				
With male or female condom	N/A	N/A	none	See costs above
With diaphragm or cap	N/A	N/A	none	See costs above
With withdrawal or other methods	N/A	N/A	none	none
Spermicide	26.0	6.0	none	$8 for applicator kits of foam and gel $4–$8 for refils
No method	85.0	85.0	none	

Emergency Contraception

Emergency Contraception Pills: treatment initated with 72 hours after unprotected intercourse reduces the risk of pregnancy by 75–89 percent. (No protection against infection.)

Emergency IUD insertion: Treatment initiated with seven days after unprotected intercourse reduces the risk of pregnancy by more than 99 percent. (No protection against infection.)

Source: Reprinted with permission from Planned Parenthood® Federation of America, Inc. © 2001 PPFA. All rights reserved.

effective is it in preventing pregnancy? Does it offer any protection from sexually transmitted infections? How much does it cost (short- and long-term)? Who is primarily responsible for making sure it is used correctly and consistently? How difficult is it to use? How will using this method affect my or my partner's future fertility? Ultimately, no form of contraception is 100 percent effective and without any risk. The best method is one that a couple will use correctly and consistently—every time they engage in penile-vaginal intercourse.

In deciding how effective a contraceptive method is, it is important to know that there is a difference between the theoretical (perfect use) failure rate and the typical use (actual use) failure rate. Based on the first year of use, the **theoretical**

> **Theoretical (perfect use) failure rate.** An estimate of the percentage of times a method of contraception would be expected to fail to prevent an unintended pregnancy under the best possible conditions if used perfectly.
>
> **Typical use (actual use) failure rate.** An estimate of the failure rate of a contraceptive method including factors of human error, carelessness, and technical failure.

(perfect use) failure rate is an estimate of the percentage of times a method of contraception would be expected to fail to prevent an unintended pregnancy under the best possible conditions, if used perfectly and in every instance of penile-vaginal intercourse. For this reason, it is also sometimes referred to as the *perfect use* failure rate. The **typical use** (actual use) or **failure rate** takes into account that most people do not use birth control perfectly and every single time. By taking into account human error and carelessness as well as technical failure, it is a more realistic estimate of the failure rate of a contraceptive method. It is important to look at both numbers when deciding on a form of contraception. A big gap between the theoretical and actual use failure rates may signal that it is a difficult method to use correctly and consistently. Table 8.1 shows some of the most common forms of contraception, their failure rates, advantages, and disadvantages for different users.

Unintended Pregnancy

It is quite common for women and men to experience a broad range of responses to an unintended pregnancy, including fear, anger, anxiety, denial, isolation, and guilt. Depending on their personal situations, they might also experience excitement and anticipation. The way people react depends on a number of factors, including their age, their relationship status, financial and social resources, and culture. Whatever the reaction, a decision about how to deal with the pregnancy must be made as soon as possible after the pregnancy has been confirmed. Nonjudgmental support and guidance from a trusted professional can be extremely helpful in these cases. Often, a person or couple experiencing an unintended pregnancy will be afraid to tell anyone for fear of being chastised or having the decision made for them. A woman "must be careful to choose counseling that will provide her with all of the information she needs about each option and will not be biased or judgmental in helping her fully explore her feelings about the pregnancy, her partner, her future life plans, and her options" (Koch, 1995, p. 397).

In dealing with an unintended pregnancy, there are basically three options available: (1) keeping the baby (which might mean choosing single parenthood, shared parenthood with or without marriage, or having the baby raised by another family member(s) until the parent(s) can take over the responsibility); (2) adoption; or (3) terminating the pregnancy through abortion. Each option has its potential complications and difficulties. Helping a woman or couple to consider all of the options and reach a decision requires a lot of patience, understanding, and support. Questions a woman might be asked to consider for herself include:

- Which choice(s) could I live with?

- Which choice(s) would be impossible for me?

- How would each choice affect my everyday life?

- What would each choice mean to the people closest to me?

- What is going on in my life?

- What are my plans for the future?

- What are my spiritual and moral beliefs?

- What do I believe is best for me in the long run?

- What can I afford? (Planned Parenthood, 2001)

Encouraging her to talk about her feelings with her partner, a family member, or a trusted friend can help her to feel she is not alone in making such a difficult decision. In any case, while it is important for her not to feel pressured to make any particular decision, she should make it as soon as possible. If she plans to continue the pregnancy, she wants to make sure to receive good prenatal care and to make the necessary changes in her health behaviors to ensure a healthy pregnancy. This may include quitting smoking, stopping alcohol and caffeine consumption, taking prenatal vitamins with folic acid, getting enough rest and exercise. If she decides to have an abortion, the sooner she has the procedure the less complicated it is. Abortion is very safe but the risks of complications increase the longer the pregnancy goes on. Although abortion has been legally available to women in the United States since the Supreme Court decision Roe v. Wade in 1973, various states have put restrictions upon its accessibility. Some states require that minors obtain parental consent before receiving an abortion, others require a waiting period or counseling giving specific information about other options before a woman can have an abortion. It is important for anyone providing counseling to be aware of the laws in effect in the particular state, as well as locations where abortions are offered. Due to strong opposition to abortion by some groups, which have included picketing abortion clinics as well as threats of and actual violence against physicians and clinics who offer abortions, the number of people and places offering abortions legally and safely has been steadily diminishing. It is important for a woman who makes the choice to have an abortion to know where she can go to get one.

If a woman or couple decides to put the baby up for adoption, there are a few options for handling this. There are public and private adoption agencies that are licensed through the government. Independent adoptions, which are legal in some states, can be arranged through a doctor or lawyer, or an independent adoption agency, or a person may choose to have the baby adopted by a family member, which must be approved by a family or surrogate court judge. In some cities and counties, mothers who may need more time to decide between putting a baby up for adoption and keeping the baby, can put the baby in temporary foster care.

The issue of unintended pregnancy is one about which many people have strong feelings and opinions. It is absolutely critical for the counselor not to let her or his own strong biases and beliefs interfere with giving proper, appropriate counseling support to someone who is dealing with this issue by putting unfair pressure on her to make one particular decision. The only right decision is the one that is right for the person or couple dealing with the pregnancy.

Case Study

A Need for Guidance in Crisis

Rob has coached boys soccer at Central High school for 7 years. He has developed a reputation among players and other students as a trusted resource when someone has a problem. One afternoon, Rob asks one of his players, Jason, into his office for a chat. Rob is concerned that Jason seems to be very distracted lately on the field. His mind seems a million miles away. After some mumbling and stuttering, Jason blurts out that his girlfriend, Rita, is 2 months pregnant and they don't know what to do or who to talk to about it. Rob immediately asks Jason if he thinks Rita would be willing to come in with Jason to talk to him so that they can make a decision together.

The next day, Rita and Jason come to see Rob before soccer practice. Recognizing that this is a crisis situation, Rob decides that his responsibility is to provide as much information as he can and then to make sure he helps Jason and Rita to locate and receive whatever services they will need. According to the PLISSIT model, Rob decides that limited information, as well as some specific suggestions, are what he needs to provide. Rob first tells them that they need to inform themselves of all of their options and the different potential impacts on the lives of each one so that they can make an informed decision. Rob gives them information about various

scenarios that involve keeping the baby, giving it up for adoption, or having an abortion; their state's laws and statutes related to each; and a list of phone numbers for getting the help they will need to proceed with whatever decision they ultimately choose. Rob suggests a list of questions that they should ask themselves as they consider the potential impact and consequences of each choice.

Rob tells Rita and Jason that he believes this is much too big a decision for them to be making by themselves. Rob asks them to consider sharing this information with their parents and asking for their help in making a decision. When the couple tells Rob that they are too afraid to bring it up Rob offers, with their permission, to tell their parents for them. He also asks Jason and Rita if there is another trusted adult who is close to them, such as a family member, in whom they can confide and who can help them to figure out what decision would be best for them.

Finally, Rob tells them that since Rita is already 2 months pregnant, they need to make a decision relatively soon if they want to consider all of their options, and, to get proper prenatal care if they are going to move ahead with the pregnancy. Rob tells Jason and Rita that he is glad that they confided in him and that he would be checking in with them regularly to see how they are doing. Then, he makes sure to do exactly that until Rita and Jason make a decision and afterward to follow up and make sure they are okay and whether they need any additional guidance, support, or referral for services.

Sexually Transmitted Infections

Sexually transmitted infections (STIs; also called sexually transmitted diseases, or STDs) are infections that are transmitted from person to person through sexual contact. Although theoretically they can be transmitted through any form of sexual contact, including oral-genital sex, the most efficient means of passing on an STI is through vaginal or anal intercourse. Some sexually transmitted in-

Sexually transmitted infections (STI). Infections that are transmitted from person to person through sexual contact.

fections, such as HIV and hepatitis B, also are transmitted by infected blood through needle-sharing, which is common with injection drug use. (Eng and Butler, 1997) Some STIs can be passed from a pregnant woman to her fetus, from a woman to her newborn during childbirth, as well as from a mom to her infant through breast-feeding.

Sexually transmitted infections are divided into two main categories: those caused by a bacteria and those caused by a virus. Bacterial STIs, such as chlamydia and gonorrhea, can be treated and cured, in fact, completing a course of antibiotics is often all that is needed. Viral STIs, on the other hand, like genital warts (also called human papilloma virus, or HPV), herpes, and HIV, can be treated with medication to lessen the discomfort and decrease symptoms, but they cannot be cured. Some STIs, if left untreated, can lead to pelvic inflammatory disease (PID) in women. PID can cause scarring of the fallopian tubes, leaving a woman unable to become pregnant (Sexually Transmitted Diseases, 2001).

While sexually transmitted infections occur throughout the plant and animal kingdoms, including humans (Baskin, 1999), among people it has come to be seen as an issue of morality. Because of this, STIs carry with them a social stigma that keeps people from seeking treatment or informing sexual partners about possible infection. Unfortunately, this only increases the incidence and prevalence of STIs among the population. It is estimated that more than 15 million new cases of sexually transmitted infections are diagnosed each year in the United States (Cates, 1999), and approximately one-fourth of these new infections occur among teenagers (CDC, 2000). Untreated STIs lead to growth in the rate of long-term medical complications—including various cancers, infertility, ectopic pregnancy, spontaneous abortion, and in some cases, death.

While we would never blame people for having other illnesses, or say that they deserved it—even for diseases that are largely preventable—we do just that to people who have gotten their illness through sexual transmission. This reflects society's uneasiness and conflicted emotions about sexual behavior. As a result, open, honest discussion and dialogue about STIs are rare to nonexistent. Because people are not informed about the most common and potentially dangerous STIs, they are not being tested or treated for them and they are not aware of the potential serious long-terms health consequences associated with untreated STIs. So, although sexually transmitted infections are among the most common infections that occur in the United States today—they accounted for 87 percent of all reported diseases in the United States in 1995 (The Hidden Epidemic, 1996)—most men and women of reproductive age (18–44) dramatically underestimate the national prevalence of such infections and their own personal risk of acquiring one (Kaiser Family Foundation, 1998).

Another factor that impedes awareness of sexually transmitted infections is that many of these infections are asymptomatic, particularly in women. Though a person may not have any symptoms, however, the STI can still do permanent damage to his/her reproductive system and the person can still transmit the infection to other people. Many people who are unknowingly infected are putting sexual partners at risk for contracting an STI unless they practice safer sex correctly and consistently which means using a male or female condom with every risky sexual behavior or engaging only in sexual behaviors that do not pose any risk for STI transmission. Meanwhile, those people who *do* know they have a sexually transmitted infection often feel the effects of the social stigma against them and are secretive about their condition. This has led to what has come to be termed a "hidden epidemic" to describe the state of STIs in this country (The Hidden Epidemic, 1996).

With approximately 12 million new cases occurring annually in the United States, rates of curable STIs in this country are the highest in the developed world (The Hidden Epidemic, 1996). The only way to combat this hidden epidemic is to bring it out into the open. Honest, direct discussion about this major health issue will begin to break down the shame and secrecy associated with STIs and free people to seek out critically important information about testing and treatment. It will also allow sexually active individuals to feel comfortable discussing with a partner the existence of a possible infection as well as what they can do to practice safer sex and keep themselves healthy and protected from infection. See the following table.

Table 8.2
Common Sexually Transmitted Diseases (STDs): Mode of Transmission, Symptoms, and Treatment

STD	Transmission	Symptoms	Treatment
Chlamydial infection	The *Chlamydia trachomatis* bacterium is transmitted primarily through sexual contact. It can also be spread by fingers from one body site to another.	In somen, PID (pelvic inflammatory disease) caused by *Chlamydia* may included disrupted menstrual periods, pelvic pain, elevated temperature, nausea, vomiting, headache, infertility, and ectopic pregnancy. In men, chlamydial infection of the urethra may cause a discharge and burning during urination. *Chlamydia*-caused epididymitis may produce a sense of heaviness in the affected testicle(s), inflammation of the scrotal skin, and painful swelling at the bottom of the testicle.	Doxycycline, azithromycin, or ofloxacin
Gonorrhea ("clap")	The *Neisseria gonorrhoeae* bacterium ("gonoccus") is spread through genital, oral–genital, or genital–anal contact.	The most common symptoms in men are a cloudy discharge from the penis and burning sensations during urination. If disease is untreated, complications may include inflammation of scrotal skin and swelling at base of the testicle. In women, some green or yellowish discharge is produced but commonly remains undetected. Later, PID may develop.	Dual therapy of a single dose of ceftriaxone, cefixime, ciprofloxacin, or ofloxacin plus doxycycline for seven days or a single dose of azithromycin
Nongonoccal urethritis (NGU)	Primary causes are believed to be the bacteria *Chlamydia trachomatis* and *Ureaplasma urealyticum,* most commonly transmitted through coitus. Some NGU may result from allergic reactions or from *Trichomonas* infection.	Inflammation of the urethral tube. A man has a discharge from the penis and irritation during urination. A woman may have a mild discharge of pus from the vagina but often shows no symptoms.	A single dose of azithromycin or doxy-cycline for seven days
Syphillis	The *Treponema pallidum* bacterium ("spirochete") is transmitted from open lesions during genital, oral–genital, or genital–anal contact.	*Primary stage:* A painless chancre appears at the site where the spirochetes entered the body. *Secondary stage:* The chancre disappears and a generalized skin rash develops. *Latent stage:* There may be no visible symptoms. *Tertiary stage:* Heart failure, blindness, mental disturbance, and many other symptoms occur. Death may result.	Benzathine penicillin G, doxycycline, erythro-mycin, or ceftriaxone
Herpes	The genital herpes virus (HSV-2) seems to be trans-mitted primarily by vaginal, anal, or oral–genital inter-course. The oral herpes virus (HSV-1) is transmitted primarily by kissing.	Small, painful red bumps (papules) appear in the genital region (genital herpes) or mouth (oral herpes). The papules become painful blisters that eventually rupture to form wet, open sores.	No known cure; a variety of treatments may reduce symptoms; oral or intra-venous acyclovir (Zovirax) promotes healing and suppresses recurrent outbreaks.
Chancroid	The *Haemophilus ducrevi* bacterium is usually trans-mitted by sexual interaction.	Small bumps (papules) in genital regions eventually rupture and form painful, soft, craterlike ulcers that emit a foul-smelling discharge.	Single doses of either ceftriaxone or azithro-mycin or seven days of erythromycin.

(continued on next page)

Table 8.2 *(continued)*

STD	Transmission	Symptoms	Treatment
Human Papilloma virus (HPV) (genital warts)	The virus is spread primarily through vaginal, anal, or oral–genital sexual interaction.	Hard and yellow-gray on dry skin areas; soft, pinkish-red, and cauliflowerlike on moist areas.	Freezing, application of topical agents like trichloroacetic acid or podofilox, cauterization, surgical removal, or vaporization by carbon dioxide laser
Pubic lice ("crabs")	*Phthirus pubis,* the pubic louse, is spread easily through body contact or through shared clothing or bedding.	Persistent itching. Lice are visible and may often be located in pubic hair or other body hair.	1% permethrin cream for body areas; 1% Lindane shampoo for hair.
Scabies	*Sarcoptes scabiei* is highly contagious and may be transmitted by close physical contact, sexual and nonsexual.	Small bumps and a red rash that itch intensely, especially at night.	5% permethrin lotion or cream.
Acquired immuno-deficiency syndrome (AIDS)	Blood and semen are the major vehicles for transmitting HIV, which attacks the immune system. It appears to be passed primarily through sexual contact, or needle sharing among injecting drug users.	Vary with the type of cancer or opportunistic infections that afflict an infected person. Common symptoms include fevers, night sweats, weight loss, chronic fatigue, swollen lymph nodes, diarrhea and/or bloody stools, atypical bruising or bleeding, skin rashes, headache, chronic cough, and a whitish coating on the tongue or throat.	Commence treatment early after a positive HIV test with a combination of three or more antiretro-viral drugs (HAART) plus other specific treatment(s), if necessary, of opportunistic infections and tumors.
Viral hepatitis	The hepatitis B virus can be transmitted by blood, semen, vaginal secretions, and saliva. Manual, oral, or penile stimulation of the anus are strongly associated with the spread of this virus. Hepatitis A seems to be primarily spread via the fecal–oral route, but oral–anal sexual contact is a common mode for sexual transmission of hepatitis A.	Vary from nonexistent to mild, flulike symptoms to an incapacitating illness characterized by high fever, vomiting, and severe abdominal pain.	No specific therapy for A and B types; treatment generally consists of bed rest and adequate fluid intake. Combination therapy with interferon and ribavarin may be effective for hepatitis C infections.
Bacterial vaginosis	The most common causative agent, the *Gardnerella vaginalis* bacterium, is sometimes transmitted through coitus.	In women, a fishy- or musty-smelling, thin discharge, like flour paste in consistency and usually gray. Most men are asymptomatic.	Metronidazole (flagyl) by mouth or intravaginal applications of topical metronidazole gel or clindamycin cream.
Candidiasis (yeast infection)	The *Candida albicans* fungus may accelerate growth when the chemical balance of the vagina is disturbed; it may also be transmitted through sexual interaction.	White, "cheesy" discharge; irritation of vaginal and vulval tissues	Vaginal suppositories or topical cream, such as clotrimazole and miconazole, or oral fluconazole.
Trichomoniasis	The protozoan parasite *Trichomonas vaginalis* is usually passed through genital sexual contact.	White or yellow vaginal discharge with an unpleasant odor; vulva is sore and irritated.	Metronidazole (Flagyl) for both women and men.

Source: Crooks, Robert L., and Karla Baur. *Our Sexuality,* 8th ed. Pacific Grove, CA: Wadsworth, 2002.

Important Counseling Information for People Concerned about STIs

Planned Parenthood of New York City offers some important guidelines to remember when providing counseling to someone with concerns about STIs.

- It is important for sexually active people to be checked for certain STIs at least once a year so that if they do have an STI, they can get early treatment that can avoid or reduce long-term consequences.

- Condoms must be worn correctly for every single act of intercourse in order to help prevent contracting STIs. Using a condom sometimes, or even most of the time, will not adequately protect against STIs.

- If a person contracts an STI, both that person and his or her partner need to be tested and possibly treated. If the partner is not treated, he or she may have the STI and pass it back to the first person.

- Even people in a long-term, exclusive relationship should still worry about STIs. It could be that their relationship isn't as exclusive as they think. Or they or their partner may have a pre-existing STI that they do not know about.

- Not all STIs have obvious symptoms. Further, only some STIs are tested for in a routine pelvic exam. To get a complete STI exam, an individual must go to an STD clinic. Hepatitis B, which can be tested for at an STD clinic, can be very difficult to diagnose. Herpes also may be difficult to diagnose, unless a person has an outbreak at the time of their clinic visit. Also, it can take up to 6 months for HIV to show up on a test. For these reasons, it is always best to use a condom (female or male) with every act of sexual intercourse (Sexually Transmitted Diseases, 2001).

HIV/AIDS

HIV (human immunodeficiency virus), the virus that can lead to AIDS (acquired immune deficiency syndrome) requires lengthy discussion be-

cause it has given rise to more concern among sexually active people of all ages than any other STI. This is likely because it is caused by a virus, which means there is no cure, and can eventually prove to be fatal for those infected. Also, HIV/AIDS has been in the public consciousness only since the early 1980s, and there are still many unanswered questions about the disease. HIV is transmitted through sexual contact in which infected bodily fluid enters the body through broken skin or mucous membrane such as the vagina, urethra, rectum, or mouth. The only fluids that can transmit HIV are blood, semen, vaginal secretions, and breast milk. Anal and vaginal sexual intercourse without the proper use of a condom are the most efficient sexual ways to transmit HIV. HIV can also be transmitted through the sharing of IV needles, which is a common practice among injection drug users; from an infected mother to her fetus in utero; or from an infected mother to her baby through breast-feeding. Extensive studies have shown that HIV cannot be transmitted through hugging or caring for someone with HIV (Fischl et al., 1987), through mosquito bites (Lifson, 1988), or on toilet seats. In fact, unlike the virus that causes the common cold, which can survive outside the human body for some time, HIV is quite fragile and cannot survive outside of the body fluids listed above, in which it resides.

Currently, education is the only prevention that exists against HIV. Even though there has been a massive worldwide effort to develop effective vaccines, they are still quite a number of years away and there is still no agreement that HIV will ever be successfully prevented in this way. People must be encouraged to practice safe, healthy behaviors, like using a condom (male or female) correctly and consistently—*every* time they engage in sexual behaviors that put them at risk for HIV or other STI transmission.

Although there is no cure, there are treatments for HIV that have been shown to keep the virus in

HIV (human immunodeficiency virus). The virus that can lead to AIDS, that is transmitted through the body fluids blood, semen, vaginal discharge, and breast milk.

check, allowing infected people to live longer and healthier lives. Today, the amount of time from when a person becomes infected with HIV to when they begin to show symptoms of AIDS and begin to get sick can be up to 15 years or longer. New antiviral therapies known as cocktails are enabling people to treat HIV as a chronic disease more than a terminal one. Long-term success of these treatments, however, is still unclear.

Tests for HIV

When HIV enters the body, it begins to attack certain white blood cells called T4 lymphocyte cells (helper cells), sometimes also referred to as CD4 cells. The immune system then produces antibodies to fight off the infection. Although these antibodies are ineffective in destroying HIV, their presence is used to confirm HIV infection. HIV tests look for the presence of HIV antibodies; they do not test for the virus itself. In order to obtain a reliable test, a person must wait for his/her immune system to produce enough antibodies to be detectable. Although a person may test positive for HIV within several weeks of infection, the Centers for Disease Control and Prevention (CDC) recommends waiting at least 3 months from the date of exposure in order to get a reliable test. A negative result before then may just mean that the body has not yet produced enough HIV antibodies to show up on a test. The only way to find out is to get tested after the 3-month "window period" has passed (Florida Department of Health, 2001).

The most common types of HIV antibody tests are blood tests. Urine and oral-fluid (Orasure©) HIV tests offer alternatives for anyone reluctant to have blood drawn. Urine testing for HIV antibodies, however, is not as sensitive or specific as blood testing.

To Get Tested or Not?

It is not uncommon for people to have questions about whether or not to get tested for HIV. Unfortunately, there are still a lot of misconceptions about HIV and the people who contract it, so there is stigma attached to getting tested. People may be concerned that they will lose family or friends, be the victim of job or benefits discrimination, or be stereotyped if people find out they were tested. Because there is no cure, others just don't want to know if they are infected or not. Only the person who is questioning his/her own HIV status can make the decision about whether to get tested.

If a person does decide to get tested, it is a good idea to take the test at an anonymous testing site, where no one ever knows his or her name. People coming in for testing are assigned a number only which is used to identify their test. The person being tested is the only one to know the results of his/her test and to decide with whom, when, and if to share those results. Some sites do confidential, not anonymous testing. The difference is that while a person's name is kept private, it is connected to the test and to the results. That presents the potential for someone getting that information. Health-care providers, the person's insurance company, and, in some states, the health department will have access to an individual's test results. Most states offer both anonymous and confidential testing sites. Depending on where someone lives, he/she can get tested at any of several places. Testing may be offered at the following local sites:

- STD clinic
- family-planning clinic
- community health center
- doctor's office
- hospital

In making the decision to get tested, it is critical for a person to choose a site that provides counseling both before and after the test.

Home testing kits, also referred to as home blood collection systems, are also an option. These contain HIV/AIDS literature and materials that allow a person to take his/her own blood sample and mail it to a testing facility where his/her HIV status will be determined. Results are accessed by an anonymous identification number and are given over the telephone several days later. Home testing kits are sold in drugstores and health clinics throughout the country and are available by mail.

Case Study

Providing Valuable Information

Fatima is a health educator at State University's Wellness Center. Brianna and Steve come in one day to talk. They tell Fatima that they have been together for 6 months and have decided they are ready to have sexual intercourse but want to make sure that they are both sexually healthy and free of STDs. Fatima thanks them for coming in to see her and supports their efforts to be responsible to themselves and one another. Fatima recognizes this visit as a search for information and proceeds to share with the couple some important guidelines.

First, Fatima tells Brianna and Steve if either one of them has been sexually active before with another partner in a way that involved the exchange of bodily fluids or contact with genitals, they may have been exposed to a sexually transmitted infection (STI). The first thing each must do is to get tested for STIs. Fatima gives each of them a list of clinics that provide STI testing.

Next, Fatima tells the couple that they need to get tested for HIV. She reviews with them what HIV testing is and their various options while suggesting to them that anonymous testing is always a good choice. She explains to them about the 3-month window period for the development of antibodies. This means, she says, that if either one has engaged in any risky sexual behavior within the last 3 months, they must wait for 3 months to pass before getting tested. After being tested, it would be a good idea to wait another 3 months to get tested one more time to be sure. During that time, if either engages in any risky behaviors they will have to reset the clock for another 3 months. After that, assuming both tests come out negative, they can feel confident that they are both free of HIV.

After she finishes, Fatima notices the looks of concern on the young couple's faces. "This is a lot to think about, I know" Fatima acknowledges. And, in fact, she tells them that it brings up some important issues about trust and communication in their relationship. All of the testing in the world will not replace honest communication about outside relationships and experiences. And once both get a clean bill of health, they must be sure that both are remaining monogamous with each other or the potential for new exposure enters the relationship. It is important to be tested so that if there is an infection, it can be properly treated. Still, however, Fatima encourages the couple to practice safer sex, using a male or female latex or polyurethane condom every time they engage in sexual behaviors that put them at risk for and infection. This way, she tells them, they can enjoy one another without experiencing worry or fear which can interfere with their ability to experience pleasure and intimacy.

Fatima repeats her support for the couple's decision to seek out information. Taking the steps to protect their sexual health demonstrates commitment and mutual respect that are wonderful signs for a healthy relationship. Brianna and Steve thank Fatima. They now feel more in control of their sexual health and of the stability of their relationship.

Sexual Dysfunctions

Not every sexual encounter is satisfying and pleasurable. Almost everyone will experience some dissatisfaction with their sexual experiences at different times of their lives. Though media portrayals of sexuality might lead us to believe that sex is always great for everyone involved, that it goes on and on for hours, complete with simultaneous orgasms, in reality, this is far from the truth. Just as eating an ice cream cone may be more enjoyable under certain conditions, for example when the weather is hot, the person eating it is hungry, is feeling well, the quality of the ice cream is good, the flavor is one that the person prefers, and so on, the same is true for sexual experiences. How we are feeling (tired or awake, healthy or sick), who we are with, the level of stress we are experiencing in our lives, all have an impact on how we experience our sexual encounters and how satisfied we are with them. As one textbook about Human Sexuality puts it:

Because our sexuality is an integral part of ourselves, it reflects our excitement and boredom, intimacy and distance, emotional well-being and distress, health and illness. As a consequence, our sexual desires and activities ebb and flow. Sometimes they are highly erotic; at other times, they may be boring. Furthermore, many of us who are sexually active may sometimes experience sexual difficulties or problems. (Strong and De Vault, 1994, pp. 588–589)

In general, people's sexual satisfaction is related to their overall satisfaction in life and in relationships in particular. One major research survey, for example, found that people who report that they are not happy also are more likely to report that they are less interested in sex, and do not find sex pleasurable. They are also more likely to report that when they do have sex they have trouble having orgasms or have pain during sex (Michael et al., 1994). Furthermore, most people report that having an orgasm is not the only component to having satisfying sexual experiences, and in fact, some people who have frequent orgasms are dissatisfied with their sex lives.

A **sexual dysfunction** is usually an ongoing or chronic disturbance or disorder related to sexual functioning that keeps a person from being able to behave sexually the way she or he would like to. Because sexual dysfunctions can be the results of physical, psychological, social, and spiritual factors, a sexual and medical history taken by a professional counselor is important before a course of treatment, either counseling or therapy, can be decided upon. Most people, however, experience occasional dissatisfaction with their level of sexual functioning at different times of their lives, whether it is related to their level of desire, their orgasmic response, or physical discomfort during sexual behavior. While the problem or concern may be temporary and may not clinically be considered a sexual dysfunction, it is serious and troublesome to the individual.

Although we have little scientific data on the prevalence of sexual disorders and dysfunctions, professionals in the field agree that, in their milder forms, most of them are believed to be relatively common. Because of this, it is important for the sexuality educator/counselor to be knowledgeable about the most common causes for concern. Counseling that offers reassurance, support, and some basic information can often be extremely beneficial to the person or couple who has a sexual concern. If such counseling is not sufficient, appropriate referral to a sex counselor or therapist needs to be made.

One sexual dysfunction that is experienced by both males and females is called **Hypoactive Sexual Desire Disorder** or **Inhibited Sexual Desire (ISD)**. ISD, basically, is a lack of interest in sexual activity. People with ISD do not initiate sexual activity, and may engage in sexual relations only to please or placate their partner. They do not seek out sexual stimulation and are not bothered by the lack of opportunity for sexual activity. This condition is also characterized by a lack of sexual fantasies, dreams, or thoughts. Problems with sexual desire are the most common complaint for which people enter into sex therapy, with more men than women complaining of this problem. It is also the most common sexual complaint among lesbian couples (Nichols, 1989). It is important to note, however, that because there is an enormous range of the levels of sexual desire that people experience, sometimes what might be interpreted as inhibited sexual desire is actually a discrepancy between the sexual desires of two people involved in a relationship. If one person in a couple wants to have sex three times a day, and the other is satisfied with engaging in sexual behaviors once a week, the couple might consider that the once-a-week person has a sexual desire disorder. In fact, the problem lies in the differences in the couple's levels of desire, not with one person. If a couple engages in sex twice a month, or twice a year, and

Sexual dysfunction. Disorders that can be physical or psychological, based on values and beliefs, stress, fatigue, anxiety, or a combination of factors that inhibit sexual expression.

Hypoactive Sexual Desire Disorder or **Inhibited Sexual Desire (ISD).** A lack of interest in sexual activity, in males and females.

both are sexually satisfied and happy, then there really is no problem. Inhibited sexual desire is considered a sexual dysfunction when the lack of interest in sex is a source of distress and unhappiness for the person. This lack of interest may be caused by physiological factors related to hormone levels or some chronic illness. Most often, however, it is due to psychological factors such as depression, shame regarding one's body, or some earlier traumatic sexual experience such as rape.

Male Dysfunctions

The most common sexual dysfunctions for males are erectile dysfunction and premature ejaculation. The first is considered to be an arousal disorder because it occurs during the arousal phase of physiological sexual response. The second is an orgasm disorder because it occurs during that phase of sexual response.

Erectile dysfunction (previously called impotence) is the persistent or recurrent inability of a man to attain or maintain an erection in order to engage in satisfying sexual activities requiring this response. This is accompanied by a lack of subjective sense of sexual excitement, or being turned on, and lack of pleasure during sexual activity. Erectile dysfunction is the most common complaint of men who seek sex therapy. Erectile dysfunction can often be the result of physiological factors including circulation system problems, aging, or drug or alcohol abuse. The most common psychological cause is what is labeled performance anxiety which is the fear of not performing well or up to expected standards during sexual activity. Guilt about various aspects of one's sexual behaviors can also lead to erectile difficulties.

While this disorder can have both physiological and psychological causes, cultural expectations can also play a part raising men's concerns over their erectile abilities or behavior. In American culture the vision of the sexually healthy male, a vision that is reinforced by the media, is a male who can get an erection any time he wants, and maintain it for as long as he wants or needs. There is a generalized expectation that once a penis becomes erect it is supposed to stay that way throughout a sexual experience until the man is satisfied, typically by ejaculation and orgasm. In fact, it is part of normal sexual functioning for a male to have an erection, lose it, and get it back again a few times within a single sexual encounter. Also, almost all men will experience, from time to time, the inability to have or maintain an erection as long as they would like. That too, is part of normal sexual functioning.

Premature ejaculation is when a male has a persistent or recurrent experience of ejaculation with minimal sexual stimulation before he or he and his partner wish it. This is a subjective definition because there is no objective or scientific determination of how much time a person or a couple needs to be sexually satisfied. Again, while there might be a perception that a man should be able to engage in sexual activity for hours at a time, in fact, that is not necessary for satisfying sexual experiences. As a noted sexologist wrote:

> Good sex is not determined by clocks. You can make great love in two hours, in twenty minutes, and even in twenty seconds. The key is not how long it takes, but how good you both feel about yourselves, each other, and what you are doing. (Zilbergeld, 1992, p. 475)

Although premature ejaculation can have physical causes, including surgery, trauma, or disease, it is almost always caused by the inability of the mind to control the body's ejaculation process. Sometimes premature ejaculation is related to an extremely high level of sexual arousal in the male which can cause orgasm before he wants it. This occurrence is not atypical and is not considered to be a dysfunction. Premature ejaculation is almost

---

Erectile dysfunction (impotence). The persistent or recurrent inability of a man to attain or maintain an erection in order to engage in satisfying sexual activities requiring this response.

Premature ejaculation. When a male has a persistent or recurrent experience of ejaculation with minimal sexual stimulation before he and his partner wish it.

always due to a lack of knowledge, attention, or skill (Koch, 1995). With sexual experience, better communication techniques, and aging, most men learn to delay their orgasm. While some men experience this disorder in all situations, others find it happens only when they are in new relationships or are experiencing anxiety about their sexual interactions. Fortunately, this disorder, the most common dysfunction among heterosexual men, is also one of the easiest to overcome. Information, knowledge about his own body and how it responds to sexual stimulation, and specific sex therapy techniques can all help a male to delay the onset of orgasm and ejaculation.

Female Dysfunctions

The most common concerns about sexual functioning affecting women are Female Sexual Arousal Disorder, Female Orgasmic Disorder (inhibited orgasm, anorgasmia, preorgasmia), and Sexual Pain Disorder—dyspareunia, vaginismus. **Female Arousal Disorder** is a persistent or recurrent inability to attain or maintain sufficient vaginal lubrication and swelling to engage in satisfying sexual activities. It is also a persistent lack of a subjective sense of sexual excitement, feeling turned on, and pleasure during sexual activity. The arousal stage of sexual response requires a physiological process known as vasocongestion, which helps to cause erections in males and vaginal lubrication and expansion and swelling of the external genitalia in women. If vasocongestion does not occur in a female, the vagina and external genitalia do not become engorged with blood sufficiently, her vagina does not lubricate sufficiently, her genitals do not fully expand, and as a result penetration becomes difficult, which could lead to painful intercourse. Female Arousal Disorder can cause

difficulty within relationships and may lead some females to avoid sexual relations.

There are a number of biological, psychological, and sociocultural factors associated with arousal disorder in females. Shame, guilt, or fear associated with sexual behaviors can interrupt a female's arousal response. A relationship that is poor in other areas, or an inexperienced, inept, or insensitive lover, can contribute to the onset of arousal disorder. When estrogen levels are lower, such as during menopause or breast-feeding, vaginal lubrication is naturally decreased. During such times, the use of a water-based lubricant, such as K-Y jelly, can help with penetration during sexual activity. Quite often, sexual activity progresses to penetration before a woman has received enough stimulation to excite her and trigger her arousal response. Good communication and effective sexual stimulation can help to prevent this problem.

Female Orgasmic Disorder—inhibited female orgasm—is persistent or recurrent delay in, or absence of, orgasm following sexual arousal and excitement, when orgasm is desired (Koch, 1995). It is the most common sexual complaint among women seeking sexual therapy. Because there is tremendous variation in the amount of sexual stimulation people enjoy or require before having an orgasm, it is difficult to know whether a woman who does not experience orgasm has a dysfunction or is not getting enough sexual stimulation. One factor that contributes to women not having orgasms is the emphasis in our culture on penile-vaginal intercourse, particularly, the male-on-top position, as the ultimate sexual experience. In fact, most women experience orgasm primarily through stimulation of their clitoris. The penetration and thrusting involved in sexual intercourse often does not provide sufficient clitoral stimulation for a woman to experience orgasm. Most women who do not experience orgasm from intercourse alone are able to experience orgasm from

Female Arousal Disorder. Persistent or recurrent inability to attain or maintain sufficient vaginal lubrication and swelling to engage in satisfying sexual activities; can also be a persistent lack of arousal, excitement, or pleasure.

Female Orgasmic Disorder (inhibited female orgasm). Persistent or recurrent delay in or absence of orgasm following sexual arousal and excitement, when orgasm is desired.

clitoral stimulation through oral sex (cunnilingus) or masturbation. Females who experience orgasm only through stimulation of the clitoris are not considered dysfunctional.

It is also important to remember that because people respond to stimulation differently—some more slowly, others more quickly—the idea of a simultaneous orgasm—coming at the same time—is not only not necessary, but not typical. One partner may have an orgasm and then continue to provide stimulation in a variety of ways to the other person until she/he too has an orgasm if one is desired.

Lack of orgasm (**anorgasmia**) in females usually has psychological causes. Sexual inhibition, lack of knowledge concerning her own sexual response, and reluctance to ask for and receive sexual stimulation that gives her the most pleasure can all lead to lack of orgasm. **Preorgasmia** is a term for females who have never experienced an orgasm. Because capacity for orgasm increases with age, experience, and sexual confidence, the term preorgasmia suggests that all women are ultimately capable of experiencing orgasm.

Sexual Pain Disorder—Dyspareunia is recurrent or persistent pain occurring in the genital area during sexual stimulation or intercourse. While dyspareunia can be experienced by both men and women it is more common in females. It may be felt before, during, or after sexual intercourse and can range from mild discomfort to strong pain. There are many potential physical reasons for pain during sexual intercourse. In men, pain can be caused by the foreskin being too tight over the glans or from smegma collecting under the foreskin in addition to other infections or diseases. Among women, who experience dyspareunia much more commonly than men, pain can be the result of infections, disease, or sexual or surgical trauma. Certain positions in sexual intercourse can cause the ovaries or uterus to be jarred, causing pain. When estrogen levels are low, vaginal lubrication decreases, which can lead to painful intercourse. People experiencing pain during sexual activity must get a physical examination to determine the cause. Psychological or relationship causes should also be explored. If pain is due to lack of vaginal lubrication, better and/or prolonged sexual stimulation might be needed or the use of additional lubricants such as K-Y Jelly. Sometimes changing sexual positions can be helpful.

Vaginismus is the persistent or recurrent involuntary contraction of the perineal muscles surrounding the outer third of the vagina, making it difficult or impossible for penetration to take place by a penis, finger, tampon, speculum, or other object. Symptoms of vaginismus can range from mild discomfort and tightness to severe contractions and cramping (Blonna & Levitan, 2000). Vaginismus is more common among young women than older women and is often first discovered at the first gynecological exam or the onset of sexual intercourse. It is a primary reason for a marriage not to be consummated and can interfere with the development of sexual relationships. While vaginismus can prevent penetration, however, many women who experience this are still sexually responsive in other ways that do not require penetration. They may still have a capacity for arousal and orgasm.

Vaginismus is a conditioned response to fear, anxiety, or pain and the situations that were the cause of those reactions must be eliminated. There are specific techniques, including Kegel exercises, that can help a woman to learn to relax her vaginal muscles.

Anorgasmia. Lack of orgasm in females which usually has psychological causes.

Preorgasmia. A term for females who have never experienced an orgasm.

Sexual Pain Disorder—Dyspareunia. A recurrent or persistent pain in the genital area during sexual stimulation or intercourse.

Vaginismus. The persistent or recurrent involuntary contraction of the perineal muscles surrounding the outer third of the vagina, making it difficult or impossible for penetration to take place.

Table 8.3
Sexual Dysfunctions by Gender and Age

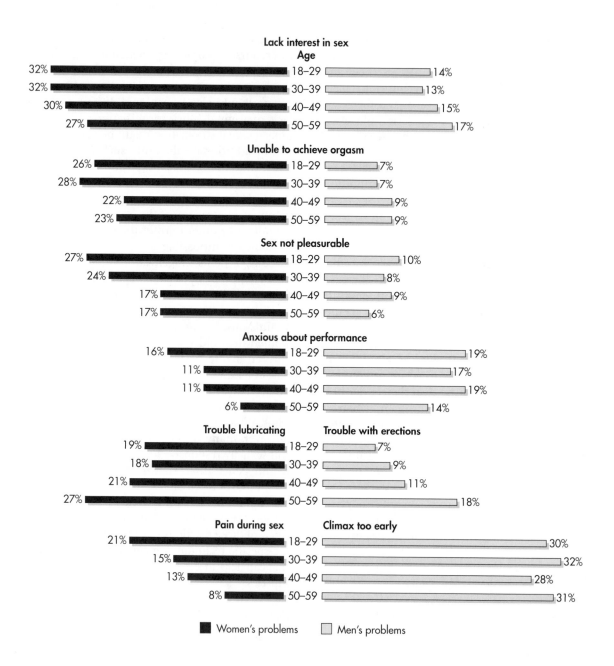

Source: From "National Health and Social Life Survey, 1992" in *Social Organization of Sexuality: Sexual Practices in the United States* by E. Lauman, J. Gagnon, R. Michael, and S. Michaels, 1994. Reprinted by permission of The University of Chicago Press.

Causes

The table above looks at sexual dysfunctions by gener and age. Sexual dysfunctions and disorders can have many underlying causes. There can be physical or medical causes, ranging from cardiovascular disease, sexually transmitted infection, endocrine disorders, diabetes, cancer, neurological problems, injuries, allergies, and other ailments to the side effects of legal and illegal drugs. Psychological factors can be the result of prior learning—the fundamental attitudes, values, and beliefs about sexuality we develop throughout our childhood—or immediate causes such as ignorance, performance anxiety, communication problems, or stress and fatigue. Culture also plays a part in creating and/or exacerbating dysfunctions by affecting our expectations for ourselves, sexual partners, and sexual experiences. Quite often, sexual dysfunctions are caused by a combination of different factors. Successful treatment is often the result of determining the underlying cause.

Sexual Assault/Abuse

Sexual assault or **sexual violence** is any unwanted sexual attention, touching, or coercive action or behaviors. The terms sexual assault and sexual violence can include several types of behaviors and/or crimes including rape; incest; sexual, verbal or physical harassment; child molestation; marital rape; indecent exposure; and voyeurism. National statistics reveal that one in three women and one in 10 men is the victim of sexual assault (Sexual Assault Victim Advocate, 2001). Sexual assault is *not*: an expression of love, passion, or sexual desire, and it is *not* ever the fault of the victim. The exact criminal definitions of these acts vary from state to state.

> **Sexual assault/sexual violence.** Any unwanted sexual attention, touching, or coercive action or behaviors, including rape; incest; sexual, verbal, or physical harassment; child molestation; marital rape; indecent exposure; and voyeurism.

Some important facts about sexual violence are:

- Victims of sexual violence do not invite or cause the assault to happen. Only the person initiating the sexually violent act is responsible.

- Sexual assaults are committed primarily out of anger and/or a need to feel powerful, to control and dominate another person.

- Victims of sexual violence are forced, coerced, or manipulated to participate in unwanted sexual activity.

- Victims are usually traumatized by the assault. Friends and family members may also experience trauma reaction.

- Sexual assault is a reportable crime. It is important for adult victim/survivors to consider reporting so sexual offenders can be identified by the system and the community.

Reporting Cases of Sexual Assault

Each state has its own guidelines about the circumstances under which professionals are mandated to report a sexual assault to law enforcement or child protective services. Some of the more common circumstances include:

- If the victim is a child

- If the victim goes to the emergency room

- If the victim was assaulted by someone in a position of authority or trust (that is, coaches, psychotherapists, scout leaders, teachers, priests or rabbis, and so on)

- If the victim is physically, emotionally, or mentally disadvantaged

Impact of Sexual Assault

Sexual assault, whether it happens to oneself or someone you know, is a major life event. It can create roadblocks to normal life at home, at work, or at school, with friends, family or coworkers. Common emotional responses to sexual assault can include: sleeplessness, lack of concentration, overeating or loss of appetite, nightmares, loss of self-confidence, stress-related illness, feelings of grief and despair, fear of being alone or being with people, fear of various settings or various people.

Every person reacts differently to sexual assault. In general, though, there are five stages of recovery which almost everyone will experience to some degree. It is not unusual for different people to experience these stages in different orders, however, or even to repeat some stages several times.

Stages of Recovery

- **Stage 1: Initial Shock**—Shock following an assault can take on many forms. A person may feel emotional as well as physical shock, which in turn may be expressed as very controlled and/or withdrawn, or highly expressive, including crying, screaming, or shaking. The person may or may not feel comfortable communicating these feelings to others.

- **Stage 2: Denial**—This stage may be characterized by the person attempting to go on with normal routine, wanting to forget about the assault. This denial or rationalization of what happened is an attempt by the victim to deal with her/his inner turmoil.

- **Stage 3: Reactivation**—This stage involves a re-experiencing of the feelings from Stage 1, usually brought on by the triggering of memories of the assault. Feelings of depression, anxiety, and shame increase. Other symptoms can include nightmares, flashbacks, a sense of vulnerability, mistrust, and physical complaints.

- **Stage 4: Anger**—The victim/survivor may experience feelings of anger—often toward her or himself, friends, significant others, society, the legal system, all men/women, and so on. With skillful support this anger can be directed more appropriately toward the assailant.

- **Stage 5: Integration (Closure)**—As the person begins to integrate the thoughts and feelings stemming from the assault into her/his life experience she/he will begin to feel "back on track." As a result of support, education, and the passage of time, she/he will feel strengthened. (Sexual Assault Victim Advocate, 2001)

Helping a Victim/Survivor of Sexual Assault or Violence

There are things that a professional with some good counseling skills can do when faced with a person who has been the victim of a sexual assault that can help to give her/him back some sense of control and stability in her/his life. Pat Koch, sexuality educator, offers the following guidelines for helping someone who has been raped:

- Express your happiness and relief that the person who was raped is alive and has survived!

- Believe the survivor. Do not call into question any of her decisions (for example, Were you walking alone? Why did you date that jerk? Why did you drink so much? Why didn't you fight back?)

- Provide a physically and emotionally safe environment whenever the survivor needs it: Make sure the survivor is out of danger.

- Do not tell the survivor how to feel or act. It's normal for a survivor to experience a variety of emotions and reactions. The survivor's feelings and actions may be very different from those that you might have in the same situation.

- Do not react violently to her rape (for example, I'll kill him!). The survivor has just been through a violent experience and does not need to deal with any more expressions of violence.

- Be a supportive listener. Allow the survivor to tell you anything or everything about the rape and retell it to you as many times as she feels the need. However, do not grill her on the experience. Try to minimize the number of times she must retell the details of the experience to others. Respect her silence as well as her talking.

- Do not tell anyone else about the rape without her consent.

- Assist her in getting the immediate and long-term medical, legal, and psychological help she wants and needs.

- Avoid making decisions for the survivor. Her own power and control over her own life was taken from her through the rape experience. Help her take back control of her own life through making her own decisions. Ask her what you can do to help.

- Let her know what your limits are. Be realistic with the time, energy, and commitment you can give to her.

- Do not touch or hug her unless you are sure she is comfortable with your physical contact. Ask her what she would feel comfortable with.

- Recognize that it will be difficult for the survivor to reestablish trust and intimacy with other people.

- Realize that supporters need support too. Seek help with your own reactions from others, such as family, friends, professionals, or support groups.

- Remind her it was not her fault.

- Remember there is no set timetable for recovery. Healing is not a smooth, linear process and is unique to each individual. (Koch, 1995, pp. 346–347)

Although this point has already been made, it is important to repeat it here: While a skilled educator with some good counseling skills can be very helpful to a victim of sexual assault, *educationally based counseling is not a replacement for a professional counselor who is trained in the area of sexual assault*. It is important for the educator to know his/her limitations in this area and to encourage

victims/survivors to seek professional help. Having local referrals, and helping the individual to get help—calling to make an appointment, accompanying her/him to the first visit, following up to make sure she/he has gone—are critically important to helping someone to begin the process of healing and recovery. Victims of sexual violence will sometimes feel embarrassed or ashamed of what has happened to them. They may feel responsible in some way. Because of these feelings, often victims are afraid to seek professional help. They may feel that, with time, they can get past the trauma and heal themselves. While these are common feelings, most often they are not accurate. Time can help to ease the pain a victim of sexual assault experiences, but rarely is time enough. The repercussions of sexual assault can last for years and have a devastating impact on a person's life. Survivors of sexual assault can and do go on to lead happy, normal lives. The more support understanding and professional help a person receives, the more quickly and completely the healing process will be.

Summary

Many sexuality-related concerns and problems can be helped significantly through education-based counseling that provides information, permission-giving, support, and understanding. Due to the personal nature of the topic, an effective, nonjudgmental, approachable sexuality educator may find him/herself in great demand by people needing guidance. With some basic counseling skills and knowledge about the most common issues for which people seek help, the educator can serve a very important function as counselor. It is critical to understand one's strengths and one's limitations in providing any kind of sexuality counseling. The educator must be able to identify a problem that requires a specifically trained counselor or therapist, make the proper referral, and then follow up to make sure that the person received the appropriate help. The PLISSIT model for sexual counseling offers helpful guidelines for the counselor to determine both the level and the type of counseling that would be most appropriate for a given situation.

Key Terms

anorgasmia, 161
coming out, 146
Erectile dysfunction, 159
family planning, 147
Female Arousal
  Disorder, 160
Female Orgasmic
  Disorder (or inhibited
  female orgasm), 160
HIV (Human
  Immunodeficiency
  Virus), 155
Hypoactive Sexual
  Desire Disorder (or
  Inhibited Sexual
  Desire [ISD]), 158
PLISSIT, 141

premature
  ejaculation, 159
preorgasmia, 161
sexual assault or
  sexual violence, 163
sexual dysfunction, 158
sexual orientation, 144
Sexual Pain
  Disorder—
  Dyspareunia, 161
sexually transmitted
  infections (STI), 151
theoretical (perfect
  use) failure rate, 149
typical use (actual
  use) failure rate, 149
vaginismus, 161

Questions for Discussion

1. What do you consider to be the most important characteristics of a person providing sexuality counseling?

2. What is the best response to someone who is worried that his/her behavior may not be normal?

3. How does the view of a continuum of sexual orientations affect the way one can provide counseling on the subject?

4. What are some issues a counselor might encourage a person to consider when they are making a decision about whether or not to "come out" at school?

5. How can a counselor's personal beliefs about unintended pregnancy affect his/her ability to provide appropriate counseling to someone facing this issue? What are some things the counselor can do to make sure the person seeking help/advice receives the best possible counseling?

Related Web Sites

http:// www.siecus.org
The Sexuality Information and Education Council of the United States is a national nonprofit organization that promotes comprehensive education about sexuality.

http://planned parenthood.org
Provides sexuality education through a network of affiliates nationwide, offers online brochures.

http:// www.sexuality.org/wc
The Sex Education Web Circle. A ring of Web sites which offer varied contributions to Internet sex education, with the focus on sites that provide factually positive and pleasure-positive materials.

http://www.guttmacher.org
The Allan Guttmacher Institute. Features articles, research, publications, e-lists around the areas of abortion, law and public policy, pregnancy and birth, sexual behavior, sexually transmitted diseases, youth. Links to periodicals such as the Guttmacher Report on Public Policy and Perspectives on Sexual and Reproductive Health.

http://www.sexuality.org
Home page of the Society for Human Sexuality. Links to guides and reviews, essays, and sex-positive community resources.

CHAPTER 9

Aging: Myths and Challenges

LUIS MONTESINOS, PH.D.

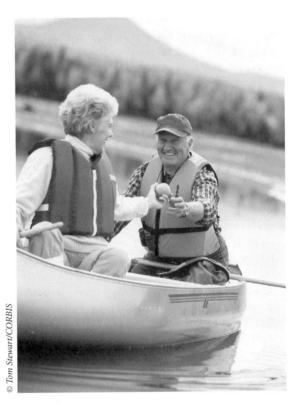

© Tom Stewart/CORBIS

OBJECTIVES

By the end of the chapter, the reader should be able to:

- Describe the impact of changing demographics and epidemiological trends on society

- Discuss the definition and theories of aging

- Relate some of the myths about aging that counselors are likely to encounter

- Name two critical components of "successful aging"

- Describe some of the ways in which health counselors can best serve elderly clients

Demographic Changes

During the past few decades, we have witnessed impressive demographic changes in the world's population. The elderly (individuals over 65 years old) are the segment that is growing most rapidly, increasing to 380 million (a 14 percent increase) between 1990 and 1995. It is expected that between 1996 and 2020 the number of persons over 65 years of age will increase by 82 percent worldwide (110 percent in developing countries and 40 percent in industrialized countries). In not fewer than 10 countries, at least one out of five people will be over 65 years old by the year 2020. In industrialized countries like the United States, people over 65 years old represented 4 percent of the population in the early 1900s. They increased to 11.3 percent by 1980 and it is expected that by 2030 they will represent 21.1 percent of the population. The growth of the group of individuals older than 85 years is even more dramatic. This group has been increasing at rates much higher than any other segment in American society. It is estimated that people who reach 65 years old in the United States can expect at least 12 more years of independent life. Those over 85 years old can expect that at least 50 percent of the rest of their lives will be independent. Because of this and other reasons some authors have suggested the use of the label "young elders" to refer to those individuals over 65 and under 75 years old, and "old elders" for those persons over 85 years old. This makes sense in light of the different life experiences that these groups have had and because patterns of aging might differ between the two groups.

The reduction in infant mortality (due to a better peri- and prenatal attention, better sanitation, and immunization), the decrement of mortality among middle-age individuals, a better control of infectious diseases, and a reduction in birth rates have been signaled as important factors in this demographic change (Gordon, 1987; Perlmutter & Hall, 1985).

There are several important characteristics of this population that will have an impact on future disease prevention and **health promotion.** First, the number of women is and will continue to be larger than the number of men among this segment of the population. It was estimated in 1992 that, among women, mortality rate was 23 percent less than among males. In fact, we can say that aging has become an issue of primary interest to women. Accordingly, the gender factor needs to be considered in any intervention or research program with the elderly.

The second characteristic of this elderly population is that they are well educated, have better access to health services, and have more economic power than previous cohorts. The third characteristic is the great diversity that is found among the

elderly population in terms of attitudes, behaviors, and health status. Aging is infinite in its variety; there is never one pattern that applies to everyone.

The increased interest in this segment of the population has been marked, unfortunately, by an emphasis on the assumed impact that they will have on the costs of health-care services that they will require (due to the expected increase in chronic conditions) and the need to provide support services. It is estimated that by the year 2040 in the United States people over 65 years old will consume almost half of all health resources. Some believe that increases in life expectancy will be unavoidable followed by increases in the prevalence of disability and decreases on quality of life that are associated with chronic conditions in spite of the decline of the incidence of these chronic conditions among the elderly (Spillman & Lubitz, 2000). Health promotion and **disease prevention** efforts with the elderly population are rather recent in contrast to other strategies such as those intended to reduce the incidence of cardiovascular disease (Lovett, 1989). This may be due to certain persistent stereotypes about aging that deemed such efforts unnecessary.

Epidemiological Trends

In the industrialized world infectious diseases are, for the most part, under control (although this statement is argued by some who point to the increasing incidence of tuberculosis, Hepatitis B, and HIV-AIDS). In industrialized countries chronic conditions, especially cancer, cardiovascular diseases, dementia, respiratory problems, and musculoskeletal conditions, are the most prevalent today. These conditions tend to occur later in life. As life expectancy increases, it is expected that their prevalence will increase (World Health Organization, 1987).

In developing countries dramatic increases in life expectancy combined with lifestyles changes

Health promotion. Actions directed to achieve and maintain health through the empowerment of individuals and communities.

Disease prevention. Any efforts, activities or information whose purpose is to prevent diseases and promote good health.

(particularly the adoption of behavioral patterns of the Western countries) may result in global epidemics of cancer and other chronic conditions within the next two decades. This phenomenon has been termed **epidemiological transition** and describes the change in health habits by which developing countries, not only adopt the economic development model of the industrialized countries, but also inherit its high incidence of chronic conditions, unhealthful behavioral patterns (such as smoking, alcohol, and other drug abuse) and the common results of these, which are unintentional injuries, suicide, and increased violence.

Defining Aging

The maximum length of time that an individual has lived has been recorded as 120 years; Shirechiyo Izuni, a Japanese, reached 120 years and 237 days in 1986. He died from pneumonia, escaping from the diseases that often kill individuals in their 60s and 70s. Most gerontologists believe that the secret of longevity lies in the interaction of inheritance, environment, and lifestyle, and Izuni is a perfect example of this.

It is important to distinguish between **primary aging** (the one that occurs as a consequence of the passage of time and it is unavoidable) and **secondary aging** (which occurs because of environmental events and the adoption of certain behavioral patterns). Secondary aging could be avoided if those factors and behaviors were changed. It is highly possible that the great part of

---

Epidemiological transition. The change in health habits by which developing countries not only adopt the economic development model of the industrialized countries, but also inherit its high incidence of chronic conditions and unhealthful behavioral patterns.

Primary aging. Aging that occurs as a consequence of the passage of time and is unavoidable.

Secondary aging. Aging that occurs because of environmental events and the adoption of certain behavioral patterns, and which could be avoided.

---

the decline that is observed among some old persons is due more to this second type of aging than to the aging process itself. This distinction is relevant because sometimes primary aging, which may include some memory decreases, can be confused with early manifestations of diseases such as Alzheimer's, which is not a natural consequence of aging.

Since aging indicates the prospective end of our lives, it is a terminal process (we start to die as soon as we are born, it has been said). Nevertheless, the central issue of aging has been whether there is a biological limit, a maximum duration of life that cannot be overcome no matter how optimum the environment is or how favorable our genetic endowment. In most species, the maximum observed lifespan is equivalent to six times the time elapsed between birth and maturity. In the case of humans, assuming that maturity is achieved at 18–20 years of age, the **maximum range of life** possible would be between 108 and 120 years.

Sanitary improvements, the use of antibiotics, and to a certain extent better medical care have resulted in an increase of the median age of life and an increase in life expectancy. The improvement in the treatment of chronic conditions has made some believe that life expectancy will be extended even more. Diseases that at one point were seen as an inseparable part of the aging process are seen now as preventable or at least controllable through lifestyle changes. For instance, lung diseases can be prevented if people do not smoke or quit smoking, and cardiovascular diseases have been reduced since people have quit smoking, reduced ingestion of saturated fats, and begun to exercise more. On the other hand, there is no evidence that the maximum lifespan of human beings has changed during the last thousand years. However, the scientific advances in genetics and the better understanding of the aging process have reinvigorated the question of maximum lifespan. What *has* increased during the past decades has

---

Maximum range of life. The number of years a species can be expected to live; generally, six times the time elapsed between birth and maturity.

been **life expectancy,** the number of years that on average we can expect to live.

The fact that most species seem to have a maximum range of life suggests a genetic basis for aging. This is supported by certain family clusters that tend to live longer and by the fact that the capacity of human cells to divide is limited.

Very interesting studies have been conducted on caloric restriction. In the study the animal (mostly rats and more recently some primates) is fed with a diet that, although nutritious, is well below the caloric level that was previously ingested. Results from these studies show that animals treated this way are better equipped to deal with diseases and that they have a rate of longevity 60 percent higher than the maximum expected. Rats fed this way lived almost the double amount of time than a control group that was fed as usual. Several studies have found that caloric restriction delays the appearance of chronic conditions (especially cancer) and delays the weakening of the immune system (therefore improving the ability to fight infections). It also improves the capacity to withstand extreme temperatures and diminishes the changes that occur in the intestine and liver as we age, improving glucose metabolism (delaying or preventing the occurrence of diabetes) and increasing muscle strength. In other words, an impressive antiaging effect is seen.

Two Basic Principles of Aging

The Baltimore Longitudinal Study started in 1958 (Shock, 1984) to study the aging process in more than 2,000 people between 20 and 90 or more years old. The earlier sample was composed mainly of white males, but since 1978 women were incorporated and most recently, minorities have been recruited for the study. In the current sample, 13 percent are African Americans. Subjects are evaluated every one or two years in the Center for Gerontological Studies of Baltimore where they

Life expectancy. The number of years that on average we can expect to live.

are medically examined and assessed in terms of their strength, reaction time, body-fat composition, and respiratory capacity. They are also administered memory, learning, and personality tests as well as tests to determine their ways of dealing with stress. The main limitation of the study is that these are volunteers who might be more interested in their health than other segments of the elderly population. The results of the study suggest two basic principles of aging: variability and loss compensation.

Variability

Aging varies dramatically between people and this variation increases as we age; pulmonary function, handshake strength, glucose metabolization, all vary greatly as we age. Even within the same individual there is **variability** in the aging of different organs. It seems that each of the organs has its own internal clock.

Weakening or Decreases in Bodily Function Related to the Development of Diseases. Some weakening thought to be part of the aging process occurs only if a person suffers from certain diseases; testosterone levels, for example, diminish significantly only in very old individuals and only if they are sick. Another interesting aspect of this is that if weakening of normally stable functions occur, this weakening might indicate the likelihood of imminent death. In general, the decrement in the number of lymphocytes, no matter if the person reports any problems or appears healthy in the medical exam, is an indicator of imminent death. The group of individuals who presented a significant decrement in the number of lymphocytes in one control was more likely to have died by the next control. Death was due to a variety of causes.

Loss Compensation

Variability. One of the two basic principles of aging—that aging varies dramatically between people and this variation increases with age.

Another general principle is that if there are any losses in function or capacity of organs or body systems there will be a tendency to make up for it somehow. This is called the principle of **compensation.** For example, in general the loss of neurons is compensated for by the growth of dendrites and new connections.

Theories of Aging

In spite of there being several **theories of aging,** they all basically fall under two approaches: those that assume the existence of a set "program," and those that assume that the process of aging occurs because of "mistakes or accidents."

Random Damages

Random damages refer to the accumulation of failures in the ability of the cell to produce proteins. These proteins provide the support for all cellular functions and reactions. DNA, the genetic material in each cell nucleus, synthesizes RNA that after several steps serves as the mold from which the proteins are formed. In this process, the theory is that the DNA suffers some structural changes, mutations that occur because of environmental and other factors. If these mutations are damaging enough or too numerous they will result in the cell's death. Cells have some corrective mechanisms to repair these damages but as we age mistakes are more frequent and the corrective mechanisms become less efficient. Consequently more errors are accumulated in the DNA and more damaged proteins are produced, which results in more cells working poorly and eventually dying.

> **Compensation.** One of the two basic principles of aging—If there are any losses in function or capacity of organs or body systems there will be a tendency to compensate for it somehow.
>
> **Theories of aging.** The rationale for how and why we age; usually either assuming the existence of a set "program" for aging or assuming that "mistakes" or "accidents" cause aging to occur.

The Free Radicals. Cells produce some waste that is excreted. These substances can permeate and cover other cells' membranes, impairing their functioning and causing their death. They can also produce some internal damage affecting the DNA. Free radicals are molecular fragments that are secreted by cells. There is evidence that antioxidants (vitamins C and E) that neutralize these substances can prolong life in animals and prevent further disability in humans.

Programmed Theories

This approach assumes that there is an organized, predictable way in which changes occur as we age. Furthermore, as we pointed out before, the fact that all species seem to have a maximum range of age possible also gives support to the notion that aging and death are genetically programmed.

The aging clock might be located in each cell, affecting the protein production through the DNA, or be centralized in a system responsible for the coordination of a great amount of body functions. If this were the case, the most likely candidates would be the hypothalamus and the immune system.

The hypothalamus is a small structure responsible for the coordination of activities like eating, sexual behavior, body temperature, and emotional expression. It serves a fundamental role in the regulation of physical growth, sexual maturity, and reproduction, because of its central role in hormone production. Its responsibility in the aging of at least one body system is clearly demonstrated, controlling estrogen production by the ovaries which precipitates menopause and prevents conception.

Another area of interest for researchers relates to the effect that certain hormones have on the immune system. Estrogen levels affect IL-2, and if one of these decreases the other one decreases as well. IL-2 (Inter-Leukin-2) also known as T-Cell Growth Factor (TGF) is secreted by stimulated Helper T-Cells, CytoToxic T-Cells (CD8+) and Large Granular Lymphocytes (LGL). IL-2 promotes proliferation (colonal expansion) and differentation of additional CD4+ cells. Pituitary hormones (growth and prolactin) also affect the system. Pituitary cells implanted in old rats induce the thymus to grow to its juvenile size and increase the number of helper T cells.

The Immune System. The disappearance of the thymus has been speculated as a pacemaker of aging, because its disappearance signals an important weakening of the immune system with vast consequences.

The ability to distinguish foreign substances that must be attacked diminishes as we age, which explains why elderly individuals have more difficulty recuperating from infections and are more prone to cancer. It is believed that cancerous cells are produced all the time and that if our immune system is working appropriately it should be capable of detecting and destroying them. It is also believed that immune system deficiencies can result in the incapacity to recognize the body's own cells, confusing them with foreign elements and attacking them (as in the case of lupus).

It is well known that the body's defenses diminish with age. Within the complex immune system, lymphocytes are of special interest for gerontologists. They fall into two categories: (1) B cells that mature in the bone marrow and which have as one of their functions the secretion of antibodies in response to infectious agents or antigens; (2) T cells develop in the thymus and diminish as we age. They are divided into Cytotoxic T cells that attack infected or damaged cells directly and Helper T cells that produce lymphokines that mobilize other substances and cells of the immune system.

As we age, the number of T cells remains constant, but they functionally decline with age. One of the T cells products, interleukins (messengers that take signals that regulate the immune response), vary with age. Some of them, like interleukin 6, increase with age, which is thought to interfere with the immune response. Others, like interleukin 2, which stimulates the proliferation of T cells, tend to diminish with age.

Aging Mythology

I would like now to address some common myths and beliefs with respect to the elderly. I believe it is important that the health-care practitioner be aware of these myths because they might affect his/her perceptions of the clients and consequently the actions he/she recommends.

Myth: Being Old Is Being Ill

The first myth refers to the expectation that to be old means to be ill (Verbrugge, 1984). In spite of the prevalence of chronic conditions among the elderly (arthritis affects approximately 50 percent; hypertension and cardiovascular diseases near 30 percent; diabetes almost 11 percent; auditory problems 32 percent; cataracts 17 percent, and other forms of vision problems affect 9 percent), several studies have demonstrated the falsehood of this statement. First, it must be considered that there has been an important reduction in the risk factors associated with almost all of these conditions. For example, with hypertension, levels of cholesterol and rates of smoking have decreased. Second, the incidence of arthritis, arteriosclerosis, and dementia has diminished, and dental health has improved markedly. Finally, the most important aspect is the impact that these diseases are having on the quality of life of persons affected by them, in their capacity to remain self-sufficient and independent. Factors of independence include the capacity to engage in personal-care activities (dress, bathe, go to the toilet, eat, walk), and nonpersonal activities or home-management problems (prepare foods, buy groceries and other necessities, pay bills, use the phone, clean the house, read, and write).

These studies strongly suggest that a great number of people will age successfully and will not be demented and/or disabled. In fact, in the United States, the number of people living in nursing homes has decreased over the past decades (from 6.3 percent in 1983 to 5.2 percent in 1997) (Kastenbaum, 2000). Some of the reasons for this decline include lower levels of disability as well as the availability of other alternatives (Bishop, 1999; Flowers, 2000). This has prompted some authors to suggest that it is very likely that in the future we will observe a bimodal distribution among the elderly, with a segment suffering chronic conditions and being unable to live independently while the other segment will enjoy good health and will be able to live independently probably until their death.

A survey conducted in 1994 found that among persons 65 to 74 years old 81 percent did not present any level of disability. For those between 75 and 84 years old the percentage was 73 percent, and 40 percent among those over 85 years (Rowe & Kahn, 1998).

We must remember that among the elderly, disability results from the impact of one or more diseases, and from factors related with lifestyle and biological changes. In estimating disability (the effect that chronic conditions might produce in the levels of independence) the crucial factor is the person's perception. In spite of having one or more chronic conditions and several limitations, a person might still rank their health status as good or very good. In the same survey mentioned above (Rowe & Kahn, 1998), 39 percent of individuals over 65 years ranked their health as very good or excellent vis-a-vis 29 percent who considered it regular or poor. Among those over 85, 31 percent ranked their health as very good or excellent vis-a-vis 36 percent who ranked it as regular or poor. It is likely that these percentages will change as younger adults adopt healthier lifestyles that could avoid or delay the occurrence of chronic conditions. Also related is the finding that the levels of perceived stress diminish as people age.

Myth: Learning Stops with Age

The second aging myth is related to the existence of limits in our capacity to learn. Certainly as we age there are some restrictions in the amount as well as the pace of our learning. Tasks that require perceptual speed, physical coordination, and strength are more difficult and sometimes impossible to complete. In spite of this the elderly brain is able to make new connections, absorb new data, and learn new skills. There is a growing evidence that an enriched environment can affect the way neurons behave, resulting in the growth of dendrites even in very advanced ages. The fact is that the capacity to learn is preserved and can even improve, particularly in areas that are of interest to the person. Physical activity has been

found to be essential in the maintenance of our cognitive capacities; a healthy cardiovascular system is important because it supplies the brain with oxygen. In fact there is a very clear association between cardiovascular diseases and mental-activity impairment. Moreover, those individuals who keep a physically active life tend to experience weakening of their cognitive skills much later in life, if at all.

Learning capacity might also be affected by sensory changes (vision and audition). This requires a change in the pace of teaching, the use of multiple modalities, new activities, interesting methods that make some sense in the context of the person's life. In fact, the differences that have been found between young and older individuals might be a result of the time limitations and the anxiety produced by the testing situation rather than of age.

At least three factors have been identified as predictors of a lesser decrement of cognitive abilities as we age. The first and best predictor is educational level: the higher the educational level, the lesser the impairment. This is probably related to the fact that those who have higher educational levels also tend to be healthier. The second predictor is the pulmonary capacity, strictly related with regular physical activity, which most likely permits a better circulation and oxygenation of the blood that flows to the brain. The third predictor is the level of self-efficacy, the belief in one's personal skills of being able to influence what happens in daily life (Albert et al., 1995; Greider, 1996).

Myth: Memory Loss Is Inevitable

Loss of memory is neither a necessary part of the aging process nor a predictor of incipient dementia. A great number of studies have demonstrated that short-term memory can be improved by writing lists and memory training through different activities. In fact there is growing evidence that if an organ is not used its capacities are lost—"use it or lose it" (Burack, 1996). It seems that memory works in different ways as we age. There are three types of memory. The first is *sensory,* which deals with the perception of sounds and images that although perceived are not stored for future use (the aging process seem not to affect this type of memory). The second type, *short-term,* refers to those things that are remembered momentarily and then forgotten, while others (those that are relevant for the individual) are stored in the long-term memory. This last type, *long-term* memory, seems to have a limitless capacity and to not be affected (it might take longer to scan it) by age. What happens as we age is that short-term memory becomes less efficient, causing storing and retrieval to be impaired. The way in which the information is stored becomes relevant. If it is stored in ways that are important for the person, then the capacity of remembering increases. Likewise, the context in which remembering is attempted will make a difference in the capacity to remember.

The potential of learning among the elderly has slowly began to be understood by educational institutions that are in increasing numbers offering programs in different modalities for elderly individuals. It is likely that the demographic revolution, which the increased number of elderly individuals represents, will trigger a revision of the content and forms in which higher education is provided.

Myth: Weakness Is to Be Expected

A fourth belief or myth is that aging will necessarily be associated with a continuous and progressive weakening. This myth originates in cross-sectional studies that found that after 20 years of age, performance starts declining and worsens as elderly groups are tested. The trend was more obvious in reasoning scales that required the capacity to solve nonverbal problems very rapidly. In verbal tests the impairment was much slower and occurred dramatically only after age 65. Longitudinal studies, however, found that results in verbal tests were relatively stable and that there was even an improvement during middle adulthood (35–54 years). With respect to nonverbal tests, these studies also found that there was a weakening, although not as pronounced as that reported by cross-sectional studies.

In an attempt to explain these findings some authors have suggested that there are two types of intelligence, the crystallized and the fluid. *Crystallized intelligence* reflects the way in which we have absorbed the accumulated knowledge in our own culture, the amount of knowledge that we have accumulated throughout our lives. This is the type of intelligence that verbal tests assess. *Fluid intelligence,* on the other hand, refers to the capacity of reasoning in a correct and quick way when trying to solve new problems. It is thought that fluid intelligence follows the course of physiological deterioration while crystallized intelligence, being based in our accumulated knowledge, can remain stable or even improve as we age.

The Seattle Longitudinal study confirmed the difference reported by previous studies with respect to verbal and nonverbal abilities. The interesting additional finding was that at 60 years of age all participants experimented some loss in one aspect of their intelligence (Schaie 1996). In spite of this and even among individuals 80 years or older there was not one individual who presented losses in all five intelligence aspects assessed. This means that changes in intellectual abilities are multidirectional and specific for each individual, and that instead of making generalizations we should be focusing on the conditions and contexts that promote intelligence during the aging process.

Of course, intellectual deterioration will be mediated by diseases, especially cardiovascular diseases. In fact, some studies have found that abrupt changes in the typical pattern (dramatic deterioration of crystallized intelligence) may be an indicator of imminent death. This has been labeled *terminal fall hypothesis* and has been confirmed in studies in Germany, Sweden, and the United States. In the Seattle study it was found that dramatic changes in crystallized intelligence were associated with mortality. It is possible that since the usual pattern is stability, when there are dramatic changes it may indicate very negative happenings in the organism.

Although some functions can be lost as people age, most of them can be recuperated or even improved. It is never too late to engage in healthy habits and enjoy the benefits of those changes. In a couple of months the ex-smoker will feel the benefits; in 5 years the risk of having heart problems is similar to that of someone who has never smoked, and in 15 years the risk of having lung cancer is similar to that of individuals who never smoked (Hermanson, 1988). With respect to obesity, especially the "apple" shape that is associated with cardiovascular disease risk, it can be reversed by adopting a healthy diet and engaging in exercise.

Finally it is important to point out that in spite of a decrement in the nervous system function, the respiratory capacity, vision and audition, and the weakening of strength, the body of a 65-year-old person is perfectly capable of dealing with the demands of daily life. Most decrements in physical capacity are avoidable and reversible. Physical exercise increases muscle size, strength, and fitness. An active mental stimulation and maintaining social relations with friends and family has also been associated with better physical functioning.

A fourth belief relates to genetics as the determinant factor in the way we age. However, in spite of the significant relationship between genetics and life expectancy (longevity among fraternal twins is more variable than among identical twins), a strong influence of psychosocial factors has also been reported. It has been found that for most disorders the environment in which the person lives and the behaviors in which she or he engages have a powerful impact on the development of chronic conditions (World Health Organization, 1997). It is estimated that only 30 percent of physical aging can be attributed to genetic factors; moreover, it is believed that genetic relevance diminishes as we age. The way in which we live and where we live are the most important factors that determine the changes in our hearts, immune system, lungs, bones, brain, and kidneys.

The fifth myth refers to difficulties in the sexual response. In general there is a decrease in the frequency and strength of the sexual response with age but there is a great variability in this area. In women the production of progesterone and estrogen diminishes and eventually ceases completely. As estrogen diminishes the uterus shrinks, the vaginal walls lose elasticity, get dryer and thicker, and changes occur in the breasts and skin.

Estrogen replacement therapy has beneficial effects in the control of hot flushes, the lessening of the risk of developing cardiovascular diseases, and seems to help in the prevention and delaying of osteoporosis. On the other hand it seems to increase the risk of developing breast cancer. Those estrogen meds that do not contain progesterone have been associated with an increased risk of ovarian cancer. This means that women need to be informed before deciding whether to take estrogen replacement therapy. In addition, there are constantly new developments and findings in this area which can complicate the decision process.

For many women menopause is a welcome change and some will report a higher level of sexual satisfaction. As with menarche there is a great variability among women.

In the male, changes are related to the erection, which is not as firm and takes a longer time to occur. This might increase anxiety and fear and avoidance responses may occur. There is a nonsignificant decrement in testosterone and in spite of a reduction in the number of spermatozoids, the male continues being able to procreate until a very advanced age. Testosterone replacement has been explored as an alternative to help individuals with problems but the associated risk of prostate cancer makes it only an experimental treatment.

The other big change that occurs in the male is related to the prostate. Approximately 80 percent of individuals 60 years old experience an enlargement that compresses the urinary tract and restricts urination. This might require a surgical intervention with the risk of damaging some adjacent nerves and the consequent problems with erection and urination.

In general the sexual activity of the male diminishes, but again there is a great variability between subjects. Chronological age seems not to be a critical factor. Those individuals who have been sexually active all their life are likely to continue being so during their elder years. This obviously requires a certain level of fitness, so those who engage in exercise and keep a healthy diet have a greater likelihood of having an active sexual life.

In males it is the presence of chronic conditions and medication that explains the alterations in sexual response. In females, regularity of sexual activity is more related with the accessibility to a partner. For instance, females' sexual response is more affected when their partner dies than males are.

It has also been stated that sexual repertoire increases as we age. It seems that elders practice a broader number of sexual behaviors where caressing, hugging, and feeling loved are more important than penetration or achieving orgasm (Segraves & Segraves, 1995), preferring a sexual activity oriented more to the whole person and not just the genitals. Maybe because of this satisfaction, sexual activity increases among couples that have been together for long periods of time.

Some authors have speculated that the rate of females to males resulting from the increase in longevity will affect sexual behavior in at least two ways: first, is possible that homosexual activity will increase among women (especially among those individuals from the baby-boom generation that tend to be more liberal in these matters). Second, it is also likely that serial monogamy (common among younger generations today) will be adopted as a normal pattern among the elderly.

The sixth myth is related to the notion that elderly people are a heavy load for the rest of society since they do not participate in productive tasks. In part this erroneous belief is born by a misunderstanding of what is defined as productive work. If all the nonremunerated activities in which the elderly participate were to be considered, this view would change dramatically. Elderly people participate in numerous activities socially relevant (volunteerism, taking care of family members) (Morgan, 1986). We must promote the notion that all activities that are socially relevant should be considered productive and that therefore individuals performing those tasks should be considered productive. This has relevance not only in overcoming the biased perception of the elderly but also in how resources are assigned in a society (Rowe & Kahn, 1998).

The truth is that the majority of the elderly are prepared and willing to work, that a great number of them *do* work, and that there is continuing discrimination when it comes to hiring or promotion. More recently the notion of the need to employ gerontologists in business and industry

has been advanced. The elderly could play a great role as providers of factual information about aging to employees, as well as educators, counselors, and researchers for aging employees (Langer, 2001).

Successful Aging: A Quality-of-Life Issue

We have suggested that the emphasis should be placed on quality of life (**health expectancy**) and not life expectancy. This is defined as the number of expected healthy years, the number of years that the person can expect to live in a positive state of self-sufficiency. Although this is a difficult concept to assess, it seems to be more appropriate than life expectancy.

Successful aging is conceptually and philosophically opposite to what is commonly understood as "normal aging." Successful aging is determined basically by a low risk of disease and disability, good cognitive and physical functioning, and an active participation in society. These three elements are closely related to being free of disease and disability, which makes it more likely to maintain physical and mental functioning and to participate actively in society (Rowe & Kahn, 1998).

The low risk of developing diseases or disability as a consequence implies the absence or reduction of risk factors. Most chronic conditions are preceded by signs of future problems; these are unfortunately ignored by a good number of physicians who attribute them to the aging process. Slight increases in diastolic pressure, of abdominal fat, of sugar levels, and decrements in lung, kid-

Health expectancy. The number of years that a person can expect to live in a positive state of self-sufficiency.

Successful aging. Maintaining a low risk of disease and disability, good cognitive and physical functioning and an active participation in society throughout all stages of life.

neys, and immune system functioning are clear precursors of future more serious problems. One of the possible reasons why these signs are ignored is because they can be very subtle and gradual. Moreover some of them have only recently been pointed out as risk factors after some longitudinal studies and technological advances have taken place.

Very few things produce as much fear as the idea of having to depend on others for our basic needs, of not being independent. Not being able to live in a personal space, or take care of oneself, to dress, wash, do things around the house, buy, prepare food, and in some countries to drive is seen as highly undesirable and horrifying by many. However most of these fears are exaggerated. For example, the fear of developing Alzheimer's disease is not consistent with the fact that only 10 percent of individuals over 65, are likely to suffer from it. Moreover it is likely that there are different degrees of the disease; it has been found that even if there are brain changes consistent with the disease many individuals are able to maintain their cognitive abilities intact (Snowdon, 1997). With respect to the genetic components in the disease, although being very strong in those cases of early occurrence, even identical twins who develop the disease do not do it at the same time. This calls for the research of environmental and nutritional factors that could be avoided or altered.

There is obviously some weakening of cognitive abilities as we age, but as pointed out, when referring to intellectual abilities, rarely are all areas affected. The majority of them only occur rather late in life and a great number of people are never affected by these changes at all (Schaie & Willis, 1986).

Today we know that most of the changes that were previously considered intrinsic to the aging process are in reality a consequence of extrinsic factors (like not exercising or not engaging in mental activities). The problem then is that individuals over 65 years old do not engage in any kind of physical activity (less than 7 percent of people over 65 years old participate in some type of exercise to improve resistance) and much less in activities that stimulate their cognitive capacities.

Some time ago the stereotype (fortunately not so prevalent today) was that the main task of elderly people was to retire and leave their place for the new generations. It is increasingly clear that maintaining an activity level in tasks that are meaningful and keeping significant relationships with others are basic for the preservation of health throughout life.

People over 65 are taking more control of their lives by adopting healthier lifestyles. The most significant study in this area was done during the 1960s in Alameda County, California. Its objective was to study the effects of different lifestyles on morbidity and mortality. Thousands of residents in that San Francisco suburb were surveyed with respect to their health conditions, gender, social class, and race as well as health practices and social relationships. Specific behaviors were explored (physical activity, smoking, weight maintenance, drinking, sleeping, having breakfast, and social relationships) and were found to be associated with morbidity and mortality. The effects were found even at very advanced ages. In the next sections we will examine some of these behaviors in more detail as they relate to the elderly population.

The Relevance of Physical Exercise

The control of infectious conditions has been achieved thanks to public health interventions and medical advances (immunizations, better treatments). This model of action has proven to be less effective and efficient when dealing with chronic conditions. The management of these conditions needs to emphasize prevention of early occurrence, delay of development in adult life, reduction of detrimental effects, and the provision of a supportive social environment for those who are disabled by them. These diseases are for the most part caused by multiple factors. Biological, psychological, and social variables have been implicated in their etiology. Predisposing inherited factors and lifestyle (smoking, excessive drinking, unhealthy diet, and lack of physical activity) are known risk factors. Some of these factors can be controlled by informed individuals, but others, like the effects of poverty, genetic predisposition, and occupational hazards, may be things over which the person has little or no control (World Health Organization, 1997).

Among the chronic conditions, cardiovascular diseases are the most important at a global level. It has been clearly demonstrated that there are some specific behaviors associated with the incidence of those conditions. It has also been demonstrated that most of these factors start operating in childhood. Hypertension, smoking, eating habits (specifically the consumption of saturated fats), high levels of low-density lipoproteins, lack of physical exercise, obesity, and diabetes are major risk factors. The person could minimize these risks by adopting specific behavioral patterns

Among those specific behaviors, exercise is potentially the most modifiable and the one that can have the greatest impact on risk factors. A general decline in physical capacity is accepted as a normal part of the process of aging; however, that is not necessarily the case and the progressive decline of our physical capacity does not need to occur. On the contrary, it can be prevented by the adoption of a lifestyle that includes regular **exercise** throughout our lifespan. Both aerobic exercise and weight lifting have proven to be effective in improving physical well-being. Even older individuals can improve their aerobic capacity by just walking 45 minutes three times a week. Weightlifting increases the size and strength of muscles. In both cases, the critical aspect is the frequency, intensity, and duration of exercise. Both types of exercise increase metabolism and help in reducing excessive weight and dealing with depression. Physical exercise increases strength, decreases the risk of death, improves mood (helps coping with stress), improves aerobic capacity, and reduces the impact of other risk factors. This protective effect of exercise occurs even at advanced ages and for individuals who have never before engaged in physical activities or who are suffering from chronic conditions (Hickey et al., 1995). Motivat-

Exercise. Planned physical activity designed to improve physical fitness.

ing individuals to engage in physical activity has been the subject of several studies. Among them, the use of physician-delivery counseling to promote physical activity has been found successful with the elderly (Goldstein et al., 1999).

Exercise has demonstrated to be beneficial not only in the prevention of coronary diseases, but also in the prevention and reversal of hypertension (where it is used as an adjunctive treatment to medication), as protection from colon cancer, in the prevention of diabetes, in the treatment of arthritis, in the prevention of osteoporosis (exercises that put some weight on the bones such as jogging, walking, and weight lifting, have been found to strengthen bones and therefore prevent osteoporosis).

Improved muscle tone and greater strength can also help to prevent falls and maintain independence and the ability to engage in daily life activities (most of which will require some resistance capacity, like getting up from a chair). Moreover, physical activity neutralizes the malignant effects of other risk factors such as smoking, and high sugar and cholesterol levels. As mentioned before these effects make physical activity the most important protective behavior in which an individual can get involved (King, 1991).

In addition, physical exercise not only has an impact on quality of life but also can increase life expectancy. A follow-up of 40,000 postmenopausal women found that those who exercise regularly had a 20 percent less chance of dying over a period of seven years (Rowe & Kahn, 1998). Another study found that exercise could strengthen muscles, improve mobility, and reduce frailty even in people over 90 years old.

Case Study

Maggie

Maggie, at 64 years old and a smoker for over 10 years, had begun to feel run down and exhausted for no reason. She was about 20 pounds overweight and drank 10 or more cups of coffee a day. Anne, the health counselor, learned that although Maggie wanted to feel better in general, she had no intention of giving up coffee or cigarettes. Maggie did strongly want to lose weight however, and was not adverse to incorporating an exercise program into her life. Rather than aggressively try to persuade Maggie that she needed to give up coffee and cigarettes, Anne decided to focus on exercise and nutrition, since she knew that both smoking and excessive coffee drinking could deplete the body of essential vitamins and nutrients. Anne referred Maggie to a nutritionist and helped her to devise a plan for modifying her eating and physical activities throughout the day. Anne did, of course, stress the increased benefit of quitting smoking and reducing caffeine intake, but she did not push the point since her client was already defensive about these habits. Anne knew that becoming more physically fit and active often naturally leads to a decreased desire to use harmful substances and behaviors. Since losing weight was Maggie's greatest motivation, as well as diminishing chronic fatigue, the health counselor decided to focus her strategy on the client's immediate goals. She also had to be sensitive to Maggie's age and life experiences, and not attempt too drastic a change that might be unrealistic. Assessing the client's goals helped her plan how best to respond.

The Impact of Social Support

Social support is defined as information that permits the person to believe that he/she is loved, cared for, and belongs to a network of relationships with rights and obligations. The association between social relationships and longevity, the discovery that social support is at the base of these associations, and the special role that social support plays in the aging process has only recently been addressed (Unger et al., 1997). On the other hand, it has become clearer that loneliness has serious adverse effects in the elderly (Cohen, 2000). As mentioned before the seminal article in the area was the one conducted in Alameda County, Cali-

Social support. The assistance received by the others in one's life, which may be emotional, financial, spiritual, practical or informational in nature.

fornia (Berkman & Breslow, 1983) that found a very strong association between social isolation and life expectancy. An indicator of social network was built based on marital status, contact with friends and family, and church attendance. It was found that those who were more socially isolated had twice the mortality rate than those who were more connected. The effect was found even in the most advanced ages. The study also found that more than the quantity it was the quality of relationships (they were to be selected by the person, provide him/her with emotional support, and be available in times of stress) that was responsible for the protective effect.

The lack of social relationships is an important risk factor for poor health. Social support (emotional or tangible) has positive effects on the health of individuals. It can reduce or diminish the effects of the so-called "normal aging." Elderly individuals who maintain an independent life attribute it to their friends who permit them to be active and emotionally secure.

Individuals who have less and weaker relationships have a risk of dying that is four times higher than that for individuals with a higher level of social support. This has been found to be true independent of age and other factors such as socioeconomic status, physical health, smoking, use of alcohol, obesity, and use of health-care services.

The interaction with persons whom we believe care for us and esteem us and the feeling of belonging to a group is related with a lower risk of arthritis, tuberculosis, depression, and alcoholism. People with higher levels of social support tend to use fewer painkillers and recover more rapidly after surgical procedures. They also tend to adhere better to prescribed treatments.

Emotional social support (direct expressions of love, affection, and respect) is essential for successful aging (Sabin, 1993). Instrumental social support (direct assistance when sick, transportation, money) seems not to be as important. This may be because sometimes the one providing that type of assistance threatens the independence of the one receiving it. Instead of increasing self-efficacy this kind of help may sometimes result in "learned helplessness" (Adams & Blieszner, 1995).

A recent study using elder Myocardial Infarction survivors as peer advisors found that the benefits of social support might be not only for the receiver but also for the one providing the support. Peer advisors were as likely to benefit from the interaction with their advisees as those receiving the support. It was found that helping, mutual sharing, committing, and benefiting were characteristics of the experience (Whittemore et al., 2000). Because of their personal experience of recovery these individuals were in a unique position to offer a form of social support that complemented very well the work of health professionals.

Dying with Dignity

Because of the increasing number of individuals of advanced age and the control of infectious diseases it is likely that in the near future death will be for many people the consequence of chronic or degenerative diseases. This means that a good number of people will spend days if not weeks in the process of dying.

Thinking about **death and dying** can either be a cause of anxiety or, as Eriksson suggests, a positive experience when it is accepted as a natural event after having lived a fulfilling life. Medicine with all its positive impact has nothing to offer in this area. A recent study found that in their last days 40 percent of terminal patients who were hospitalized suffered pain that could be avoided, and 80 percent suffered severe fatigue. Pain can (and should) be controlled with drugs, and fatigue with well-prescribed steroids. It is absolutely essential that medical schools prepare physicians to help people make decisions in end-of-life situations.

Until very recently, in most Western societies, prolonging life was the obvious response to an imminent death. Technology today permits us to prolong life even when the person is in coma or continuous pain. People are kept alive by the combination of five different techniques: cardiopulmonary resuscitation, mechanical lungs, dialysis, intravenous feeding, and antibiotics. The results of this, according to some, is an ignominious and degrading death. Some have suggested that instead of trying to prolong life we should try to help people die with dignity, that the dying person should have a choice. In this way, the dying person would have some degree of control over the way they die. This approach has resulted in the renewal of the hospice movement, where no technology to prolong life is used but where affect, care, and relief from pain are provided. The emergence of hospice care has provided a valuable alternative, enabling more people to end their lives in their own home or in that of a family member (Kastenbaum, 2000).

In order to use these services the person must relinquish all medical treatment and a physician must estimate that the individual will die within the next 6 months. Chemotherapy, blood transfusions, or the use of artificial lungs or intravenous feeding will be suspended. Most of the individuals who use this kind of service have cancer (71 percent) and more than 70 percent are over 65 years of age.

The service is delivered in either the home or a specialized agency and it does not end with the death of the person. A very important component is the counseling provided to the family during the hospice period and after death. The emphasis goes beyond just accepting death; it is what some call the good death, dying well and with dignity.

This is obviously not for everyone. As people die they can become incontinent, might require help in the most private things, might not want to express some emotions (anger, anxiety, sadness) out of fear of depressing others. However, it is thought that if the appropriate support services are provided for the individual and the family, death can be a growing experience for a great majority of individuals.

Some hospice providers are opposed to assisted suicide (they view it as an easy escape from a complex situation), while others believe this is not an incompatible alternative. The discussion has centered on the question of whether the person (with a terminal disease with unbearable pain) has the right to suspend treatment, or require assisted suicide or euthanasia (Kelner, 1995).

Death and dying. Death is a process of transition that starts with dying and ends with being dead. Also refers to the point at which a person is declared physically dead. Dying is the irreversible and progressive period in which the organism loses its viability.

One of the most common problems of dying with dignity is that people do not establish clearly what kind of treatment they would like to receive when and if they are in this type of situation. This is important because it has been found that both physicians and family members are not good at predicting what the person would like to do if extraordinary resuscitation measures were required. Physicians tend to underestimate while spouses tend to overestimate the preferences of the dying person (Uhlmann et al., 1988). There is some evidence that indicates that elderly individuals when they are healthy express a preference for having control over the time, way, and circumstances of their death. However, when seriously ill they are much less inclined to make their own decisions (Kelner, 1995). It has been suggested that it is important that people have a living will where they clearly stipulate what they want to do in case they are incapacitated and cannot make a decision.

Death is a natural process and when there is no cure, the best alternative is to try to provide a good death. (Corr & Corr 1992) has described several criteria that make a good death.

1. Free of pain; no one wants to die in severe pain.

2. Reduce fear anxiety and increase feeling of control.

3. Emphasize significant social relationships, be surrounded by those whom we care about.

4. Have a sense of integrity and accomplishment in our lives.

5. Not feel that we are an economic burden for our family

Case Study

Assisting in Nursing Homes, Assisting Families

When Max, a father and grandfather in his mid-eighties, could not recover from the pneumonia that put him in the hospital, his family was faced with the difficult decision of putting him in a nursing home. His Alzheimer's which had been slight before, suddenly grew much worse and he could not remember his family except on occasional moments. Soon it became a regular aspect of the family's life to visit the nursing home. His wife especially needed support emotionally and sought the help of the on-site counselor to work through her conflicting feelings of guilt and fear for the future. The nursing home had directed her to local support groups, but she felt not ready to take that step. She was also in her eighties and was overwhelmed and feeling uncared for and unsupported herself. She was terrified by the prospect of being left alone, and also by the prospect of having to care for her husband at home should he have to be brought home due to financial reasons. Clearly she needed to sort out her options realistically with someone who could understand her emotional dilemma. She was falling into a serious depression.

Sharon, the health counselor at the nursing home, helped the wife express her feelings and assess her situation clearly. It was decided through therapeutic conversation that the wife would be physically unable to care for her husband at home without full-time help. Her husband's Alzheimer's was something that the wife felt unequipped to deal with emotionally on a daily basis, with no in-home help. Additionally, the wife was clearly suffering from grief and depression. She was already taking so many medications for various conditions that she did not want to take an antidepressant. Sharon asked her about her social support network, friends, and so on, and found that the wife had virtually no support system outside her family, who were only present intermittently since they all lived some distance away. Sharon emphasized the need for the wife to get out of the house and establish connections with other women her age, since the wife could drive and expressed a longing for human connection. In addition, Sharon worked up a very gentle exercise plan with the wife, which had a twofold purpose. First, exercise would directly affect the wife's state of mind and take her mind off her present situation. Secondly, it would strengthen her and keep her mobile, which would ease her fears about her own future incapacitation. The yoga-based stretching exercises would calm her mind and promote relaxation. One of the obstacles Sharon faced was the wife's sense of guilt that she should think of herself at all with her husband in the state he was in. Sharon explained to her that if she wanted to be there for her husband, and if she wanted to gain better peace of mind in order to make important decisions, she needed to take care of herself. This validation seemed to be exactly what the wife was needing to hear.

She still had a difficult road up until her husband's eventual death, but she did not let herself sink into a depression, and sought out the counsel of Sharon many times for health and psychological issues that she faced, as well as for nutritional and other support regarding her husband. Sharon had clearly filled a gap in this setting that otherwise must be filled with support groups only. In the difficult context of nursing homes where families are deciding the lives of their loved ones, health counselors can be a tremendous asset. Medical personnel for the most part do not have the time to spend with families and individuals in need of mental-health or health-related counseling.

Summary

The increase in the number of individuals over 65 years of age in most parts of the world is having a great impact. Historically in the study of aging, the perceptual and cognitive changes have been emphasized. However, due to demographic changes and to the improvement of research methodology this limited view of this particular developmental stage has been changing. The persistence of myths and stereotypes such as that aging will necessarily translate into disease, that elderly people are conservative and do not like to change, and that working with them is very depressing are slowly giving ground to a new way of viewing the elderly. Several studies conducted during the past few decades have demonstrated the fallacy of these statements; among these studies, the Baltimore Longitudinal Study on Aging has been seminal in the field (Shock et al., 1984).

Aging does not necessarily mean that the person will unavoidably slide into a stage of disability, loneliness, and physical and mental impairment. It has been established that most of the functional losses that were thought to be part of the aging process such as mobility and memory problems can be prevented or delayed (Schaie,

1994). Efforts in these areas will necessarily be multidisciplinary. The goal of any intervention with this group should be to increase the quality of life as opposed to increasing life expectancy—health expectancy as opposed to life expectancy. This same idea is what the World Health Organization has termed DALE (Disability Absent Life Expectancy), to refer to the number of years a person is expected to live without any problems that impact substantially on their quality of life (World Health Organization, 2000).

The health-care professional preparing to work with the elderly must be aware of the process of aging and be able not only to help those in need of services but also to implement interventions to promote health and prevent or delay the occurrence of disease in the elderly.

For the last few decades, the number of articles and conference presentations devoted to the elderly has increased enormously, and we should expect this trend to continue in the near future. Likewise, the role of health professionals in health promotion, disease prevention, and coping with chronic conditions among this segment of the population will also increase. It is also expected that the use of counseling services among the elderly will see some changes. Although older adults have historically underutilized these services, it is likely that the number of older adults seeking counseling and therapy will increase (Lewis, 2001). Giordano (2000) has suggested that future counselors should be trained in age-sensitive communication skills that are intended to preserve self-esteem and support self-determination while at the same time generating more accurate information to help the client.

Most if not all the problems that are associated with aging are behavioral in nature. A serious problem in the delivery of services to the elderly is that the health-care professions have focused mostly on the management of acute and chronic conditions with little or no emphasis on health promotion and prevention (Rowe, 1999). By paying more attention to these factors, chronic conditions that are highly prevalent among the elderly—such as diabetes, cardiovascular diseases, and arthritis—could be prevented or delayed.

Key Terms

compensation, 171
death and dying, 180
disease prevention, 168
epidemiological
  transition, 169
exercise, 178
health expectancy, 176
health promotion, 168
life expectancy, 170

maximum range
  of life, 169
primary aging, 169
secondary aging, 169
social support, 179
successful aging, 176
theories of aging, 171
variability, 170

Questions for Discussion

1. Discuss the impact of demographic changes in our understanding of aging. What are your beliefs and values when it comes to aging?

2. What do we understand by successful aging? Do you have examples of successful aging in your life?

3. Discuss three of the myths associated with aging. Provide evidence that prove them incorrect. What other evidence can you find that illustrates American society's views of aging and of old age?

4. What are the changes that occur in the sexual response of the female and the male as we age?

How would you respond to an elderly male or female who complained of feeling no sexual desire anymore, differing from his or her spouse?

5. Discuss the major issues surrounding death and dying. How would you discuss quality of life with a chronically ill or bedridden patient?

Related Web Sites

http://www.aoa.dhhs.gov
The site of the U. S. government Administration on Aging office. Provides statistical and governmental reports on aging.

http://www.aarp.org
The site of the American Association of retired persons, an organization dedicated to shaping and enriching the quality of life of aging individuals.

http://aging.ufl.edu/apadiv20/apadiv20.htm
The site of Division 20 (Division of Adult Development and Aging) of the American Psychological Association. Strives to advance the study of psychological development and change throughout the adult years.

http://www.geron.org
The site of the Gerontological Society of America, an interdisciplinary organization interested in all aspects of aging.

http://www.nih.gov/nia/health/
The National Institute of Aging provides scientific information on different aspects of physical aging.

CHAPTER 10

Mental-Health Counseling

JOSEPH DONNELLY, PH.D.

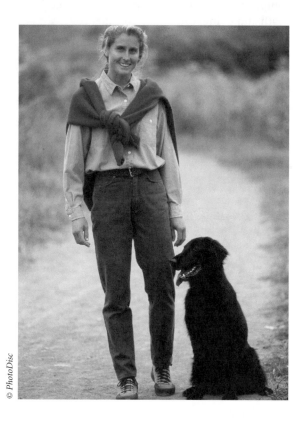

© PhotoDisc

OBJECTIVES

By the end of the chapter, the reader should be able to:

- Describe the history and development of mental-health counseling

- Provide a definition of comprehensive health

- Cite at least five different forms of psychologically based intervention

- Describe the stages of intervention

- Discuss what is meant by holistic mental health and how this relates to the job of the health counselor

Questions regarding physical health are often casually discussed: Are you feeling okay? Did you go to the doctor? People usually feel comfortable discussing circumstances around physical ailments anywhere from a broken arm to a cancerous tumor, but what people are less likely to discuss is their mental health. These issues (for one reason or another) may be considered "too personal." What is it that makes questions regarding mental health any more personal than questions regarding physical health?

Stigmas associated with mental illness have made the topic somewhat taboo, and many people are uncomfortable talking about it. For a long time, mental illness was related to patients from the movie *One Flew Over the Cuckoo's Nest* or serial killers. It is only recently that seeing a psychologist has gone from taboo to almost fashionable. Popular TV shows like *Frasier,* and *The Sopranos* feature characters who portray or who go to psychologists. This visibility has expanded the public's perception of mental-health problems. Today more people understand that ordinary people are affected by mental-health concerns and sometimes need help. Still, people are more hesitant to disclose that they are seeing a psychologist than, for example, a nutritionist. In a recent survey regarding the causes of mental illness, 71 percent of the respondents believed that mental illness is caused by emotional weakness, 65 percent believed that it is caused by bad parenting, and 43 percent believe that mental illness is brought on by the individual (National Mental Health Association Web site, 2002). These statistics show that although the public is more accepting of mental-health problems, there is still a stigma attached to mental illness.

Millions of people's lives are affected by mental-health issues, which range from poor self-esteem to severe depression or schizophrenia. Human beings experience a wide range of emotions, which include sorrow, anger, stress, and anxiety. Experiencing these emotions is a normal part of life, in fact a wide range of expression can be the sign of a healthy person. Yet there are times when these negative emotions are persistent and begin to disrupt a person's life and well-being. A person's relationships, work, self-esteem, and even physical health can suffer from an undiagnosed and untreated mental problem. The National Mental Health Association (2002) states that one in five adults has a diagnosable mental disorder. In addition, even people who function well and maintain the flow of their lives may sometimes need direction, emotional support, or help in clarifying their goals. Mental-health counseling can be a tool for empowerment and self-understanding rather than a treatment for an "illness."

Holistic mental-health counseling is based on the knowledge that the total health and well-being of a person is physical, mental, and emotional. A human being is an intricate and subtle system in which illness in any one part affects the whole. For example, a depressed person is likely to not exercise and to eat poorly, which in turn creates poor health and low energy. Likewise, many people who suffer from anxiety and stress (see Chapter 11) find that their mental state is greatly improved by beginning a regular program of vigorous exercise. There is evidence that risky health behaviors such as drug use and sexual promiscuity may be related to mental-health issues such as poor self-esteem or depression. Health problems such as anorexia and bulimia, which affect many adolescent girls, are clearly physical disorders which result from mental/emotional problems (see Chapter 6). Health and wellness can no longer be discussed without taking into account the *body-mind connection.* Indeed, the future of health education will no doubt be characterized by the integration of physical, mental, and emotional aspects of health. Health counseling is the natural outcome of this integration and new understanding. Mental health and physical health are interdependent and intertwined.

The purpose of this chapter is to provide an overview of the history and current practice of mental-health counseling in the context of an integrative model of health. The processes of assessment and prevention/intervention will be explored, as well as important counseling theories and approaches.

History of Mental-Health Counseling

Although mental illness has always existed, it has been viewed in various ways, according to the historical and social context in which individuals lived. Before the late 1700s, mentally ill people were treated as criminals, and were kept in prisons where the conditions were cruel and inhumane. Many of these people were kept in chains and were beaten and tortured. The general public had no understanding of mental illness. It was regarded as either a sign of the devil's presence or as a hideous defect which made the individual unfit to live in society. The first hospital to begin admitting mentally ill patients was the Pennsylvania Hospital in Philadelphia (Library of Congress Web site, 2001).

The hospital began admitting mentally ill patients after 1752, which was evidence of a gradual shift away from punishment of the mentally ill to treatment of the symptoms. Dr. Benjamin Horner (1797—1881), a doctor at the hospital, was a pioneer in the use of narcotics in the treatment of the insane.

Dorothea Dix was another social reformer who worked to improve society's treatment of the insane. Throughout the mid-1800s, she founded 32 mental hospitals and 15 schools, and tirelessly advocated for the humane and compassionate treatment of the insane (Viney & Zorich, 1982).

In an 1898 article found in the archives of the American Medical Association, J. H. McCassey, the Former Superintendent of the Kansas State Insane Asylum at Topeka, argues for the annihilation of the mentally insane. He argues, "It is high time to improve the method of preventing overproduction of defectives and criminals." He goes on to cite examples of "uncivilized" nations who, nevertheless, seem to have a more reasonable approach: exterminating the "defectives" of society (McCassey, 1898).

Eventually, the mentally ill were recategorized from "insane" to "sick." This new definition of mental health represented a whole new perspective. Sympathy and science were introduced as it was discovered that mental illness was the result of a brain disease, not a demon's presence. This established new forms of treatment for these sick, suffering individuals. Treatment revolved around hospital stays characterized by the use of drugs and isolation. Public sympathy was also aroused by the publication in 1908 of Clifford W. Beers's autobiographical account of his experiences as a patient in mental institutions (Brooks & Weikel, 1986). Around this time, an organization was formed which would later become the National Mental Health Association.

After World Wars I and II, the definition of mental health came to include occupational and vocational concerns, particularly the use of standardized tests to measure aptitudes and abilities. Later, interest in measuring personality came about by the publication of the Minnesota Multiphasic Personality Inventory by McKinley and Hathaway in 1940 (Smith & Robinson, 1995). In the 20th century, the definition of mental health continued to be refined by such important theorists as Sigmund Freud, Carl Jung, Carl Rogers, and Fritz Perls. The Community Mental Health Centers Act of 1963 represented a holistic, community-based approach to mental health. Mental illness was finally accepted as a legitimate and treatable disease, and one which could be dealt with within the community, rather than in an isolated environment.

Clair Turner (1951) cited the World Health Organization's definition of health as "a complete state of physical, mental, social and emotional well-being and not merely the absence of disease or infirmity." Here is where true holistic health is recognized. Metaphorically, holistic health can be thought of not as ingredients in a salad, but instead as ingredients in a broth—different pieces melted into one, instead of different elements thrown in together, but not really a part of one another. The idea of a *healthful broth* will be referred to often as a way of understanding what holistic health means.

When a narrow definition of mental health is taken and reduced to something as specific as "the absence of an anatomical or biochemical defect" (Szasz, 1987) it is an example of **reductionist thinking.** To limit any definition of health, mental or otherwise, to merely deciding whether there is disease or not is overly simplistic.

Since it is easier to think of the concrete example of physical health, consider the following example. If a person becomes sick because he does not get enough nutrients in his diet and expends no energy exercising, is he physically healthy? A person need not suffer from a terminal illness to be characterized as physically unhealthy.

Now apply that same philosophy to mental health. Is someone mentally healthy if they are not schizophrenic but cannot maintain a healthy social relationship? Must a diagnosis of a brain

Reductionist thinking. An overly simplistic way of looking at something or thinking, reducing its complexity or subtlety.

disorder be determined before a person with no sense of direction seeks help? This broader definition of mental health can apply to anyone who is looking to improve his or her life by removing self-defeating behavior at the root.

Because of the history of treatment of mental health there is a stigma that is associated with those who are looking for help in improving their mental health. This will be addressed further on in this chapter.

Physical, Mental, Social, Spiritual and Emotional "Broth"

As stated earlier, comprehensive health involves more than just physical health. In this section the five main components of holistic health will be explained.

Physical

The body's physical makeup is composed of six main systems: the nervous system, the skeletal system, the muscular system, the integumentary system (skin), the endocrine system (hormones), and the circulatory system. It would seem that with all of these complicated systems it would be difficult to keep it all running smoothly. This is not the case because all systems answer to one centralized control center, the central nervous system, or the brain.

Mental

"Our ability to manage stress, cope with emotional responses, and perhaps even produce the chemicals used in mental functioning involves aspects of the physical dimension of health" (Donnelly, Eburne, & Kittelson, 2001). **Psychoneuroimmunology (PNI)** components involve results of a direct relationship between body and mind. For exam-

ple, if a person believes that they will get a headache from peanut butter, almost every time that person eats peanut butter a headache will occur. It is arguable that peanut butter does legitimately cause headaches for that individual. But what if merely smelling or looking at peanut butter caused this person's head to throb? What would this mean?

The brain is the most complex and remarkable organ, so much so that scientists still do not know all of its capabilities and functions. What is known, however, is that the brain can overcome obstacles involving all facets of life. Think about the cliché, "If you think you can, you will; if you think you can't you won't." That is an accurate, albeit simplistic, way to describe the brain's relationship with the body.

This is also the basis behind **placebos,** which are used in medicinal experiments. *Placebo* is derived from a Latin word which means, "I will please." The placebo is used as a drug that is supposed to regulate the results of scientific testing of drugs by presenting a control group. A placebo is a substance that contains no catalystic effects. It is used in experiments to see if a person reacts to side effects of a drug, or if they react to these side effects because they were told they may. Typically two groups of subjects are used for these types of experiments. One group is given the actual experimental drug, the other group is given a placebo, usually a sugar pill. The researchers will clearly explain what this drug is supposed to do and some of the side effects the drug may cause. None of the subjects are aware whether they are taking the drug or the placebo. Researchers record results of the drug, both in its intended remedy and its possible side effects. It is remarkable to see how many people complain of side effects from a drug they are not even taking!

There are interesting statistics about people who have "thought" their cancer away, or "thought" themselves into depression. While the

---

Psychoneuroimmunology (PNI). The scientific investigation of how the brain affects the body's immune cells and how the immune system can be affected by behavior.

Placebo. A substance that contains no catalystic effects, that is used in medicinal experiments; literally mean "I will please" in Latin.

occasions aren't frequent these miracles are recorded every year. This is not to suggest that this is an easy or proven method to recovery, but it is certainly something to consider. Take a look at the following story about a little boy who was suffering from leukemia:

Case Study

Dave

Dave loved airplanes. His father used to take him to see the small jet planes at Teterboro Airport in Fairfield, New Jersey. Dave loved this because not only did he get to see the planes land and take off, but often famous people boarded and landed at this airport. Commonly the Kennedys would come in here, and the New Jersey Devils Hockey Team often left from this terminal. Dave asked his father where the planes went when you couldn't see them anymore. His father explained they went up to the clouds so far away no one could reach them. His young son couldn't wait until he could one day go up there in the clouds.

This is where Dave's family took him to break the news that he had leukemia. He was only 8 years old. His mother and father immediately took him for chemotherapy and he lost all his hair. Then they pulled him out of school so he could have round-the-clock hospital care. Still his condition worsened. After several months of drug therapy and radiation the doctor gave a grim prognosis; Dave had 3 months to live. Dave's parents were heartbroken, but Dave didn't believe the doctor's words.

This little boy continued to hold onto life, smiling to visitors and talking of airplanes. A couple of months later his mother asked him, "Honey, would you like to see Teterboro again? I could arrange it with the nurses." "No," Dave replied, "I can wait until I get out of the hospital." In tears, his mother smiled and left the room. In the hallway she pleaded with her husband to talk to the boy, to get him to understand the severity of his condition. The father went into the room.

"Son, wouldn't you like to see the planes one last time?" "One last time?" asked Dave, "Where

are they going?" "They are going up to the sky, so high that you can't see them." "Oh, no," said Dave, "I don't want to go there, that's where the cancer is."

His father was confused and asked him what he meant. "I dreamt last night that all the cancerous blood shot out of my ear and drifted up into the sky, so high that no one could ever get it. I don't want anyone to have this thing I got rid of." His father left the room in tears.

The very next day the doctor came in and took more blood from the boy. He was amazed to see that the cancerous blood cells were reducing and his T-cell count was up. The boy was healing himself! Dave is alive today and doing well at the Marine Academy of Science and Technology (MAST) at Sandy Hook, studying to become an astronaut.

This account was circulated on the Internet and therefore is not scientifically corroborated but is highly believable due to the number of similar cases in which a spontaneous remission or healing has been recorded in a terminally ill patient. Many doctors have documented cases of seemingly miraculous phenomena. One message that can be gleaned from this story is, if you think you'll fail, you will. If you think you will succeed, you will as well, maybe even with your life! The fact that the reason for these sudden healings cannot be found conclusively has caused many in the medical world and the mainstream to regard the mind–body connection as worthy of more serious and open-minded explorations.

Social

Placebos are not the only nondrugs that can significantly alter health. Social relationships can play a large part in enhancing or disturbing one's health. Consider the effects of being in love. The phenylalanine released in the brain gives off a euphoric feeling of calmness and elation. But when the relationship comes to an end, the brain might be flooded with cortisol, a major stress hormone which can leave a person depressed, inattentive, and anxious (Robbins, 2000). This too, ultimately, may be a simple biological conclusion to a complex chain of reactions leading to an end result. **Endorphins** (the natural chemical responsible for good feelings) are released through human intimacy, affection, and love. They are a natural opiate which is bound up with acts of social comfort (Levinthal, 1988). These emotional and social statuses can ultimately have dramatic effects on overall health. Goleman (1995) suggests that emotional responses are experienced as perceptions and environment before they are ever dealt with intellectually. This can explain why people tend to feel that they can "conquer the world" when they are happy and are tempted into "passion-based crimes" when they are severely depressed. Our emotional and social health has a direct result not only on our actions, but on what happens to and with others.

Spiritual

Oftentimes spiritual beliefs can help a person triumph over depressed or inadequate states. They can also promote feelings of wellness which often extend to others. Whether spiritual beliefs are oriented within Christianity, Buddhism, Islam, or Judaism, or whether one is simply at peace with oneself, any sort of spirituality will sustain a person in difficult times. In his book *Love, Medicine & Miracles*, Siegel (1986) expressed the opinion that spirituality has great potential to heal and promote a very positive state if expressed openly and freely. A famous First Lady once said, "The greater part of our happiness or misery depends upon our disposition, not our circumstances." Martha Washington was extraordinarily insightful to determine that we, *not our* circumstances, are the ones who determine our state of mind. Spirituality can be a powerful tool in meeting the challenges of life with resilience and hope.

> **Endorphins.** The natural chemical responsible for good feelings; a natural opiate released in the body.

Emotional

Eisenberg (1997), in discussing world mental health, noted the interconnectedness of health problems. Examples he gave of the interconnectedness of health problems with psychological states and conditions included: depression, heart and lung disease, and sexually transmitted diseases with certain attitudes and behavior patterns; the psychosocial pathologies such as violence, alcoholism, and abuse of women and children with underlying social conditions such as war, poverty, and discrimination. He described this interconnectedness as a self-perpetuating spiral.

The Cost of the Solution

The United States has determined there is an immediate need to address mental health. While advocating for increased attention to mental-health care, former first lady Roselynn Carter (1996) noted that mental illness creates an immeasurable cost to quality of life. Negative outcomes of mental illness include premature death from suicide, loss of productivity in the workplace, the cost of support of the mentally ill homeless, undue burdens to the criminal-justice system, and the cost of medical care due to physical illness. The cost of all of these exceeds the cost of direct treatment of mental illness.

It is a complicated process to calculate the exact costs of addressing mental health. Because of the aforementioned interconnectedness many ailments that are a result of mental-health illness are often treated as isolated incidents and the correlation is often not made that mental-health intervention is required.

Perhaps due to this interconnectedness, the federal government has established an agency called the Substance Abuse and Mental Health Services Administration (SAMHSA). This branch of government focuses on mental health, and alcohol and other drug abuse services, abbreviated MHAOD. When this government agency calculates the costs associated with services in this area they often factor drug, alcohol, and mental-health issues together (Donnelly, Eburne, & Kittelson, 2001).

Some recent statistics that illustrate current trends are:

- MHAOD expenditures were 8.8 percent of the $942.7 billion in national health expenditures (SAMHSA, report, 1998).

- A National Institutes of Health (1997) report states that the total spending for MHAOD is close to that expended for either heart disease or for injuries and trauma, and exceeds the amount spent on both diabetes and cancer.

- The consulting firm of Harris, Rothenberg International (1999) suggests that dependency and mental illness combined cost U.S corporations over $100 billion each year.

- The Surgeon General suggests that the cost to the nation for mental health is $178 billion per year (National Institutes for Mental Health, 2000).

Mental and Emotional Problems

So far we have addressed mental health in terms of how it relates to our bodies and overall quality of life. The question remains: How are mental problems determined? It has been said that most people should spend time improving their mental health, but how can a real problem be identified? Should we only be concerned with "problems" in our minds, or should we attune our awareness to a whole new level?

Just as one would not consider him or herself physically fit after working out just one time, restructuring the mind does not happen overnight either. Even if a person is mentally well this does not mean that he or she should not be aware of his or her mental state. For example, a piano must be conditioned and reconditioned on a regular basis in order to be considered in tune, and it is the same with our mental health. If a piano is out of tune it needs to be tuned several times before it is considered in tune, and then it's advised that a piano have a regular check-up two times a year.

Perhaps we should consider adopting a similar attitude with our mental health.

Basic standards of mental health and illness are based upon the American Psychiatric Association's publication *Diagnostic and Statistical Manual of Mental Disorders Fourth Edition* (DSM IV; see also Chapter 6). This publication is used as the foundation for defining deviations from mental health and is generally accepted in the United States and many other countries as the "psychiatrist's bible" (Donnelly, Eburne, & Kittelson, 2001).

According to the DSM IV, specific criteria must be present for a problem to be considered *mental illness.*

1. **Behavioral or psychological syndrome**—Is a group of symptoms (that tend to occur together) causing the present distress?

2. ***Cannot*** **be a cultural response to an event**—For example, is the present depression a result of a divorce? The loss of a child?

3. **Current behavior is a "behavioral, psychological or biological dysfunction in the individual"** (American Psychiatric Association, 1994)—Is the current situation considered highly abnormal in the individual's society, so much so that it is preventing normal interaction?

4. **Interruption in lifestyle**—how long has the problem been an interruption and is it getting worse or better? Has the interruption occurred in the past and how extensive was it?

5. **Medication**—Is physical illness or medication use associated with the present problem?

6. **Pattern of Illness**—Is there a history of a similar problem in the person's genetic makeup? (Genetic predisposition, however, is a tricky connection that is still being studied.)

Source: From Diagnostic and Statistical Manual of Mental Disorders, Fourth Edition, Text Revision. Washington, D.C., American Psychiatric Association, 1994. Reprinted with permission from the Diagnostic and Statistical Manual of Mental Disorders, Fourth Edition. Copyright 1999 American Psychiatric Association.

The DSM IV is very specific for good reasons. If therapists were to evaluate patients without taking into consideration these six factors, people might be misdiagnosed and treated for a chemical,

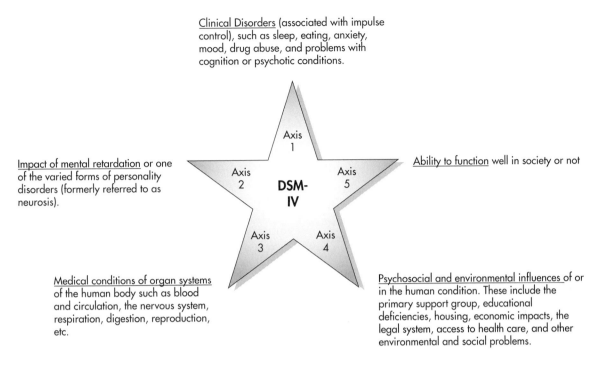

Clinical Disorders (associated with impulse control), such as sleep, eating, anxiety, mood, drug abuse, and problems with cognition or psychotic conditions.

Impact of mental retardation or one of the varied forms of personality disorders (formerly referred to as neurosis).

Ability to function well in society or not

Medical conditions of organ systems of the human body such as blood and circulation, the nervous system, respiration, digestion, reproduction, etc.

Psychosocial and environmental influences of or in the human condition. These include the primary support group, educational deficiencies, housing, economic impacts, the legal system, access to health care, and other environmental and social problems.

Figure 10.1
Multi-axial Model

genetic, or chronic problem when, in fact, it may only be a temporary issue. The converse, however, is true as well. Therapists do not want people to go untreated too long when a substantial improvement in quality of life is available.

The DSM IV utilizes a multi-axial model where each axis corresponds to an area of life that might be affected by a mental disorder. Figure 10.1 illustrates their relationship.

This multi-axial approach is the embodiment of the multifaceted nature of comprehensive mental health. Figure 10.1, perhaps more than the analogy to a broth, shows the correlation between mind and body

Assessing a Need

At times, most people could use support and assistance. Being aware of all the services available within the mental-health field creates an atmosphere where people can recognize when they need assistance and know how to get it. This is important knowledge for students who wish to become mental-health counselors, but also for anyone who may decide that it is time for them to access help.

Knowing when to access help is a key element in achieving good mental health. People seek out mental-health services for a variety of reasons, ranging anywhere from a stressful school environment to major depression with suicidal thoughts. Gaining insight as to what problem exists is the first step in developing effective coping strategies. Not everyone must consult the DSM IV to assess their problem in terms of need. Generally speaking, a problem can be determined by several factors:

- Thoughts or actions interfere with a person's daily functioning.

- Thoughts or actions have caused others to suffer.

- Thoughts or actions deviate strongly from a person's normal routine.

■ Thoughts or actions will drastically jeopardize long-term objectives.

Realistically almost everyone needs a shoulder to cry on, literally. Venting anger in a controlled way, talking about one's sorrows with a concerned listener, and discussing the patterns of one's behavior are healthy ways to release daily tensions. **Stressors** are any and all pressures that are faced in daily life. A culmination of unaddressed stressors leads to what is commonly known as *stress*. Too much stress can cause anxiety attacks, chronic nervousness, ulcers, and other health problems. When these small, daily stressors are not managed in a healthy way they can create much bigger problems.

Certain relaxing hormones are released when a person cries; this is nature's relaxer. Men tend to have more unreleased stress, because in many cultures it is common for men to avoid showing and releasing emotion. Women may cry more than men because of higher levels of the hormone prolactin. "Women have sixty percent higher levels of prolactin than men" (Current Health, 1995). People who don't cry impede the body's natural defense system against stress.

Most people have a certain degree of emotional/mental difficulty in their lives. It is when these difficulties interfere with one's life or goal pursuit in a patterned or lasting way that assistance is warranted. Any person, at any time, can make the decision that they need help. It is also appropriate for certain people (such as teachers at a school, or a close friend) to refer a person to access help.

Steps to Accessing Help

Ideally, a counselor would like to intervene before a client's problem becomes a crisis. The first level of prevention is called **primary prevention.** This stage is essentially about education and providing appropriate information for individuals to cope, deal with difficulties, and simply manage his or her stress. Having the knowledge to recognize problems and distinguish between the resources available is important so that counselors and patients can make informed decisions. Primary prevention does not eliminate difficulties, but it does allow one to manage and successfully cope with stressors. A common example of this would be a university wellness center that provides peer counseling, pamphlets, hot lines, and references for further counseling if the patient deems it necessary.

The second level of prevention is titled **secondary prevention.** In this stage a problem has been isolated and a specific focus identified. An individual may reach the point where he or she feels like they are about to unravel. This does not necessarily imply breakdown, but the difficulties are beginning to control them or cause personal, professional, or social problems in interaction. Oftentimes, people do not feel the need to seek out a counselor at the primary level for the simple fact that it is not necessary. At the secondary level, however, it is becoming more apparent and important for this person to seek help. Perhaps this means seeking out someone who can assist them in resolving stressors, managing conflict, or simply lending an ear. This secondary level does not minimize the importance of professional counseling, but it may or may not be needed or accepted at this stage of the person's perception. Crisis intervention and counseling become crucial at this stage in order to keep the problem from escalating. For example, if a student has behavior problems in school she might first be referred to the vice principal (primary intervention), who might then send her to the school counselor (secondary). If the counselor is unsuccessful with the student she may then be referred to a psychiatrist/therapist where serious, intense counseling can take place. This leads to the final level, tertiary prevention.

Primary prevention. The first level of prevention characterized by education and the provision of appropriate information.

Secondary prevention. The stage of prevention when a problem has been isolated and a specific focus identified. The client's need for assistance is more apparent and important.

During **tertiary prevention,** intense counseling is necessary. Keep in mind, these are levels of *prevention*, not *treatment*. Ironically, this is when most people seek help because their illness has become so extreme that it is actually harmful to their normal lifestyle. Individuals are not fixed in each of these stages. They might revert to previous stages, and weave in and out of several stages quickly.

It is imperative to look at the stages in which a problem can develop. It is best to catch a problem in its earliest stages, not only because it is easier to cure at this stage, but because the problem will not interfere with daily routines in drastic ways. Prevention is worth a hundred sessions of therapy! Take the famous piano player Liberace. He had said if he went two days without practicing, *he* was able to notice the change in his performance. If he went four days without practicing, *his manager* noticed his performance. Finally, if even the famous Liberace went one week without practicing, *the audience* was able to hear the difference.

Liberace's example can be looked at within the stages of prevention. First, notice that he approached primary prevention by having the knowledge to recognize his problem (lack of practice) and distinguish that this was inappropriate for his lifestyle (he needed to exemplify perfection). In entering the secondary prevention stage he had isolated the problem (practice suffered due to too much time socializing) and a specific focus was spent on its detection (he was playing the wrong notes) and intercession (he canceled Thursday's dinner party). Lastly, because his audience could hear the difference due to his lack of practice (a pianist's worst nightmare!) he entered the tertiary stage. His behavior had become harmful to his normal manner of life (excellence) and he began the initial stage of therapy, change. He returned to practicing every day.

Reverting back to the topic that started off this chapter, many of the problems that deal with counseling mental illnesses involve the reluctance

Tertiary prevention. The third level of prevention, when intense counseling is necessary.

of people to admit a problem exists. How this stigma started is unclear. It may very well be from the initial ignorance in recognizing the disorder, and further, in treating it properly. Wartik (1997) has offered several possibilities but assures that whatever the cause, if mental illness continues to go untreated, like any disorder, it will grow worse.

The omission of accurate information about mental health is a problem in most primary and secondary education curriculums. This stems from the fact that many people who suffer from mental disturbances cannot be called mentally ill. Think about it in simpler terms, as a physical illness. Let's say Carolyn has a broken leg. Would she be defined as a disabled person or is she considered unhealthy? Carolyn is merely in a temporary state of repair. But think about what would happen if she were too embarrassed to say that her leg was broken, and therefore never had a cast put on. The bone would probably heal wrong and after time, she *would be* permanently disabled. As long as the notion exists that seeking help regarding mental-health problems represents a personal failure, mental-health management will remain difficult.

Stages Assessment

Clinical assessment is often implemented once tertiary prevention has been applied (see also chapter 2). This is the point where clinicians narrow the problem down and then assess how they are going to work together to implement a solution. This step is not as involved as a counseling session but it is the precursor that lays the work for the therapist. The mental-health counselor is expected to meet the challenge of discerning the particular personality traits of an individual and how those traits interact in the individual's social environments.

This is usually done through an interview-style process. The interview may be more or less formal, depending on the situation and the clinician. The main goal of the clinician is to talk with the client in order to get basic information on the presented problem, background, and the individual's social/emotional functioning. Since a person is not an isolated entity it is essential to gather as

Table 10.1
Types of Testing used by Clinicians

Personality Test Type	Structure/ Instruments	Evaluation Methods	Desired Outcome	Common Types
Objective	more controlled and objective in interpreting behavior rating scales, adaptive behavior scales, personality scales, and scales to assess specific disorders	a self-report technique, the client has to answer true or false	gives clinicians specific information about how a person is functioning in a particular area (such as social attitudes, moral attitudes, psychological states, and physical conditions)	Minnesota Multiphasic Personality Inventory (MMPI)
Projective	unstructured tasks, picture cards, oral prompts, or other ambiguous stimuli	the client has to respond to pictures or ambiguous stimuli instead of verbal questions or rating scales (a psychoanalytic perspective)	client will project their own characteristics, problems, motives, and wishes onto that situation	Thematic Apperception Test (TAT), the Rorschach Test, and sentence-completion tests

Source: Clark, 1995; Waiswol, 1995

much information as possible about him or her in order to conduct a thorough assessment. See Table 10.1 for types of testing used by clinicians.

Psychologically Based Intervention

Another type of assessment is psychologically based intervention. This type of intervention is done in a similar matter in a more intense setting. Often these therapists are trained at the doctoral level and have extraordinarily effective communication skills. There are several different types of therapy that are predominantly used by therapists. Some of the most used are: Psychodynamic Therapy, Cognitive-Behavioral Therapy, and Humanistic/Experiential Therapy. Specific descriptions will be given as to the function, purpose, methods, and style for each type.

Psychodynamic Therapy

The psychodynamic-therapy approach focuses on an individual's personality dynamics through a psychoanalytic perspective. Psychoanalysts focus on drawing out an individual's repressed feelings from childhood by seeing what defense mechanism the person is utilizing. **Defense mechanisms** are subconsciously used by individuals to battle the daily plights of life. By relating what defense mechanisms a client is employing a therapist can gain better insight into the client's inner motivations and desires. Once this is done the counselor will be able to turn the client's energies toward integrating their personality into a more productive manner.

Psychodynamic therapy was evolved from Sigmund Freud's *Psychoanalytic Theory* (1935). Psychoanalysis is based on the idea that humans are in constant internal conflict to resolve aggressive and sexual impulses that occur during daily life. **Determinism,** or the belief that prior experience directs

Defense mechanisms. Strategies, usually subconscious, that a person uses to protect or defend her or himself against anxiety and perceived psychological threat.

Determinism. The belief that prior experience, not free will, directs the course of our lives.

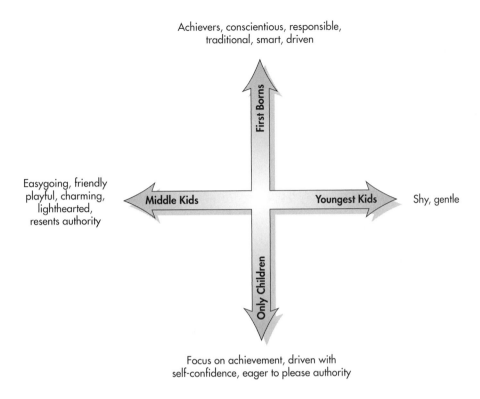

Achievers, conscientious, responsible,
traditional, smart, driven

First Borns

Easygoing, friendly
playful, charming,
lighthearted,
resents authority

Middle Kids　　　　　　　**Youngest Kids**　　Shy, gentle

Only Children

Focus on achievement, driven with
self-confidence, eager to please authority

Figure 10.2
Adler's characteristics attributed to birth order

the course of our lives, was an original theory of Freud's. In this idea free will is determined an illusion that humans have developed, and the effects of internal conflicts about sexual and aggressive impulses are the only determining factors of our behavior (Carson, Butcher, & Mineka, 1996; Freud, 1935; Wallace, 1986).

Psychoanalysts have borrowed another technique used by Freud called **free association,** where the client is instructed to say anything that comes to mind. The client free-associates while the counselor takes extensive notes or records the session with the hope of extricating unconscious information that the client may have repressed. This can be

Free Association. A technique originally developed by Freud, where the client is instructed to say anything that comes to mind, in hopes of extricating unconscious information.

a frustrating process since clients often are unconsciously reluctant to provide information that can truly be useful in therapy. Counselors are also aware of this resistance, and try to break down the client's defenses to get to the true problem (Carson, Butcher, & Mineka, 1996; Freud, 1935).

Freud's theories and techniques formatted the basis of psychology, more specifically psychoanalysis, and it has fallen under significant criticism since its inception. Opponents mainly disagree with his overemphasis on sexual and aggressive urges. Alfred Adler, for example, followed the same school of thought as Freud but highlighted a different emphasis. Adler focused on the role of the individual and where that individual fell in birth order. The individual is composed of seven entities that he or she attempts to attain, develop, or thwart in a lifetime. These entities are grounded in motivation and fulfillment. They are as follows:

- Will for power

- Social nature

- Inferiority

- Style of life

- Strive for superiority

- Fictional finalism

- Creative self

According to Adler, these units are based upon a child's birth order. See Figure 10.2 for the characteristics attributed to this relationship.

Adlerians are known for their belief that any method that solicits interest from the client can help them improve their train of logic and personality quirks, and amend destructive behavior. Adler began the use of paradoxical directives, a technique that exaggerates undesirable behavior to increase awareness. This technique is often used in marital and family counseling. Using Adler's techniques the individual is really in control, the rewards are theirs, but most importantly the individuals are masters of their own fate (Dinkmeyer, Pew, & Dinkmeyer, 1979).

Cognitive-Behavioral Therapy

Cognitive-behaviorial therapy (see Chapter 4) is based on the idea that mental illness stems from a person's illogical and formless thinking. The main goal of cognitive-behavioral therapy, therefore, is to replace faulty thinking and negative self-statements with more positive ideas. Hopefully this will restructure unstable behaviors and emotions into more helpful conduct. This process is appropriately coined **cognitive restructuring.**

One type of cognitive-behavioral therapy is transactional analysis, developed by Eric Berne.

Transactional analysis (TA) focuses on the interactions between individuals. In his theory, Berne identified three ego states, which he defines as a coherent system of thoughts and feelings that manifest themselves in patterns of behavior. Figure 10.3 illustrates these three ego states.

Humanistic-Experiential Therapy

Different from the cognitive behavioral approach is humanistic-experiential therapy. These theorists believe that there is a need to look at the full potential of human beings by examining self-concept versus free will. Theorists believe that if a client can see what they want versus what they have, the clients will discover for themselves why they fail to find meaning in their lives. The client needs to become more aware of their uniqueness and "wholeness" as a person. Professionals in this school of thought, as in the others, believe the client should be responsible for the success and direction of therapy through the facilitation of the therapist. That is the basis behind Carl Roger's "client-centered" therapy.

Yet another closely related therapy, is Victor Frankl's existential therapy. He developed a concept called **logo therapy** that focuses on individual power and freedom. As in client-centered therapy, the existential therapist sees people as basically good and rational, but existentialism takes this idea one step further to the notion of complete freedom. By this Frankl means each of us is free to decide how we live and give meaning to our lives. An existential therapist would agree with the quote from Martha Washington citing that we can't blame others for our unhappiness. We must create our own happiness internally (Frankl, 1979).

Transactional analysis. A form of cognitive behavioral therapy developed by Eric Berne; it focuses on the interactions between individuals through different ego states.

Logo therapy. A kind of existential therapy developed by Victor Frankl, that focuses on individual power and freedom to create our lives.

Cognitive restructuring. A type of cognitive behavioral therapy that attempts to restructure faulty thinking and negative self-statements into more positive ideas.

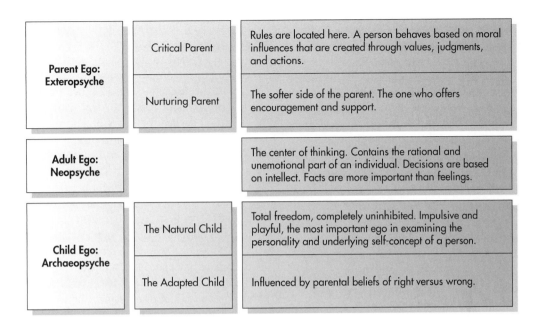

Figure 10.3
Egos states of transactional analysis
Source: Hollenbeck, Donnelly, & Eburne, 2001

Everyday Life Issues

Health counseling can be utilized within a variety of areas. Of course, within most schools there is a school counselor or psychologist, but sometimes the student may simply not be comfortable speaking with this professional or the professional is not easily accessible. In most schools the main psychologist is only present when the school is dealing with a known tragedy (such as the death of student). Or the psychologist is only available sporadically because, usually, school boards hire one psychologist for an entire district (which may comprise of over 20 schools!) So what does a 13-year-old girl do when she finds out she is pregnant? Or her 18-year-old boyfriend for that matter?

Whether it has to do with social stigmas, parental rules, or fear of punishment, children may not feel comfortable to address the "proper authorities." That is when they rely on their favorite English teacher, or perhaps, their health teacher. This is a perfect, perhaps extreme, example of where counseling know-how is necessary and useful for the health educator.

This does not imply that the teacher acts as the student's counselor, but the teacher must be capable of and comfortable with listening to these problems. He or she must be prepared to provide skillful advice. While it may seem easiest to not get involved, it is necessary for the health educator or teacher to be aware of the most appropriate ways of helping a student while not overstepping his or her professional role and legal responsibilities.

Where to Find Help

As stated earlier, a problem need not be present for a person to access help. Some people may not be looking for help per se but rather just someone to talk to. At many colleges and workplaces there is a counseling or wellness center on-site where people can go to reflect on their present experiences and seek advice on how to manage their professional or personal lives in a more productive manner.

Many communities have mental-health centers where people can get short-term inpatient and outpatient care, emergency services, community consultation, and educational programs. When people are released from psychological counseling at a hospital they often utilize the outpatient programs in their communities. This should not be a replacement for hospital care, but rather a supplement to it. Sometimes insurance companies stop providing coverage for people who are seeking psychological treatment in hospitals because they only cover a segmented amount of time (such as 30 days). A mistake in removing someone from inpatient care too soon could be lethal. A New Jersey teenager committed suicide just weeks after being sent home from a hospital that treated her for depression. A June 2000 newspaper article in *The Bergen Record* recalls the tragic story of a girl whose death might have been prevented (see box).

Case Study

A Suicide

Keri Sohlman left the hospital in early January, six weeks after sinking into a depression so profound that a therapist called an ambulance.

The Saddle Brook teenager's descent had begun six years earlier, with the sudden death of her father. A brother's suicide in April 1999 had pushed her deeper into despondency. After that, she fell apart, drinking and smoking marijuana so much that her friends asked her mother to do something.

Keri spent the weeks at Holy Name Hospital under medication and in therapy. She received electroshock treatments and wrote in her journal. She also slashed her wrists with a bottle, the first time she had hurt herself to that extent. Her psychiatrist at Holy Name described her as "extremely fragile." Her "cutting behavior" was a bid to discharge tension and get help, the psychiatrist said.

But now, according to Oxford Health Plans, it was time for Keri to go home.

Hospital care was no longer necessary, the insurer's medical director said. Guided by a combination of length-of-stay criteria, symptom assessments, and the bottom line, the managed-care plan instead decided to pay for a "partial hospital" or day-treatment program. Keri's psychiatrist argued against the discharge. Keri's mother argued that her daughter wasn't ready to deal with the outside world and needed the safety of a hospital.

Their pleas made no difference.

Sometime later, Keri walked onto an overpass across the Garden State Parkway. She jumped, falling 30 feet onto the cement barrier below.

Keri's suicide ended not one, but two troubling stories. The first, was her own painful journey through family loss, grief, and despair.

The second was the story of her treatment in the age of managed care, a tale of fragmentation in the mental-health system, limits on coverage, financial pressure, and disagreement between the insurance company and the professional treating her. Keri's story, though, illustrates a larger tale: It shows how much medical care today depends not on what is available or what is best, but on what insurance will pay for.

"The key thing for these patients is continuity," [Gladys Halvorsen, the Holy Name psychiatrist] said. "There was no continuity" she added, as Keri was passed from a private therapist to Bergen Regional Medical Center to Holy Name Hospital, and then to Carrier.

"Given the opportunity, I would have continued to see her, so she could have had that one bond, that one very strong bond. The point is, I was pressured tremendously to release her. I treated her two weeks without any pay." Halvorsen added.

Dr. Lawrence Goldberg of the Carrier Clinic commented: "It sounds like this patient received very serious, quality, state-of-the-art treatment. . . . I think the only conclusion you can draw is that despite the best efforts of contemporary standards of treatment, some patients will commit suicide."

Dr. Alan Muney of Oxford Health Plan stated: "Regardless of diagnosis, some patients are going to have bad outcomes. Do we feel that we interacted appropriately with the physician, and followed criteria? We're comfortable with that. Ultimately, she was under the care of a physician." (Lindy Washburn. (2000). "Did She Have to Die?" *The Bergen Record*, June 25.)

Support groups and "self-help" groups are available regionally for several situations. Some of the most common are:

- parenting skills

- stress management

- domestic violence

- addictive problems (gambling, alcohol, drugs, and so on)

Local groups in the community gather to share feelings and talk about their situation. Knowing that one is not suffering alone is one of the biggest comforts a person can have.

These building blocks to mental health are formatted in stages where people can find help and can manage their lives better. When all of these preliminary steps are taken and there is no relief or improvement, many people consult a psychiatrist. A psychiatrist is a medical doctor (M.D.) who has the skills to communicate with a client to help figure out the problem and work with the client to find a resolution. A psychiatrist differs from a psychologist, who has a Ph.D., because the former is certified to provide prescription drugs to aid in the recovery process. It is important to reinforce the fact that drugs prescribed to patients are not intended to replace therapy or to keep patients from facing the reality of life. Drugs should be used as a supplemental aid to help regulate stress, hyperactivity, depression, or other emotions that might cause a setback to a healthy and productive lifestyle.

Current Issues in Mental Health

The example of the young woman who committed suicide highlights not only the challenges within the current system of managed health care but also one of the most important issues facing society at large: Depression and anxiety disorders are the two most common mental illnesses, affecting 19 million American adults annually (National Institutes of Mental Health, 1999). And it is estimated that of the 54 million Americans who have a mental disorder in any given year, fewer than 8 million seek treatment (SGRMH, 1999). Therefore anyone in the mental-health or health-counseling field can expect to be touched by these problems.

Depression has been linked with serious health problems such as high blood pressure and heart disease. It has been found that people with depression are four times more likely to have a heart attack than those with no history of depression. Heart problems also can add to and cause depression in people. While 1 in 20 American adults experience major depression every year, the number goes up to about 1 in 3 for people who have survived a heart attack. Other researchers have found that most heart patients with depression do not receive treatment. Many physicians miss the diagnosis of depression, and even when it is recognized, they do not treat it adequately (National Institutes of Mental Health, 2001).

The rates of depression are even higher for women than they are for men. Women experience depression at roughly twice the rate that men do. This statistic holds true for teenage girls and boys. The urgency of giving attention to this problem becomes more dramatic for certain groups who are less likely to seek or receive treatment for mental-health disorders. Seventy percent of children do not receive mental-health services, and only 10 percent of older Americans affected with late-life depression receive treatment. Among minorities, unmet mental-health needs are even greater. Adult African Americans experience depression and anxiety disorders at the same rates as Caucasians, but are less likely to receive treatment based on socioeconomic factors. Half as many African Americans had health insurance in 1998 and 1999 as did Caucasians (National Institutes of Mental Health, 2000). Clearly the problems of depression and anxiety are affecting Americans across all socioeconomic strata. Health counselors should be aware of the pharmacological and therapeutic treatments that clients/students may be undergoing, or be prepared to refer the client who is demonstrating signs of depression to appropriate sources for help, if the need is out of the range of a health counselor's abilities.

Studies have confirmed the short-term efficacy and safety of treatments for depression in youth (National Institutes of Mental Health, 2000). Since health counselors are concerned with the holistic well-being of clients/students, they can use statistical information which reinforces positive lifestyles and has been shown to help depression. For instance, participation in an exercise training program has been shown to have a comparable effect to treatment with antidepressant medication (a selective serotonin reuptake inhibitor) in older adults diagnosed with major depression (National Institutes of Mental Health, 2000). Therefore, when facing a client with minor symptoms of depression, a counselor might inquire as to their daily or weekly exercise quotient. While the root of a mental disturbance may still need to be identified and dealt with, a health counselor can address the symptoms of depression in straightforward and simple ways such as encouraging a regular exercise program to the client.

The prevalence of depression and anxiety disorders in today's society highlight the need for a better understanding of how mind and body work together in creating health or dysfunction in the individual. Many other diseases, such as cancer, have been examined in relation to attitudes and personal beliefs as well as to behaviors and environmental factors. Society at large is looking to psychology, and in some cases, to spirituality, for answers as to why some persons get some diseases and experience differing outcomes in treatment. The notion of what creates overall health has expanded to include mental health as well as physical health. The wisdom of prevention is becoming increasingly popular, even within the medical establishment. That the state of the mind influences the state of body, and vice versa, is a principle that health counselors can apply when faced with client issues regarding such widespread conditions as anxiety and depression.

Summary

Mental-health counseling plays an important part in achieving a new understanding of health and well-being. A holistic model of health incorporates the physical, mental, emotional, and spiritual aspects of life, and recognizes that these elements are interdependent. Mental health and illness vary along a continuum, from everyday stress to serious depression or personality disorders. Those facing serious mental-health problems should be treated with respect and understanding. Society still has work to do in overcoming the stigmas associated with mental illness. Increasingly, many people are realizing that their own mental state, beliefs, attitudes, and emotions have a significant impact on their lives. It is becoming more common to see ordinary people seeking help with stress relief, goal setting, relationship problems, and self-esteem. Improving one's mental health is a necessary and important part of a healthy lifestyle. The integration of body, mind, and spirit will no doubt become the hallmark of health counseling in the 21st century.

Key Terms

cognitive restructuring, 196	primary prevention, 192
defense mechanisms, 194	psychoneuroimmunology, 187
determinism, 194	reductionist thinking, 186
endorphins, 189	secondary prevention, 192
free association, 195	tertiary prevention, 193
logo therapy, 196	transactional analysis, 196
placebos, 187	

Questions For Discussion

1. List six symptoms (signs) that someone is suffering from a mental-health problem.

2. A person comes to you and describes a psychological difficulty they've been having. They are wondering whether to seek help for it. What factors would you evaluate in order to respond?

3. What are specific programs that could be implemented for each of the three levels of intervention?

4. Distinguish between Adler's, Berne's, and Frankl's theories and approach to therapy. Which do you agree with most? Why?

5. What potential client situations might necessitate the assistance of a psychologist? psychiatrist? health counselor?

Related Web Sites

http://www.apa.org
The home page of the American Psychological Association, including its newspaper, links to information, journals, employment, public practice, education, and so on.

http://www.athealth.com
Designed to connect mental-health professionals and those they serve with the power and resources of the Internet.

http://www.shef.ac.uk/~psysc/psychotherapy/index.html
Features search capabilities of all the major mental-health resources on the Web. Connects to all 857 psychology, psychiatry, neuroscience, and social science journals and journal search engines.

http:// www.cmhc.com
A comprehensive guide to mental health online, this site features information on depression, anxiety, panic attacks, chronic fatigue syndrome, substance abuse, and professional resources in psychology, journals, and magazines.

http:// www.nimh.com
The Web site of the National Institute of Mental Health. Features many links to information, research, publications, statistics, and resources.

Stress and Health Counseling

JERROLD S. GREENBERG, PH.D.

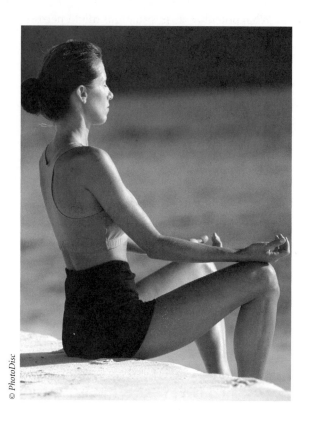

© PhotoDisc

OBJECTIVES

By the end of this chapter, the reader should be able to:

- Define and differentiate between stressors, stress reactivity, and stress

- Cite changes in the body resulting from stress and the relationship between those changes and illness and disease

- Describe a model of stress and a concept of intervening between stressors and negative consequences based on this model

- Define the stress-management-related constructs of attitude of gratitude, locus of control, self-esteem, anxiety, life events, hassles, occupational stress, Type A Behavior Pattern, and social support

- List three relaxation techniques and describe how they can be used

- Feel confident in counseling students who present with stress-related issues

Case Study

Jack's best friend put a gun to his head and pulled the trigger. Aside from feeling a deep sense of loss, Jack was angry and disappointed. "I was his best friend. Why didn't he talk to me about this? Why did he have to kill himself?" It seemed that much of Jack's day was preoccupied by such questions. His schoolwork and his job outside of school were both affected.

Kim was a student from Taiwan who was sent, at great expense to her family, to the United States to attend college. With the difficulty she had with studying in a second language and the pressure she felt to succeed in school, (her parents sacrificed to send her to school in the United States), she was just keeping her head above water. She barely passed several course and had to take incompletes in others. Her concern and frustration about her schoolwork overflowed into her social life. She found herself being angry and argumentative with friends and devoting so much time to her studies that she soon had no friends. Alone and lonely in a foreign country, not doing well in school, Kim was experiencing a great deal of stress.

Bill was a mail carrier who was attending college at night to prepare for another career when he retired from the postal service. He was having problems with his marriage, his job, and his schooling. There never seemed to be enough time for any of these. His wife and daughter complained that with work and school he was seldom at home, and, when he was, he was always doing schoolwork. His supervisor at the post office claimed he always seemed tired and grouchy, and this was affecting his job performance. His professors told Bill that he was not turning in his work on time, nor was it of sufficient quality to pass his courses. When Bill finally left his family (his domestic problems became more and more serious), he brooded so much that he had less time, instead of more, to concentrate on other aspects of his life.

These are but a few of the students enrolled in this author's stress-management class during *one semester*. They came in during office hours to discuss their problems and to get guidance regarding how to manage them. They recognized they needed assistance in managing the stress they were experiencing and sought counsel in doing that. Furthermore, they wanted to prevent the unhealthy consequences of stress that had been discussed in class.

It is not unusual for instructors to encounter students and others who seek this type of help and, therefore, this chapter is devoted to preparing health educators and health counselors to be able to provide this assistance. Before beginning, however, a clear understanding of stress and stress-related constructs is necessary.

Stress: The Concept

Stress consists of a stressor and stress reactivity.

The Stressor

A stress response is initiated by a **stressor.** A stressor is a stimulus with the potential to elicit the flight-or-fight response. The threats for which our bodies were evolutionarily trained were threats to our physical safety. The caveman who saw a lion looking for its next meal needed to react quickly. The flight-or-fight response, then, was vital for survival. Today's stressors often threaten our psychological and emotional health. Students may be "stressed out" over having to give a speech in their speech class, or asking someone out on a date. The threat is often to one's sense of self-worth, fearing rejection will uncover our unworthy selves.

Stress Reactivity

When the stressor elicits a stress response we term that **stress reactivity.** This response is discussed later in this chapter. Suffice it to say here, the stress response prepares the individual to do something physical, to fight or to take flight. Oftentimes it is appropriate to do something physical. However, when it is not, such as having to give that speech in class, the stress by-products are not used and the result can be illness and disease.

A Conceptualization of Stress

Stress then is the combination of a stressor and the stress reactivity it produces. Although we will discuss stressors in detail later in this chapter, at this point recognize that not all stressors need to result in a stress response. There are numerous techniques to prevent that from happening or, if it does occur, for the stress reaction to be minimized.

Stressors. The small everyday pressures and hassles of life that can accumulate and lead to stress.

Stress reactivity. Changes in the body in response to a stressor that include increased heart rate, blood pressure, and respiratory rate.

Stress. The combination of a stressor and stress reactivity.

For example, Kim, the Taiwanese student mentioned in the opening of this chapter, could have used self-talk or other cognitive restructuring techniques presented later in this chapter to reduce her physiological arousal (heart pounding, tense muscles, perspiration). Health counselors who help their clients understand that they are in control over their stress reaction, and who teach clients to exercise that control, have gone a long way in helping clients manage stress.

Stress Psychophysiology

Stress psychophysiology can be understood as a kind of chain reaction that occurs. When the brain perceives a stressor, it activates endocrine glands which, in turn, secrete hormones that target various body organs. For example, as a reaction to a stressor, the hypothalamus releases corticotrophin releasing factor (CRF) that stimulates the pituitary gland to secrete adrenocorticotropic hormone (ACTH). ACTH activates the adrenal glands (in particular, the adrenal cortex) to secrete glucocorticoids (such as cortisol) and mineralocorticoids (such as aldosterone). Cortisol increases blood glucose so we have the energy to fight or flee. Aldosterone increase blood volume so we are able to transmit more food and oxygen, once again to be able to fight or flee. In addition, a direct nerve connection between the hypothalamus and the adrenal medulla results in the secretion of epinephrine (adrenaline) and norepinephrine (noradrenalin) which lead to an increase in heart rate, dilation of coronary arteries, an increase in oxygen consumption, and an increase in the force in which blood is pumped from the heart. All of this is by way of preparing the body to do something physical. This is what was occurring in Bill, the postal carrier mentioned in the opening of this chapter.

> **Stress psychophysiology.** The physical chain reaction to a stressor, which involves the secretion of hormones, and the increase of heart rate and oxygen consumption.

In addition to the adrenal glands, the thyroid gland releases the hormone thyroxine which accelerates heart rate, increases blood pressure and the rate and depth of breathing, and increases free fatty acids in the bloodstream. Further stress reactivity results in greater muscle tension, a decrease in white blood cells, and secretion of hydrochloric acid in and just outside the stomach.

Stress-Related Illnesses and Diseases

Illness and Diseases Associated with Stress

As a result of changes in the body when a stress reaction occurs, we are susceptible to a range of illnesses and diseases. For example, we discussed how aldosterone, secreted by the adrenal cortex in response to a stressor, results in an increase of blood volume. We also discussed how epinephrine and norepinephrine, secreted by the adrenal medulla, results in an increase in the force that blood is pumped from the heart. More blood, pumped with greater force, in the same-size blood vessels will inevitably increase blood pressure. If chronic, this can lead to hypertension. Hypertension, in turn, can lead to coronary heart disease or stroke.

The stress response also results in a decrease in white blood cells. White blood cells consist of phagocytes and two kinds of lymphocytes (T cells, B cells) that fight foreign substances in the body such as bacteria, viruses, and substances to which people are allergic (allergens). If stress results in fewer white blood cells, the immunological system will be less effective in responding to these foreign substances. Studies have verified the relationship between stress and illnesses and diseases resulting from a decreased effectiveness of the immunological system. For example, college students' levels of salivary IgA, an antibody that fights infections, were lower during final exams than at other times (Princeton Study, 1989). In another study (Rein, Atkinson & McCraty, 1995) subjects were asked to induce positive moods by "experiencing care and compassion." When researchers measured salivary IgA during these positive moods, they were increased. Researchers concluded that not only can stress result in a decreased effectiveness of the immunological system and illness and disease, but positive moods could enhance immunosuppressive effects thereby preventing disease.

Psychosomatic Illnesses and Diseases

Psyche is the Greek word for mind, and *soma* is the Greek word for body. Therefore, psychosomatic illness and diseases are mind–body conditions. Unfortunately, the lay public too often thinks of psychosomatic conditions to be "all in the mind." To understand how inaccurate that perception is, imagine people allergic to pollen. They may listen to the pollen count reported by the local weather forecaster in order to gauge whether they need to take their medication that day. If the pollen count is low, they can be assured they will not have an allergic reaction. However, if the count is above a certain level, they will react with a runny nose, tearing eyes, or coughing. The level at which they will react is called their threshold level. Below the threshold level, the immunological system (the white blood cells) can manage and control the pollen. Above that level and the white blood cells are ineffective. However, we know that stress decreases the number of white blood cells, thereby decreasing the level at which the immunological system can control the pollen. The result is an allergic reaction. To sum up then, the mind perceived a stressor and, as a result, changed the body (a decrease in white blood cells) that led to a real physical reaction. This mind–body relationship is the basis of psychosomatic illnesses and disease—real physical conditions exacerbated or initiated by the mind perceiving a stressor. Other illnesses and diseases with a mind–body connection are hypertension (Benson, 2000), stroke (Manuck et al., 1992), coronary heart disease (Koskenvuo et al., 1988; Stoney and Engebreston, 2000), ulcers, migraine headaches, and tension headaches (Pelletier, 1977; Stang, Von Korff & Galer, 1998), asthma (Steptoe, 1997), rheumatoid arthritis and backache (Waning & Castleman, 1984), temporomandibular syndrome (TMJ) and posttraumatic stress disorder (Ballinger et al., 2000), and even some forms of cancer.

A whole new field of study has emerged based on the relationship between the immunological system and stress known as *psychoneuroimmunology* (Yang & Glaser, 2002). In a review of studies in psychoneuroimmunology, Keicolt-Glaser and colleagues (2002) conclude that there is "sufficient data to conclude that immune modulation by psychosocial stressors or interventions can lead to actual health changes." Concurring with Kiecolt-Glaser's conclusions, Moynihan and colleagues (2000) state, "we provide evidence that immune deviation can occur following a pychosocial stressor." Various health conditions are affected by stress and its effect on the immunological system. Among these are cardiovascular disease, osteoporosis, arthritis, type 2 diabetes, certain cancers, Alzheimer's disease, and periodontal disease (Kiecolt-Glaser et al., 2002a). Emotional health is also affected by stress and its relation to the immune system. For example, despair that results from maternal separation has been referred to as a "stress-induced 'sickness behavior' " (Hennessey, Deak & Schiml-Webb, 2001), and there is evidence that stress and social support impact certain cancers (Spiegel & Sephton, 2001). In their review of research, Cruess and colleagues (2001) provide evidence for the relationship between depression, stressful life events, coping, and social support and immune system function and disease. A study of caregivers concurred with this conclusion that chronic distress is associated with impaired immunity (Baur et al., 2000).

Stress Management

We have discussed the conceptualization of stress as the combination of a stressor and stress reactivity. Another way to look at stress is when something occurs to knock one out of balance (something to which one has to adjust), the attempt to right oneself is stress. With that latter view, stress management, then, would require preventing the event that knocks one out of balance and/or helping one to apply coping skills once the imbalance has occurred. Referring back to the opening of this chapter, Jack, Kim, and Bill each experienced life events that "knocked them out of balance," to which they had to adjust. Each of them, however, were enrolled in a stress-management course that taught them ways of reducing the effect of the stress they experienced on their physical and emotional health. Imagine you are Jack, Kim, or Bill's health counselor as you read about these techniques below. Which do you think are most likely to benefit these students?

The Goal of Stress Management

Mistakenly, many people believe the goal of stress management is to eliminate all stress. If health counselors were successful at that, clients would experience stress from not having stress. Imagine a life so routine that nothing unexpected occurred, no challenges presented themselves, and no events happened that required an adjustment. That kind of a life would be boring, unstimulating, and therefore stressful. When the relationship between worker stress and health was studied, it was found that workers who experienced a great deal of stress, as expected, also experienced a great deal of illness and disease (Weiman, 1977). However, it was also found that workers who reported very little stress experienced the same level of disease as those reporting a great deal of stress. In other words, too little stress was as unhealthy as too much stress. The goal of stress management then is to help clients maintain their stress at an *optimal* level, enough to make life interesting, but not so much that illness/disease develops.

The Stress Model

One way to help clients conceptualize stress and **stress management** is by visually describing the process. The stress model (see Figure 11.1) can be used for that purpose. The model (Greenberg,

2002) starts with a *life situation* that knocks one out of balance. The life situation could be a change in temperature, a threat from another person, the death of a loved one, or any other change to which the client needs to adjust. Jack's life situation was the suicide of his friend; Kim's was her difficulty doing well in school; and Bill's was having a full-time job and then going to school in the evening which kept him away from his family. The life situation is akin to a stressor in that one can react to it with physiological arousal or not. Whether the client reacts with arousal depends on his or her perception and interpretation of the threat posed by the **life event.** For example, imagine a student fails a course in his major and presents with stress about the likelihood of obtaining a degree and entering the profession of his choice. That student has interpreted the life event—failing the course—as distressing and will, therefore, develop emotional arousal (anxiety, nervousness, anger). Another student, though, might experience the same stressor but interpret it quite differently. She might consider failing the course a sign that this is not the profession for her, and that she is fortunate to find this out so early. In this latter case, the student will not have emotional arousal. So, again, it is not the stressor or life event that leads to negative consequences, it is the person's interpretation of that event.

Once the life event is perceived/interpreted as distressing and emotional arousal has occurred, the body responds with physiological arousal (for example, increased heart rate, blood pressure, perspiration, and so on) and if that goes unabated, illness or other negative consequences (for example, poor interpersonal relationships or poor performance at work or school) can result.

Intervention: Setting Up Roadblocks on the Stress Model

Imagine the stress model is a road map of stress, passing through the "towns" of life situation, perception/interpretation, emotional arousal, physio-

---

Stress management. The practice of obtaining an optimal level of stress in one's life, or helping a client to do so.

Life event. Change in one's life routine that can be stressful.

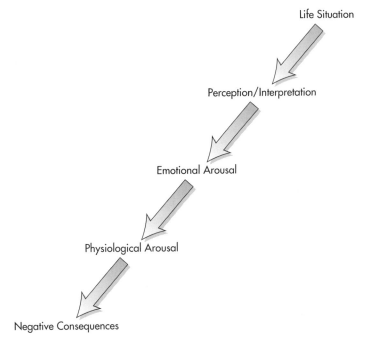

Figure 11.1
A stress model

logical arousal, and negative consequences. As with any road, roadblocks can be set up anywhere along the way. Stress management is the setting up of these roadblocks on the road of stress as illustrated in the stress model.

A roadblock can be placed even before the "town" of life situation if the stressor is avoided in the first place. For example, if a student finds speaking in front of a class stressful, she can be counseled not to register for classes that require oral presentations. If she finds herself required to enroll in one of these courses, she can change her interpretation of the oral presentation from one of a threat to one of a challenge with techniques such as cognitive restructuring (discussed later in this chapter). If she still perceives the oral presentation as a threat and winds up with emotional arousal, she can engage in relaxation as a roadblock at that level on the stress model. Relaxation techniques such as meditation, autogenics, and progressive relaxation are discussed later in this

chapter. Lastly, if the emotional arousal persists and physiological arousal occurs to prepare the body to react physically (fight or flee) to the stressor, the client can be counseled to engage in a program of regular exercise to use the built-up stress by-products.

The health counselor's responsibility is to help the client understand the nature of the perceived threat, assure the client that there are approaches that are successful in managing the stress, and facilitate the client's learning and applying these techniques.

Stress-Management–Related Constructs

Health counselors should be familiar with several constructs that pertain to stress management. This familiarity will provide health counselors with the tools to better respond to clients and/or students who present with stress-related issues.

An Attitude of Gratitude

There is a story going around about a college student who fell out of a dormitory window and landed in the bushes below. From the hospital where she was recovering from relatively minor injuries, she wrote her parents:

Dear Mom and Dad:

I had an accident at school, but am doing okay. My writing may be difficult to read because my right side is temporarily paralyzed but the good news is that I met someone in the hospital that I came to love. His name is Eric and he is a hospital orderly. In fact, we care so much for one another that we have decided to get married. Now, we guessed you would disapprove since he is of a different religion, ethnicity, and culture than we, so we decided to elope. Don't worry though, I am convinced our marriage will work out because he learned from his previous two marriages not to hit women when he gets angry with them, and the jail term he served only tended to reinforce that message.

Mom and Dad, don't worry. I did not get injured, I am not in a hospital, and I haven't met someone I love and with whom I am planning on getting married. However, I did fail chemistry, and wanted you to be able to put that in its proper perspective.

Isn't that what is most important about life—placing things in their proper perspective? I have conducted stress-management workshops for parents and grandparents residing at the Ronald McDonald House in Washington, D.C., and other cities. Parents residing at the Ronald McDonald House have children being treated at local hospitals for serious, and often life-threatening, illnesses. The Ronald McDonald House provides a residence for these families. It is often referred to as the "House That Love Built." At one workshop, two mothers spoke of their children's illnesses. One had a teenager who was dying of cancer in a local hospital and the other had a newborn who was not going to live very long. As these two mothers shared their stories, I could only think, "This is as bad as it gets." It was about then that both mothers told us that this was their *second* child that was dying!

In spite of the situation in which they find themselves, during these workshops the parents develop an **attitude of gratitude**. That is, they learn to be grateful for what they have, while not denying or ignoring the reality of their children's illnesses. In every situation there is something about which to be grateful. The mother of the teenager learned to be grateful for all the years she had with her son, recognizing that the mother of the newborn would never have the same time with her child. The Ronald McDonald House parents learn to be thankful for the health of their other children, for the days in which their children are feeling well, and that they can communicate effectively, for the expertise of the hospital staff, and for the support available to them (from other family members, church or synagogue congregants, or the Ronald McDonald House staff).

Health counselors should help clients develop an attitude of gratitude. Ask clients to imagine standing on a spot. As they look to the right they see people who have more money, are better looking, have a nicer house with more cars, have more friends, and have better jobs. Turning their heads to the left, they see people living in poverty, who are physically scarred and disabled, who are homeless and unemployed, and whose families have disowned them. If they look to the right and constantly bemoan what they do not have, they will be unhappy and, eventually, unhealthy. If they look to the left and appreciate what they do have, they will be more satisfied with their lives and be happier. No one decides for anyone else in which direction they will look and focus. That is an individual decision. Clients decide to be grateful for what they have (while still striving to improve their lives) or to envy the lives of others. Jack had other friends, Kim had a family that cared for her so much that they were willing to sacrifice financially to enhance her education, and Bill had a good job and the competence to pursue other work when he retired from the postal service. If the Ronald McDonald House parents can develop an attitude of gratitude, then health-counseling clients, and the rest of us, certainly should be able to as well.

Attitude of gratitude. Learning to be grateful for what one has, while not denying or ignoring reality.

Locus of Control

Students or clients who do not think they are able to control events in their lives are disadvantaged. They will be like a rudderless ship on the sea, tossed here and there as the currents determine. On the other hand, people who believe they can control their destinies will seek out information to take charge of their lives. The perception one has over the degree of control of events in one's life is called **locus of control.** If someone believes that events are controlled by fate, luck, chance, or powerful others, he is said to have an external locus of control. If someone believes that she controls events, that is referred to as an internal locus of control. The distinction between the two is obvious when we consider gambling. Those with an external locus of control would prefer bingo or slot machines since these games do not require any special action by the gambler and is solely based on luck. On the other hand, gamblers with an internal locus of control might prefer betting at the horse track since they can study the racing program and, based on that and the track conditions, choose a horse they think has the best chance of winning. Blackjack is another game requiring decisions by the gambler and, therefore, people with internal loci of control would prefer that game.

Although the tendency of health counselors might be to foster an internal locus of control, that is not always appropriate. Rather, the counselor's job is to assist clients to develop a *realistic* locus of control. Those clients who really do not have control of an event should not assume responsibility for how that event turns out. For example, assume a student studies well for an exam and knows all the important content but the professor writes questions based solely on the information contained in the captions under the photographs in the textbook. That is obviously an unfair exam. Students with an internal locus of control who take responsibility for failing that exam are being un-

realistic. That is an event that one is better off perceiving externally. To do otherwise can be very stressful. On the other hand, if the exam is fair, an internal locus of control would help students take responsibility for failing the exam and to identify what led to that failure. In this way, failing the exam will result in a greater likelihood of success on subsequent exams. Using health-counseling skills presented elsewhere in this book, the counselor can, therefore, help students be more successful when it is in their capacity to be so, and accept that they are not responsible for negative outcomes when they have no control over those outcomes.

Self-Esteem

People who do not think well of themselves will experience a good deal of stress in many aspects of their lives. They will not trust their own opinions and, therefore, be more prone to be influenced by others. This can lead to students engaging in activities they might otherwise not engage in if they were confident in themselves and their own decisions.

Self-esteem is learned. How people react to us; what we come to believe are acceptable societal standards of beauty, competence, and intelligence; and how our performance is judged by parents, teachers, friends, and bosses affect how we feel about ourselves. Our successes improve our self-esteem and our failures diminish it. The very essence of stress management requires confidence in oneself and in one's decisions to control one's life effectively. Counselors who facilitate client success will help enhance client self-esteem. Self-talk and cognitive restructuring (both of which are discussed later in this chapter) are also useful counseling tools for improving client self-esteem.

Anxiety

Anxiety is an unrealistic fear that manifests itself as:

- a subjective sense of fear
- physiological arousal
- avoidance or escape

Locus of control. A person's perceptions of the degree of control they have over events that affect their lives (external vs. internal).

Clients who have test anxiety, for example, become fearful when they think about having to take a test; they feel their hearts pounding, start perspiring, breath rapidly and shallow, and experience muscle tension; they may cut class the day of the test or take the test hurriedly to get out of the room as soon as possible. Clients who have agoraphobia (Rosenham and Seligman, 1995) have a fear of going out and being with a group of other people, experience physiological arousal when thinking of leaving their homes, and if forced to go out, will return as soon as feasible.

Fortunately, there are many tools which health counselors can employ to assist clients to decrease their levels of anxiety. Among these are environmental planning, self-talk, and systematic desensitization. *Environmental planning* encourages clients to rearrange the situation around the anxiety-provoking stimulus so it is less fearful. For example, clients who are anxious about medical checkups can be instructed to make a list of friends and relatives in whose presence they feel especially comfortable. Then, they can plan a visit to a medical practitioner accompanied by one of these friends or relatives. Clients who are anxious about having to speak in public can be instructed to arrive at the sight early so as to arrange the setting just the way they want, and the way in which they will feel less anxious.

Self-talk consists of speaking to oneself in an attempt to more realistically perceive the situation about which one is anxious. Statements such as the following can help clients be less anxious:

- I've done this before, I know I'll be able to do it again.

- If I have problems, I can always call on my buddy Ralph to help me out.

- Everyone feels nervous on occasions such as these. It's perfectly natural.

- What am I really afraid will happen? How likely is that to happen?

Counselors can help clients understand that their anxiety consists of an unrealistic fear, and they can help clients manage that fear by having them engage in self-talk to perceive the threat more accurately.

Systematic Desensitization, developed by Joseph Wolpe (1973) involves imagining or experiencing an anxiety-provoking scene while practicing a response incompatible with anxiety (such as relaxation). The first step is to help the client develop a fear hierarchy, a sequence of small steps (at least 10) that lead up to the anxiety-provoking event. The client is also taught deep muscle relaxation (for example, meditation, imagery, autogenics). Then the client relaxes herself and imagines the first step on the fear hierarchy for 1 to 5 seconds, gradually increasing the time to 30 seconds. After being able to imagine the event for 30 seconds, the client then engages in relaxation for 30 seconds. The client eventually moves down the fear hierarchy in this fashion until she can imagine the event without it provoking physiological arousal. As an alternative to imagining themselves performing the steps on the fear hierarchy, the client can actually engage in the event. When imagination is used, this is termed *arm chair desensitization*. When actually performing the steps, this is termed *in vivo desensitization*.

Life Events

If stress is the need to adapt to change (a life situation on the stress model), it stands to reason that the more a client has to adjust to, the greater the stress experienced. Using this theoretical framework, scales have been developed (Anderson, 1972; Holmes & Rahe, 1967) to measure the amount of potentially stressful life events a client experiences and the degree of perceived stress associated with those events. If counselors find clients are experiencing too many changes in their life events, they can help them make their client's lives more routine. For example, going on a vacation at a time of great stress may not be the wisest decision. Vacations themselves can be stressful, requiring that arrangements be made to water the plants, take care of the dog, buy clothes appropriate for the vacation spot, and adapt to a new daily style in a different environment. Life-events theory recommends not taking on additional changes in one's life if experiencing too many changes as is.

Hassles

Some researchers theorize that it is not the significant changes in people's lives that translate into negative consequences (for example, psychosomatic illness). Rather, they argue, it is the **hassles** people encounter on a daily basis that is the culprit (Kanner et al., 1981). Losing a wallet or having troublesome neighbors are examples of daily hassles that are essentially negative and of a chronic nature that can take a toll on one's health. In fact, hassles have been found to be predictive of psychological distress (Holahan, Holahan & Belk, 1984), and related to poor mental and physical health (Zarski, 1984). DeLongis and colleagues (1982) developed a Hassles Scale to measure people's susceptibility to subsequent illness and disease. Health counselors can administer that scale to clients and if the counselor finds their client experiences too many daily hassles, they should work with the client to eliminate as many hassles as is feasible.

Occupational Stress

Many people define job stress too simplistically. They think of job stress as stressors they encounter at work. Health counselors should help clients perceive **occupational stress** as comprised of more than just these stressors. Certainly sources of stress at work such as having too much work to do in too short a period of time (work overload), or being unsure about the expectations of workers held by those who provide rewards of promotion or salary increases (role ambiguity), or being asked to do several things at the same time by different supervisors (role conflict) can be stressful. However,

each of these and other stressors only have the potential to elicit a stress response. These stressors affect people differently because people vary on several important characteristics. Some workers have a low tolerance for ambiguity, others do not. Some workers have low self-esteem, others do not. Added to this mix of sources of stress at work and those stressors being viewed through individual characteristics are the stressors that workers bring to the work site from outside of work. Whereas workers can hang up their coats on a coatrack at the start of the workday and leave it there until they are ready to go home, there is no such thing as a "stress rack." Rather, workers "wear" the stressors they bring from outside the work site throughout the work day, and these stressors affect the way in which they react to the stressors they experience at work. The stressors that Bill the postal worker experienced at home had to affect him at work. When his wife argued with him about not being home enough, and he was upset about that for the rest of the day, not only his health was in jeopardy, but his job performance was as well. Figure 11.2 depicts the complexity of occupational stress.

The implication of this model of job stress is that the counselor needs to work with the client on coping with sources of stress at work, stressors from outside of work, and individual characteristics that contribute to a stress response when such a response is not desirable.

Two Alternative Occupational Stress Models

One way of conceptualizing work stress is the *job strain* model. The job-strain model conceives of stress as the result of high job demands and low job control. You can imagine how frustrating, and stressful, it would be to be expected to be highly productive, while at the same time not being able to decide how to do that. In a sense, the manner in which you are evaluated (meeting the high job demands) is dependent on factors beyond your control. How unfair that must feel!

Another way of conceptualizing work stress is the *effort-reward imbalance* model. The effort-reward imbalance model conceives of work stress as a function of too great a work effort required to do

> **Hassles.** Minor stressing events encountered on a daily basis that can take a toll on one's health.
>
> **Occupational stress.** Stress on the job that may be comprised of sources of stress at work, stressors from outside of work and/or individual characteristics that contribute to an unwanted stress response.

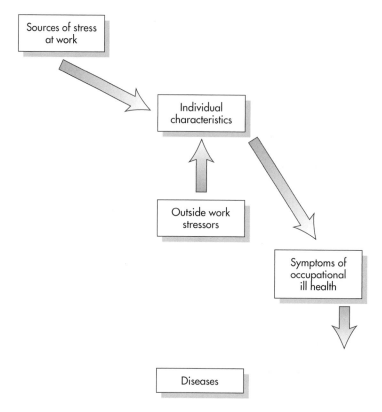

Figure 11.2
A model of occupational stress (Cooper & Marshall, 1978)

the job accompanied by low reward for a job well done. This model considers such effort as high workload on one end of the equation, and such rewards as salary, esteem, and occupational status on the other. According to the effort-reward imbalance model, "demanding tasks under insecure conditions, lack of promotion, and low wages compared to qualifications may in the long run threaten workers' health and well-being."*

Perhaps occupational stress is a combination of the factors included in each of these models. That is, high work demand, low job control, and lack of accompanying reward are all probably factors that contribute to work stress.

* "Chronic Load is Dangerous for Health and Well-Being," *Euro Review on Research in Health and Safety at Work,* 1997, p. 13.

Type A Behavior Pattern

Related to job stress, but also to other aspects of a person's life, is the pace at which one travels through the world. Researchers have found a stressful behavior pattern related to a range of illness and disease. These behaviors are called **Type A Behavior Pattern.** Type A Behavior Pattern was first described by Friedman and Rosenman (1974) as comprised of a sense of time urgency, excessive competitive drive, aggressiveness, impatience, and free-floating hostility. Subsequent research indicated that the hostil-

Type A behavior pattern. A behavior pattern comprised of a sense of time urgency, excessive competitive drive, aggressiveness, impatience, and free-floating hostility.

ity component was the most related to coronary heart disease (Shekelle, et al., 1983). However, more recent research has found Type A to be comprised of two different components that appear to be operating in opposing directions. One component is defined as Impatience/Irritability (II), and the other as Achievement Striving (AS). Only II is associated with physical health complaints (Pred, Spence & Helmreich, 1986), depression, and job satisfaction (Bluen, Barling & Burns, 1990), and marital dissatisfaction (Barling, Bluen & Moss, 1990). AS was found to be "nontoxic," having no effect on these variables.

The health counselor's role, therefore, is to assist clients to alter their perceptions of their world so as to view it as more friendly and supportive of them. The use of social support networks can be an important component of this strategy. In addition, clients should be helped to slow down their worlds. The relaxation techniques described later in this chapter can help clients accomplish that goal.

Social Support

Social support is the assistance received by others in one's life. These "others" might be family, friends, fellow parishioners, professors, or any other people who can help the client manage a stressful situation. Social support can take various forms. For example, a family member might provide the *emotional support* during a particularly stressful event. Or, a friend might provide *financial support* when bills are overdue and the stress associated with that is overbearing. Alternatively, a member of the clergy might provide *spiritual support* when that is appropriate. And, a professor might provide *informational support* when certain facts or advice can help alleviate stress (Matich & Sims, 1992).

We know that social support helps to decrease the negative effects of stress. For example,

melanoma patients who participated in a 6-week support group experienced only half as many recurrences as similar patients who did not ("Stress," 1999). It has also led to improved academic performance (Feiner, Farber & Primavera, 1983) and less combat stress among soldiers (Solomon, Mikulincer & Hobfill, 1987). The health counselor's role is to work with clients to determine the nature of social support they need and sources of that type of support available to them, and then to facilitate clients using this social support effectively.

Stress-Management Skills

Health counselors should be familiar with various stress-management skills in order to be able to assist clients in managing stress. Some of these skills are behavioral (such as relaxation techniques and time-management skills), whereas others are cognitive (such as cognitive restructuring and self-talk). Given space limitations, it is not possible to teach these techniques in their entirety. Instead, an introduction to several means of managing stress is presented. Health counselors are encouraged to research these techniques in more detail elsewhere.

Relaxation Techniques

Relaxation techniques result in the relaxation response; decreased heart rate, blood pressure, respiration, muscle tension, and various other physiological changes. Some relaxation techniques relax the mind and the body follows, others relax the body and the mind follows, and still others relax both the mind and the body.

Meditation. Meditation requires the meditator to focus on either an unchanging object (such as a spot on the wall) or something repetitive (such as

---

Social support. The assistance received by the others in one's life, which may be emotional, financial, spiritual, practical or informational in nature.

Relaxation techniques. Techniques that result in decreased heart rate, blood pressure, respiration and muscle tension, such as meditation, mildfulness, and diaphragmatic breathing.

a word that is repeated). It is recommended that meditation be conducted for approximately 20 minutes twice a day, once in the morning on rising and once halfway through the day (perhaps just before dinner).

Mindfulness. Mindfulness is focusing your attention on the present moment. It is paying attention to each moment, living in the here and now. Instead of the what-ifs and if-onlys, the focus is on the what-is. Its opposite, mindlessness, is going through life ignoring the present moment because of attention directed toward the goal rather than the experience. Mindlessness occurs when you drive to school or work and describe yourself as being on automatic pilot. All of a sudden you are at your destination without having really experienced the trip. Some people may reach the end of their lives without ever having truly experienced the trip along the way.

Mindfulness dates all the way back to Eastern and Western traditions of religion, philosophy, and psychology. It recognizes existentialist philosophy, such as that of Albert Camus, that argues who we are is more important than what we do. When patients have been taught to have this focus, mindfulness has been found effective in treating chronic pain (Kabat-Zinn et al., 1987), psoriasis (Bernhard, Kristeller & Kabat-Zinn, 1988), and anxiety disorders (Kabat-Zinn et al., 1992). Since stress is often caused by a preoccupation with the past (guilt, shame, regret) or with the future (fear of upcoming events), mindfulness is an excellent way to help manage stress.

Mindfulness can be developed in a number of ways. One is to focus on your breathing, called mindful breathing. In this way the mind is quieted and attention is drawn to the here and now.

Diaphragmatic Breathing. When distressed, breathing becomes rapid, shallow, and stems from the chest. There are several different ways that people breathe (Girdano, Everly & Dusek, 1993). When people expand the upper third of their chest they are doing *upper costal breathing* (named after the intercostal muscles that connect the ribs). Most people breath by expanding the middle third of their chest (approximately at the sixth rib

down). This is known as *thoracic breathing* or *middle costal breathing*. However, the more relaxing and healthier form of breathing is to expand the belly. This is called *diaphragmatic breathing* (Forman & Myers, 1987) since the diaphragm is expanded when breathing this way. Sometimes people make a deep sigh to relieve stress by inhaling a large amount of air and exhaling it slowly. This we call *very deep breathing* and it is quite effective as an immediate response to stress.

To help clients practice diaphragmatic breathing, have them lie on their backs with the palms of their hands placed on their lower stomach area. As they breathe, instruct them to expand their chest area while keeping their stomach flat. Encourage them to become aware that this is thoracic breathing and to recognize it as such. Next, instruct them to expand their abdomen so that their stomach rises and falls with each breath while their chest size remains relatively constant (it will expand some). Encourage them to recognize this type of breathing as diaphragmatic breathing. Have clients practice diaphragmatic breathing at various times of the day (when seated doing school work, for instance). Diaphragmatic breathing is basic to all forms of relaxation. It is difficult being relaxed if you are breathing thoracically.

To help people practice breathing diaphragmatically, Krucoff and Krucoff (2000) recommend a variation of the above:

1. Lie on your back and place a book on your belly. Make the book rise with your breathing.

2. Sit with your right hand on your abdomen and your left hand on your chest and make your right hand rise as you breath.

3. Use a second hand on a clock and inhale for 5 seconds and exhale for 5 seconds.

4. Repeat a mantra and breathe in synchrony as you say it in your mind. Zen master Thich Nhat Hahn suggests repeating, "Breathing in I calm myself, breathing out I smile."

Other Relaxation Techniques. Health counselors can employ still other relaxation techniques with their clients. Among these other methods of relaxation are autogenic training, progressive neuromuscular relaxation, biofeedback, Tai Chi, massage, acupressure, body scanning, yoga and stretching, aromatherapy, reflexology, repetitive prayer, the Quieting Reflex, the Instant Calming Sequence, and listening to music. These relaxation methods are described in more detail in a book by this author (Greenberg, 2002).

Cognitive Restructuring

Cognitive restructuring is a way of controlling the way one views a stressor so as to make it less stressful (see Chapter 4). The attitude of gratitude discussed earlier in this chapter is a form of cognitive restructuring. One purposefully focuses on the positive aspects of a situation and, therefore, becomes grateful for that aspect of the situation. Self-talk is another form of cognitive restructuring. As you read about the cognitive restructuring techniques described below, imagine how you would counsel Jack, Kim, or Bill from the Case Study at the start of this chapter to use them to manage their stress.

Self-Talk. Health counselors can help their clients to more realistically perceive the threat/risk of situations, thereby decreasing the likelihood of a stress reaction. One way to do this is to teach clients the technique of *self-talk*. Ask clients to think of the worst thing that can happen in the situation, and then to estimate the likelihood of that happening. For example, if students are anxious about having to make a presentation before their class, they can list the threats as not doing well, no one listening to them, the class laughing at their ineptitude, or the professor interrupting because the presentation is so boring. These are not desirable outcomes! However, even if these outcomes occurred, students could live through them. They would have other assignments in that class and/or tests on which they could do well and improve their grades. They would still have their friends, their health, and their families. The point is that

even if the worst things happened, that would not be tragic—not something to look forward to, but not tragic. However, the likelihood of these outcomes occurring is small. Many people catastrophize events and perceive them as more likely than they actually are. So, the likelihood is low that these reactions to a class presentation will occur. Furthermore, even if they did occur, it wouldn't be the end of the world. Now, if the feared outcomes are really not that bad, and the likelihood of them occurring is low anyhow, there really is not much to worry about. Counselors who use self-talk to help their clients perceive their fears in a more realistic light are helping them manage their stress.

Stress Inoculation. As one can receive an inoculation for influenza, one can receive inoculation for stress. At least that is what Donald Meichenbaum (1977) thinks. Stress inoculation utilizes self-talk in an organized fashion to prepare, cope, and reinforce behavior that might otherwise be avoided because of stress associated with that behavior. For example, as clients are preparing for a stressful event, they can say to themselves such a self-talk statement as: "I am well prepared and I should, therefore, do well" or "I can always call on Betty if I need help." As they are performing the stressful event, they can say: "I am doing it now. I've made it this far and it's okay." And, after they have performed the event, they can reinforce having gotten through it by such statements as "I did it! If I did it this time, I'm sure I can do it again next time." Health counselors can teach clients stress inoculation to help them as they encounter stressful events.

Time Management

Many students and other clients experience stress due to their inability to manage their time well. They feel they have too much to do in too little time, or not enough time to engage in the activities they particularly enjoy (such as spending more time with their children or skiing on a snow-covered mountain). This was especially true of Bill the postal worker in our Case Study. Although employing time-management skills will not give clients any more time, it can organize their time better so as to free up time for others things. The

> **Cognitive restructuring.** A type of cognitive behavioral therapy that attempts to restructure faulty thinking and negative self-statements into more positive ideas.

first step in time management is for health counselors to assist clients to understand that when they waste time, there is no bank from which they can withdraw time previously saved. Time is continually used up, it cannot be saved. However, it can be used more efficiently. Time-management skills are presented below.

Assessing the Use of Time. Have clients record what they are doing every 15 minutes. Then have them add up all the time they spent on various categories of activities. For example, how much time was spent socializing, studying, on the telephone, on the computer? Next, instruct clients to determine whether an adjustment is desired. Do they wish to spend more time studying, or less time on the telephone? This determination will help clients focus on the desired behavior change so their time is used more efficiently.

Setting Goals. Where do clients want to be at the end of the semester? at the end of the year? At the end of their schooling? In 10 years? Without clients having a goal in mind, it is impossible for them to determine how best to use their time to achieve their goals.

Prioritizing. Too often people perform daily activities with very little thought as to what is most important that day. To help clients spend their time on the most important activities before engaging in the less important, health counselors should instruct them to make four lists. The *A List* includes activities that have the highest priority that day. These are activities that have to be done that day. For example, a student has a term paper due tomorrow and it hasn't been typed yet. On the *B List* are activities that clients would like to do that day, but that can wait until the next day or two. Perhaps they have to return a friend's phone call. It does not have to get done today, but should get done soon. On the *C List* are those activities that need to get done but that can wait until there is more time available to do them. For example, clients may need to shop for a new pair of shoes. Although that needs to get done, it can probably

wait several weeks if need be. Lastly, the *Not-to-Do List* includes activities that clients definitely want to avoid doing. For example, if clients have been watching too much television, they might include not watching television on their Not-to-Do List that day. Providing this kind of organization and prioritizing skill for clients will help them make more sense of the way they use their time each day.

Delegating. Too often people feel uncomfortable asking for help. Especially when particularly busy, clients should be taught to delegate responsibilities. Students who have an important examination tomorrow should ask their roommates to do the dishes after dinner, or to take out the garbage. There will be a time when time pressures are not so severe that these students can pay back the favor to their roommates.

Saying No. Exacerbating the problem of not delegating is not being able to refuse requests from others when there is not enough time to meet these requests. Some clients will feel they are not being a good friend or a good employee if they don't say yes to such requests. Teaching clients to be assertive—that is, explaining they would like to help but they do not have the time at that moment—will make it easier for clients to use their time more appropriately.

Controlling Stressful Behaviors

Health counselors will encounter clients who engage in behaviors they would like to give up (for example, smoking cigarettes, biting their nails, partying too much). They will also encounter clients who wish they would engage in certain behaviors but do not (for example, studying more, exercising regularly). Health counselors can teach clients ways to manage these behaviors and, therefore, experience less stress.

Self-Monitoring. Observing and recording behavior can offer the insight necessary for changing that behavior. It can also provide the encouragement/reinforcement clients need once they start a behavior change program. For example, if students regularly come late for class, they could monitor that behavior to determine the extent of the problem and, once attempting to arrive on time, could record how successful they are at the new behavior.

Material Reinforcement. Rewarding a desired behavior results in that behavior more likely to be repeated. Health counselors can help clients list rewards that would motivate them to adopt the desired behavior.

Social Reinforcement. As material rewards are effective in helping clients change their behavior, so are social rewards. In this case, clients would not receive tangible objects as rewards (such as a new CD) but instead receive the encouragement, support, and recognition from close friends, relatives, coworkers, or others significant in the client's lives. Counselors can help clients identify these sources of social reinforcement, as well as the nature the reinforcement might take.

Contracting. One of the most effective behavior change strategies is contracting. The counselor can help the client make a behavior change contract. The contract should include a specific behavior, a time by when that behavior should be performed, the reward for performing that behavior, and the punishment for not performing it. The contract can take the form of an "if-then" rule. For example, "If I am on time for all my classes this week, then I will go to that movie I've been really wanting to see." Contracts are even more effective if they involve a friend or relative who serves as a witness to the contract. In that case, the client uses peer pressure in a positive way.

Reminders. Clients may not always remember to perform the behavior they desire. In this case, the health counselor can help the client develop reminders. Reminders can take the form of mailed postcards from the counselor to the client, notes on refrigerators or bathroom mirrors, or notations on a calendar.

Summary

Health educators/counselors can expect to be presented with clients who are having difficulty managing the stress in their lives. *Stress* is the combination of a stressor and stress reactivity. *Stressors* only have the potential of eliciting a stress response; they need not do so if the stressor is interpreted as nonthreatening. Stress leads to changes in the body—*stress reactivity*—that include increased heart rate, blood pressure, and respiratory rate. These physiological changes are a result of direct nerve intervention and hormonal secretions of various glands in the body.

Several diseases are associated with stress. These include stroke, coronary heart disease, and psychosomatic illnesses and diseases. Psychosomatic illnesses and diseases involve a connection between the mind and the body.

The goal of stress management is to help clients obtain an optimal level of stress, rather than to eliminate all stress in their lives. In this way, life will be interesting, including unforeseen occurrences and challenges for which talents and skills are required.

One model of stress starts with a *life situation* that is perceived or interpreted as distressing. That interpretation results in *emotional arousal* that, in turn, leads to *physiological arousal*. The result is *negative consequences* such as illness, poor job or school performance, or dysfunctional interpersonal relationships.

Clients' perceptions of the degree of control they have over events that affect their lives is called their *locus of control*. Clients with an external locus of control believe these events are a result of luck, fate, chance, or powerful others. Those with an internal locus of control believe they can control events in their lives. Clients with external loci of control, believing they can influence events in their lives–for example, their levels of stress—will take actions to exercise that influence.

Anxiety is an unrealistic fear that includes a subjective sense of fear, physiological arousal, and either avoidance or escape behavior. Counselors can help clients manage their anxiety by teaching them environmental planning, self-talk, and systematic desensitization.

Occupational stress is a result of sources of stress at work, sources of stress outside the work place, and the worker's individual characteristics. Health counselors can help clients manage occupational and other forms of stress by teaching them stress-management skills. Among these skills are relaxation techniques such as meditation, mindfulness, diaphragmatic breathing, autogenic training, progressive neuromuscular relaxation, biofeedback, Tai Chi, massage, accupressure, body scanning, yoga and stretching, aromatherapy, reflexology, repetitive prayer, the Quieting Reflex, the Instant Calming Sequence, and listening to music. Clients can also be taught to manage stress through the cognitive restructuring techniques of self-talk and stress inoculation. Other stress-management techniques health counselors can teach clients include time-management skills and ways to take control of stressful behaviors.

Key Terms

attitude of gratitude, 208

cognitive restructuring, 215

hassles, 211

life events, 206

locus of control, 209

occupational stress, 211

relaxation techniques, 213

social support, 213

stress management, 206

stress psychophysiology, 204

stress reactivity, 203

stressor, 203

Type A Behavior Pattern, 212

Questions for Discussion

1. What might be considered an optimal level of stress? How can you determine whether a client has too much or too little stress in his/her life?

2. How can stress management be seen as the setting up of "roadblocks?"

3. Why is someone with an "internal locus of control" more likely to experience success from health counseling? Do you have an internal or external locus of control, or a combination of both?

4. Why is self-esteem so important in stress-management efforts?

5. What are some tools health counselors can employ to help clients decrease their anxiety level?

Related Web Sites

http://www.ncptsd.org/West_haven.html
Clinical Neuroscience Division. Studies on stress and brain function as well as treatment for trauma patients. Also includes studies by international researchers and training for the next generation of researchers.

http://www.mcms.dal.ca/danat/anat_res.htm
Anatomy and Neurobiology. Provides research articles and activities regarding the human brain, its function, and responses during stress.

http://www.aomc.org/stressreduction.html
Stress: Techniques for Stress Reduction. Provides exercises and tips for coping with various stressors.

http://www.oz.sannyas.net/quotes/med03.htm
Exploration of Dynamic Meditation. Includes explanation of its purpose, technique, and instructions on its use.

http://www.ub-counseling.buffalo.edu/Stress
Stress and Anxiety. Includes information on stress and time management, test anxiety, overcoming procrastination, and study skills for students.

Ecotherapy

GLORIA PIERCE, PH.D.

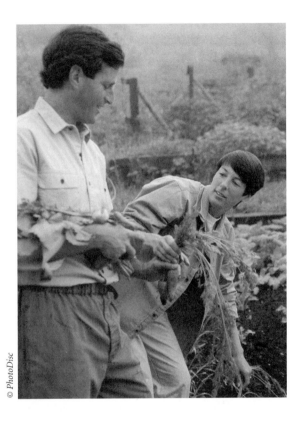

© PhotoDisc

OBJECTIVES

By the end of the chapter, the reader should be able to:

- Describe the key principles of ecopsychology

- Cite the prominent therapies that ecotherapy draws on

- Understand the difference between the concepts of androcentrism and ecological self

- Provide examples of methods ecotherapists might use to create psychological well being in clients

Effective health counseling and health education are based on what might be called "a holistic imperative." Simply stated, this means that there are many aspects to health that interact with one another. Consequently, health professionals must understand and attend to the multidimensional, systemic nature of wellness when educating their students and counseling their clients. Ecotherapy provides the holistic framework necessary for helping others to learn and develop positive, health-enhancing behaviors and attitudes. Because ecotherapy recognizes that human wellbeing consists of mental, physical, emotional, social, spiritual, and environmental factors, it seeks to incorporate these elements into its therapeutic concepts and methods. Most important, ecotherapy views the multifaceted nature of well-

219

ness in the context of the larger environment in which humans function and is thus a truly holistic approach to health. This chapter demonstrates the value of ecotherapy to the field of health counseling and education in promoting the overall health of the human being.

As recently as 1991, psychologist Ralph Metzner complained that his discipline "remained virtually untouched by any concern for the environment or the human-to-nature relationship" (Metzer, 1991, p. 147). Although theologians, lawyers, historians, economists, and politicians had begun to examine their own areas of knowledge in the context of the dire environmental news received almost daily, Metzner lamented:

> You will search in vain in the texts and journals of any of the major schools of psychology—clinical, behaviorist, cognitive, physiological, humanistic or transpersonal—for any theory or research concerning the most basic fact of human existence: the fact of our relationship to the natural world of which we are a part. (p. 147)

Such a "glaring, scandalous, and . . . embarrassing omission" (p. 147) was about to be remedied the following year with the publication of Theodore Roszak's landmark book, *The Voice of the Earth* (1992). In addition, small groups of prominent environmental activists and psychologists had been gathering to discuss what they might do to bridge the theoretical gap between ecology and psychology in order to make the profession of psychology relevant to the ecological situation of our time. The first **ecopsychology** conference, "Psychology as if the Whole Earth Mattered," was held at the Center for Psychology and Social Change at the Harvard Medical School in Cambridge, Massachusetts, in 1990, followed shortly thereafter by two conferences at the Esalen Institute in Big Sur, California, in 1993 and 1994. These meetings were tremendously influential in launching ecopsychology as a viable conceptual

framework for a new definition of psychology and a new vision of health and well-being.

Priniples of Ecopsychology

As an evolving concept and approach to health, ecopsychology is based on several key principles:

1. The earth is a living system of which human beings are a part.
2. The core of the mind is the ecological unconscious and embedded within it is an innate love of the earth and its life forms.
3. Psychopathology is rooted in human estrangement from nature and repression of the ecological unconscious.
4. Ecopsychology seeks to heal the alienation between humans and nature.
5. Mental health, sanity, and the psyche all need redefinition. The ego-bound self must be expanded to include the biosphere. The ego-centric self must evolve to the eco-centric self.
6. The reciprocal, synergistic relationship between personal and planetary well-being may be stated as: the needs of the planet are the needs of the person; the rights of the person are the rights of the planet.
7. Ecopsychology draws upon insights from non-Western indigenous cultures, **deep ecology, ecofeminism,** spiritual traditions and **depth psychology**.

Ecopsychology. Psychology that embraces an ecological conception of the human psyche, wherein the roots of modern psychological distress lie in the estrangement from nature and inadequate definitions of sanity.

Deep ecology. The philosophical idea that there needs to be a widening and deepening of the self to include all other forms of life.

Ecofeminism. A form of feminism/ecology that rejects the male-centered system of domination and control that leads to violence against women and the earth.

Depth psychology. A branch of psychology that seeks to restore emotional well-being by reconnecting human consciousness to its deepest roots, the matrix of a universal consciousness within an ecological frame of reference.

8. Ecopsychology critiques modern technocratic, consumer culture and rejects systems of domination and control based on patriarchal, androcentric, and anthropocentric worldviews.

Ecotherapy is the application of the principles of ecopsychology to the work of health practitioners. This concise definition belies the far-reaching, profound effects that an ecotherapy approach could have on the well-being of humans and their environment. This chapter will describe (1) how ecopsychology provides a much-needed, major revisioning of what constitutes a healthy person, and (2) how an ecotherapy approach can transform the practice of health counseling.

It is folly to believe that healthy persons can exist in an unhealthy environment. Such a premise may be rather easily accepted when it comes to the physical health of human beings. We know that we require clean water to drink, unpolluted air to breathe, and uncontaminated food to eat. Without such basic necessities, our physical bodies sicken and die. But what effect does the condition of the environment have on the human psyche, on the health of the mind and the soul? The emerging field of ecopsychology asks this question and its converse: how does the psychological makeup of human beings affect the earth that sustains us? By reexamining and understanding the reciprocal relationship between the human psyche and the natural world, ecopsychology hopes to heal the damage done to this relationship by contemporary industrialized society.

Contextual Backdrop of Ecopsychology

Although environmentalists have been warning about ecological devastation for decades, there existed no "adequate psychological critique of our highly scientific-materialist world view and technologically based lifestyles" (Yunt, 2001, p. 104). In fact, psychologists realized that the environmental movement too often employed tactics of fear, shame, and guilt to motivate people to change their profligate environmental habits, motivations that seldom succeed in facilitating behavioral change. Ecopsychologists see the environmental crisis as a consequence of the maladaptive behavior of people (Winter, 2000) arising from a misconception of self (Conn, 1995). Therapists can use their knowledge and skill to help change the problem behavior by changing how we see ourselves in relation to the planet: rather than seeing the earth as belonging to us, we would see ourselves as belonging to the earth (Chief Seattle, in Clinebell, 1996, p. 1). Hence, we would love and protect the ecosystem to which we belong.

The history of psychology can be seen as the gradual expansion of the *context* of health and wellness. For much of the 20th century, psychology attended primarily to individual concerns and problems; clients were helped to cope and adjust to the world they lived in. Social psychology broadened the phenomenological field to include interpersonal interactions and the dynamics of group situations (Miles, 1981). A shift to a systemic worldview occurred with the ascendance of family therapy which used the family system as the unit of analysis and treatment (Ivey, Ivey & Simek-Morgan, 1993). More recently, approaches such as feminist therapy enlarged the scope of therapeutic inquiry still further by considering the impact of social, political, and economic forces on clients' lives (Worell & Remer, 1992). Therapies that take a systems view acknowledge that humans are *creatures of culture*, a part of social systems that people have created and within which we function. Before the emergence of ecopsychology, systems theories did not fully recognize that humans are first and foremost *creatures of nature*, that we are biological beings dependent upon the earth for our very existence. Ecopsychology has now begun to place the helping relationship in the context of the biosphere as well as the social sphere.

Freudian analyst Harold Searles clearly anticipated the emergence of ecopsychology in his innovative work, *The Nonhuman Environment in Normal Development and in Schizophrenia*:

Ecotherapy. A form of therapy that assumes a connection between healing the wounded human psyche and healing the wounds inflicted on the earth.

During the past sixty years, the focus on psychiatry's attention has gradually become enlarged, from an early preoccupation with intrapsychic processes (particularly the individual's struggles with his own conflictual id, ego, and and superego strivings), to include interpersonal and broad sociological-anthropological factors. It would seem, then, that a natural next phase would consist in our broadening our focus still further, to include the investigation of man's relationships with his nonhuman environment. (Searles, as quoted in Roszak, 1992, p. 295)

Thus, the theoretical framework of the helping professional has evolved from an emphasis on the individual to perspectives that seek to understand human beings in a widening context of the larger systems within which they operate: from the single individual to family systems to social systems and now the ecosystem.

Ecopsychology gained momentum at the end of the 20th century because of a severe sense of alarm on the part of many ecologically aware psychotherapists who saw environmental degradation as inextricably linked to their clients' emotional distress. In their iconoclastic book, *We've Had a Hundred Years of Psychotherapy and the World's Getting Worse* (1992), Jungian analyst James Hillman and co-author Michael Ventura criticized the myopia and timidity of psychotherapy for turning social and environmental problems into private pathologies. The long list of environmental atrocities we have perpetrated—soil and ozone depletion; pollution of the air, oceans, rivers and lakes; numerous extinctions of entire species; acid rain; deforestation and the clear-cutting of forests; global warming; sprawl and overdevelopment; decimation of indigenous cultures (Oskamp, 2000)—takes a heavy toll on the human psyche, albeit unconsciously in most people:

The depression we're all trying to avoid could very well be a prolonged chronic reaction to what we've been doing to the world, a mourning and grieving for what we're doing to nature and to cities and to whole peoples—the destruction of a lot of our world. We may be depressed partly because this is the soul's reaction to the mourning and grieving that we're not consciously doing. (Hillman, 1992, p. 140)

Michael Cohen, who developed and directs an academic program in ecopsychology and ecotherapy at Greenwich University in Washington state, writes:

People are an integral part of nature. As we learn to assault the natural world around us, we learn to assault our true inner nature, and vice versa. The hurt from this assault feeds our disorders. Your happiness, humanity's destiny, and life on Earth as we know it depends on our ability to become involved in reconnecting with nature. (Cohen, 1997, pp. 81 & 154)

Implicit in the remarks of Cohen and Hillman is the assumption that humans have become alienated from the earth and the disruption of that crucial bond results in the emotional suffering and spiritual emptiness reflected back to us in the agony of ecological pain. It is the aim of ecopsychology, therefore, to restore the lost connection between humans and our planetary home and to heal the wounds of both.

In *The Voice of the Earth* (1992), Roszak elaborates upon the analysis of the human–earth relationship he had begun to explore in *Person/Planet* (1978). This seminal work articulates the rationale, goals, theoretical framework, and principles of ecopsychology. It suggests that the havoc which human societies have wreaked on our own habitat can be considered nothing less than madness. Psychology, at least as it has developed thus far, has failed to provide an adequate concept of psychological health. "At its deepest level, psychology is the search for sanity. And sanity at its deepest level is the health of the soul" (Roszak, 1978, p. 51). Yet, psychological theory has offered little guidance in the face of the irrationality of environmental destruction which has led to a dis-ease of the soul. Roszak, therefore, calls for a new kind of psychology—one that is grounded in an ecological paradigm that defines the self as *eco*centric rather than *ego*centric: "Ecopsychology seeks to redefine sanity within an environmental context, to reexamine the human psyche as an integral part of the web of nature" (Roszak, 1992, p. xvi). Because we are embedded in nature, when we inflict damage upon the natural world, we do deep psychological damage to ourselves. Thus, the responsibility of health professionals today is to shape new criteria for sanity, to base a new understanding of the "self" on its deep abiding connection to the earth, and to see psychological distress as a disruption of this connection.

Conceptual Foundations of Ecopsychology

Estrangement from the natural world occurred as industrialized societies became wedded to the buying and selling of material objects and to the technologies required to produce them. Not all cultures, however, have fallen into the trap of technology, nor have they exchanged their spiritual identities for a "consumer false self" (Kanner & Gomes, 1995, p. 83). Many nonindustrialized societies have endured terrible atrocities at the hands of self-proclaimed "advanced" cultures that stigmatized native peoples as "savages" in need of being civilized (Churchill, 1994). Yet, the traditions of these indigenous people stand ready to teach the commercialized contemporary culture how to regain harmony with the earth and avoid environmental catastrophe.

On the North American continent, the tribal nations of the Native Americans offer an alternative view of the environment based on a sense of connectedness, relatedness, and sacredness. To these societies, heaven is not only above us; it is beneath our feet and all around us. To Native Americans, this is neither a metaphorical statement nor a poetic image; it is the concrete reality that governs the universe. When a person is ill, for example, a Native American healer or shaman would look for the cause in a disharmonious relationship with some part(s) of the spirit/nature/social world (Eaton, 1982; Heart, 1998; Garrett, 1998; Matthiessen, 1984; Bear, et al., 1989). That Western medicine or psychotherapy should attempt to help a person suffering from emotional or physical disturbances without considering imbalances in the natural/social/spiritual order seems a very curious notion:

> In the traditional Sioux world-view, healing is accomplished by reestablishing right relationship with 'all my relations' . . . [by] rebalancing relationship with the mineral realm, the the vegetable realm, the animal realm, the human realm and the spirit realm. (Hoffman, 1998, p. 127)

Equally bizarre to the tribal societies of North America is the idea that human beings can buy, sell, and own the land. From the early days of their contact with white settlers, Native Americans were able to foresee the disastrous outcomes that their actions against Mother Earth would bring. Chief Seattle's famous letter to President Franklin Pierce (1854) is an eloquent expression of ecological consciousness and a warning of disaster that will result from violence against the earth:

> We know the white man does not understand our ways. One portion of the land is the same to him as the next, for he is a stranger who comes in the night and takes from the land whatever he needs. The earth is not his brother but his enemy and when he has conquered it, he moves on. . . .
>
> How can you buy or sell the sky, the warmth of the land? The idea is strange to us. If we do not own the freshness of the air and the sparkle of the water, how can you buy them from us? Every part of this earth is sacred to my people. . . . The air is precious to the red man. For all things share the same breath—the beasts, the trees, the man.
>
> Whatever befalls the earth befalls the sons of the earth. Man did not weave the web of life; he is merely a strand in it. Whatever he does to the web, he does to himself. For all things are connected. . . . Continue to contaminate your bed, and you will one night suffocate in your own waste. (Chief Seattle, as quoted in McGaa, 1990, pp. xi—xii)

In the Okanagan language, a four-syllable word meaning insanity corresponds to the themes of ecopsychology. Each syllable represents "some kind of disconnection from the web of life" (Conn, 1998, p. 183). The first syllable describes the splitting off of feelings and sensations as "talking, talking inside your head." The second element refers to being "scattered and having no community;" the third and fourth syllables mean "having no relationship to the land" and being "disconnected from the whole-earth part" (Armstrong, 1995). In other words, the Okanagans equate insanity with not feeling our belongingness in the world.

The belief of the Native Americans that mental and physical health emanated from a reverence for the earth and living in harmony and balance with all things flew in the face of the mechanistic view of white culture. It was, in fact, "subversive to Western society and the entire technological direction of the past century" (Mander, 1991, p. 191). Such divergent worldviews made inevitable the clash of cultures that led to the oppression and near genocide of the Native American (Churchill, 1994). Ironically, after years of attempting to eradicate Native American ways of life, white culture may be turning to them in hopes of saving ourselves and our home, the earth.

Sociobiologist Edward O. Wilson claims that the intimate connection between humans and the earth is evident in the profound, innate love of nature called **biophilia** (Wilson, 1984) which can be seen in the fascination and attraction children have to animals and their curiosity about the natural world. From this emotional bond is born our **ecological self,** an identification with the larger network of living things. Although many indigenous peoples maintained this bond and lived in harmony with the earth for generations (Mander, 1991), Western industrialized culture chose a different path: the pursuit of power over nature, rampant acquisitiveness, and an abusive attitude toward the earth.

Ecofeminists have laid the propensity to dominate and control nature at the door of androcentric (male-centered) patriarchal belief systems that overvalue masculine qualities and denigrate the feminine. Such a worldview results in arrogance and imbalance that makes it possible to exploit the earth for its resources, just as women are exploited in society:

> We cannot separate the quaint way economics has always conceptualized the environment as 'free goods' (which will always be there freely supplying your needs) from the way in which women have been considered 'free goods,' always there supplying your needs, whether as mother or as a patriarchal wife. There is just no way to separate how we have dealt with these things. (Dodson Gray, 1982, p. 109)

Ecofeminist therapists would help their clients make these connections.

From a deep ecology perspective, the paradigmatic problem is not **androcentrism** but **anthropocentrism,** a human-centered worldview which ordains all living things to be inferior to human beings, thereby justifying exploitation and abuse of the nonhuman world (Scarce, 1990; Devall & Sessions, 1985). According to Arne Naess, the Norwegian philosopher who defined deep ecology, a person is truly mentally healthy only when there is "a widening and deepening of the self so that it embraces all life forms" (Naess, 1986, p. 235).

Resonant with deep ecology theory is the Gaia hypothesis suggested by biochemist James Lovelock (1979) and microbiologist Lynn Margulis (1975) as a possible explanation for the earth's homeostasis over millennia. All the subsystems of the earth make up a self-regulating living organism that actively maintains the life-supporting conditions which make survival possible. Gaia, taken from the name of the Greek earth goddess of antiquity, soon became a powerful metaphor that caught the imagination of ecologists who "saw it as a compelling statement of the vital connectedness of all living things [and] the basis for a quasi-mystical biocentric ethic" (Roszak, 1995, p. 13). Deep ecologist Joanna Macy believes that human beings can feel the pain of the biosphere in their own bodies and hear its voice speaking through their unconscious minds: because "we are living cells in the living body of the Earth, our collective body is in trauma and we are experiencing that" (Macy, 1995a).

Biophilia. The profound innate love of nature evidenced in children.

Ecological self. A shift in perception, often through a wilderness experience, characterized by an awareness in which one feels the oneness of self and nature.

Androcentrism. Male-centered, or patriarchal, belief system that overvalues masculine qualities and denigrates the feminine.

Anthropocentrism. A human-centered worldview which ordains all living things to be inferior to human beings, justifying exploitation and abuse of the nonhuman world.

Technoconsumer Culture

In the 19th century, the term *consumption* referred to tuberculosis, a virulent disease that consumed the body and was fatal to human life. In the 20th century, consumption of the earth's resources reached proportions that could prove fatal to all life on the planet. Some health counselors in the 21st century consider it their ethical obligation to help stop the progression of the "dis-ease" of the human psyche that threatens all species. Ecopsychology is their response to the highly commercialized, technological society that divorces the psyche from its authentic emotional and spiritual needs, with deleterious consequences for all the rest of the planet. They believe that "the patterns of control, denial, abuse and projection that sabotage intimate relationships are the very patterns that endanger the world. To change these patterns is to change not just our social lives but our relationship to the planet" (O'Connor, 1995, p. 151).

A disharmonious relationship with the environment forms the prototype for disharmonious interpersonal relationships, intrapersonal disharmony, and alienation from our true selves. The disturbed psyche then turns against the world, manifesting its distress in the form of two major cultural distortions: consumerism and technology. These twin pillars of the **technoconsumer culture** are linked to several forms of psychopathology that feed the environmental crisis: addiction, narcissism, autism, amnesia, dissociation, ontogenetic crippling, and materialistic disorder (Glendinning, 1994; Kanner, 1998; Berry, 1988; Metzner, 1995; Shepard, 1982, 1995; Conn, 1995, 1998).

Unrestrained Acquisitiveness

Psychologists are beginning to unlock the door to "the all-consuming self" (Kanner & Gomes, 1995)

> **Technoconsumer culture.** In ecotherapy, the highly technological, commercialized consumer culture that is characterized by addiction, anxiety, despair, and anguish about the devastation of the planet.

that underlies the impulse to unrestrained acquisitiveness. Philip Cushman (1990) links the consumer culture to narcissism with its duality of grandiosity and emptiness. In an industrialized mobile society like the United States, a sense of community is lost, replaced by a highly individualistic self characterized by an arrogant demand for more and more material goods to which it feels entitled. Although the narcissistic false self appears "masterful and bounded," it hides an emptiness beneath it that cries out to be filled. The advertising industry that helps to sell corporations' products deluges us with commercials suggesting all manner of goods and services to alleviate this emptiness:

> These marketing efforts create not simply an impulse to buy, but far more seriously, a "consumer false self," an ideal that is taken to heart as part of a person's identity. . . . Even more disturbing, the consumer false self is false because it arises from a merciless distortion of authentic human needs and desires. . . . Having ignored their genuine needs for so long, they feel empty. (Kanner & Gomes, 1995, p. 83)

The ecological destruction resulting from unrestrained industrial/economic growth is the price paid for the futile attempt to fill the emptiness of the false consumer self. "The modern transnational corporations are operating essentially as high-tech bandits, plundering the biosphere, [without concern for future generations of human beings] much less any concern for the intrinsic value of nonhuman beings" (Metzner, 1995, p. 60).

Technological Trance

A second powerful force that contributes to the cultural distortion of industrialized societies is the "technological trance," a tacit acceptance of technology as an unquestioned good which allows us to ignore, rationalize, minimize, or deny the ominous and obvious signs of peril. This fixation spawns "technocracy," a cultural arrangement in which social, political, and spiritual traditions are subordinated to technology but, nevertheless, still coexist with technology. The present-day United States is so enthralled by technology, however, that it has moved beyond technocracy to become a "technopoly" (Postman, 1992), a society in which technology actually displaces all other traditions by redefining religion, politics, family, intelligence, and truth to conform to its own requirements. "Technopoly, in other words, is totalitarian technocracy" (Postman, 1992, p. 42).

When a culture so deifies technology, the idea of technological progress replaces the idea of human progress and becomes the shibboleth of citizens who have become servants of technology. Deferring to the demands of technology "means that the culture seeks its authorization in technology, finds its satisfactions in technology, and takes its orders from technology" (Postman, 1992, p. 71). Any complaints about its deleterious effects–the information glut it produces or the stress of an accelerated pace of life—are dismissed along with the proliferation of warnings about the stressed life-support systems of the planet. The technological imperative regarding the biosphere "can be summed up as follows: nature is an implacable enemy that can be subdued only by technical means; the problems created by technological solutions can be solved only by the further application of technology" (Postman, 1992, p. 103).

As the predominant symbol of technology, the computer's fundamental message is that human beings are machines; we refer to ourselves as being "programmed," "hard-wired," or in need of "down-time." And in an odd role reversal, we rely on computers to perform as human beings. "The computer claims sovereignty over the whole range of human experience, and supports its claim by showing that it 'thinks' better than we can" (Postman, 1992, p. 111), usurping even some human functions better left beyond the reach of technological innovation. "Technology is not merely augmenting but replacing real human contact. Already Americans are alarmingly comfortable with this idea" (Kanner & Gomes, 1995, p. 86).

A stunning example is the intrusion of cyber-counseling or computer-assisted therapy into the domain of the helping professions. The introduction of the "virtual shrink" (Kalb, 2001) raises important questions for the health counselor who is ecologically sensitive: (1) Are computer programs

legitimate, ethical forms of therapy through which healing can occur? (2) Is the use of computers in counseling counterproductive to ecotherapy's goals? (3) What are the unintended consequences of incorporating technology into our work? (4) What are the authentic, meaningful purposes of counseling and therapy in a "high tech-high touch" society (Naisbitt, 1982) that seems to be heavily weighted on the "high tech" side of the equation?

The content of *what* we use computers for may be far less significant than the fact *that* we use them. Simply spending time engaged in computer activity drives the wedge deeper between humans, and between humans and nature. The instantaneous quality of electronic technology and the computerized world has so conditioned us to the accelerated speed of modern life that we are impatient and uncomfortable with the slower rhythms and cycles of the natural world, including our own biological, emotional, and mental healing processes. Thus, "computers actually steer society in a direction that *contradicts* environmental goals" (Mander, 1991, p. 54).

Computers compete for our attention with socially based satisfactions and communion with the natural world. Hours spent playing video games (which often involve violent and rapid interactions) rob children of hours of play that involves the use of physical, emotional, mental, and social capacities necessary for healthy human development and keeps them from bonding with the "primary matrix"—Mother Earth (Pearce, 1977). In order to feel at home in the world, children must explore by touch, taste, smell, sound, and sight the physical-biological world of which they are a part. If this bond is not forged, it becomes easier to objectify the earth, to relate to it not as the mother out of which we are born and which nurtures us, nor as a living system, but as an inert collection of resources to be used without reverence or appreciation.

False Self

In the absence of a bond with the earth, we develop an insecure false self that seeks a haven in the acquisition of information and things. Rather than a sense of stewardship impelling us to protect and cherish an earth we love, we develop instead "an intelligence determined to outwit nature, an intelligence with a vast array of tools at its disposal with which to outwit and in fact, supplant nature entirely. And in that outwitting and supplanting, damage is done that is incalculable" (Pearce, 1977, p. 44). The "I–Thou" relationship humans once had with the earth and which some indigenous peoples still maintain is lost to the "I–It" relationship which fosters attitudes of ingratitude, entitlement, and abuse (Buber, 1958; Mander, 1991; Berry, 1999; Pearce, 1977; Glendinning, 1995).

Technoconsumer culture and ecodestructive pathologies are interrelated in self-reinforcing patterns described by various ecopsychologists, some of whom believe that we are suffering from a mass posttraumatic-stressdisorder, a type of dissociative disorder sustained as a result of our dislocation from our earthly home. The trauma of this painful separation leaves us susceptible to addictions and maladaptive behaviors of all kinds, including eating disorders, compulsive spending and shopping, and substance abuse. Dissociation causes us to split off elements of reality from our consciousness and to shut out entire pieces of our experience. It also explains the widespread callous disregard for the environment:

> The entire culture of Western industrial society is dissociated from its ecological substratum. . . . We have the knowledge of our impact on the environment, we can perceive the pollution and degradation of the land, the waters, the air–but we do not attend to it, we do not connect that knowledge to other aspects of our total experience . . . because the political, economic, and educational institutions in which we are involved all have this dissociation built into them. (Metzner, 1995, pp. 64–65)

Another effect of the separation trauma is a kind of collective traumatic amnesia. Modern societies have forgotten what is needed to relate intimately to the earth: respect, humility, and empathy. Our inability "to remember our former closeness with the Earth . . . is really a double forgetting, wherein a culture forgets, and then forgets that it has forgotten how to live in harmony with the planet" (Devereux, Steele & Kubrin, 1989, pp. 2–3). Thomas Berry (1988) compares our

damaged relationship with the earth to that of autistic children to their own mother; they cannot relate to her because they seem not to see, hear, or feel her presence. The voice of the earth speaks to us, but we do not hear and so do not respond.

"The sibling society," as Robert Bly (1996) refers to the pervasive dysfunction of technoconsumerism, corresponds to the cultural pathology that Paul Shepard called "ontogenetic crippling" (1982). Seen through this lens, the shock of separation from nature arrested our development at a stage of adolescence characterized by "boisterous, arrogant pursuit of individual self-assertion" (Metzner, 1995, p. 57), demands for instant gratification, and a shaky sense of self. In other words, we are a society of childish adults whose weak identity structures cannot support an intimate, caring relationship with the earth. "It seems time that our race began to think as an adult does, rather than like an egocentric baby or insane person" (Jeffers, 1977, p. xxi).

Addictive Society

As humans continue to be exposed to technology and consumerism in various permutations throughout our lives, assessing the impact on our psyches has become increasingly difficult because we fail to notice their effects or even their existence. The addictive process has progressed beyond a neurotic attachment to gas-guzzling sport utility vehicles, cellular telephones, laptops, pagers, television sets, VCRs, and personal digital assistants. "The picture is bigger and more complex," larger than a reliance on any one machine or constellation of machines (Glendinning, 1995, p. 44). Technology and consumerism are so pervasive and so completely interwoven into society that our entire lives are organized around a cultural ideology which we no longer perceive, no longer question, and are entirely dependent upon. At this point, we are in the grip of the technoconsumer culture just as addicts are in the grip of substances or processes that control their lives and over which they are powerless. Not unexpectedly, then, does the consumer technopoly reproduce classic symptoms of the addictive process: denial, dishonesty, disordered thought, grandiosity, control, and blocked feelings (Bateson, 1972; Gore, 1992; Glendinning, 1995).

The grandiosity that characterizes addiction insists on the superiority of the technoconsumer lifestyle to other forms of social organization. Grandiose thinking has fed the illusion that Western culture has not only the right, but even the obligation to subdue indigenous cultures, and impose our own industrial/commercial civilization on them. "Manifest destiny" was the rationalization for appropriation of the lands of Native Americans on the North American continent in the 19th century, just as "progress" and "development" are terms used to rationalize the abuse of ecosystems today. Unlike Native Americans who respected the land, the values that Europeans who settled in the United States brought with them led to the plundering of the vast resources of this continent. Their anthropocentric worldview continues into the 21st century as human encroachment continues to impinge upon fragile ecosystems. In our refusal to place limits on what we take from the earth and what we demand of it, the human species makes its own desires paramount and behaves with a grandiose sense of entitlement which requires the unending pursuit of the next empty "fix."

Ecological Warning Signs

Refusal to face the plethora of warning signals from an overtaxed environment is perhaps the most striking aspect of technoconsumer addiction. Sometimes the complexity of interacting factors and the difficulty of directly perceiving environmental damage, such as global warming or the hole in the ozone layer, makes it easy to slip into denial, disbelief, or rationalization when confronted with upsetting news about the environment. We are unwilling to believe that human actions in the present will endanger the well-being of future generations. We deny that consumer habits place any strain on the biosphere, that carbon dioxide emissions have any affect on the atmosphere, that species extinction is occurring at shocking rates because of human encroachment

on habitat and human disturbance of ecosystems. We rationalize that the next technological fix will solve the problems caused by previous technologies. We labor under the delusion that the next frivolous purchase will alleviate the emptiness, anxiety, and depression that returned shortly after the last shopping spree. We block out painful feelings, becoming so emotionally frozen that we cannot empathize with the suffering brought about by our "uncounted violations against humanity, animals, the plant world, and the Earth" (Glendinning, 1995, p. 51). We numb our own feelings, rendering ourselves numb to the suffering of other living beings. We continue to pursue our normal activities while underneath is a nagging sense of foreboding, "an anguish beyond naming" (Macy, 1995b, p. 243) that drains us of the energy needed to act on behalf of the environment.

Rather than developing technologies to ease the pressures on the earth's resources and ecosystems, "we strive to develop technologies, from dams to anti-aging creams, that allow us an increasing degree of control over the natural world" (Glendinning, 1995, p. 48). In an androcentric/patriarchal system, however, control over natural processes is reserved only for men who exercise their power through policy making that can adversely affect women and the environment. For example, decisions to withhold family-planning methods deprive women of the right to control their own reproductive processes, choose to have fewer children, and stabilize world population at levels that would make life on the planet sustainable for future generations. Furthermore, because patriarchy and androcentrism devalue feminine qualities, "soft technologies" such as fuel cells and solar power are deemed unworthy of serious consideration while nuclear power plants, oil drilling, and strip mining continue to scar the land and devastate the seas.

Redirection of Psychology and Therapy

Ecotherapists criticize and resist the tendency of mainstream psychology to individualize their clients' feelings about our environmental plight by interpreting them in terms of personal history and pathology. They urge a redirection of psychology which encourages therapists to listen to their clients in a different way; they would hear their clients' symptoms not only as personal problems in living but as some aspect of Gaia's pain speaking through one of her children:

> As an ecopsychologist, I would like to see a revision of the DSM that looks at individual symptoms as 'signals' of distress in our connection with the larger context or as a defect in the larger context itself. For example, I would interpret what I have called 'materialistic disorder,' the need to consume, as a serious signal of our culture's disconnection from the earth. (Conn, 1995, p. 162)

The futile effort to fill the emptiness that arises from this disconnection fuels the consumer culture which taxes the earth even more.

James Hillman and Joanna Macy became dismayed when their own therapists reframed their feelings of sorrow and despair about homelessness and the abuse of their earthly home as unresolved issues with their fathers. According to Hillman and Macy, their therapists' narrow, inadequate psychological paradigm completely missed the point of their anguish. At the very least, therapists should not attempt to delegitimize their clients' ecological sensibilities. Clients who feel heartbroken by the pillage of the planet deserve to be believed and supported. Therapy should help them work through their feelings and channel their energies into self-healing and earth-healing activities. Pathologizing feelings about the world situation may truncate the client's emotions and therefore deprive the world of their creative response. When the ecological self is stifled, the client remains entrapped by purely egotistic needs and drives that feed alienation rather than nourish the authentic needs of the person.

Ecotherapists emphasize the reciprocal nondualistic nature of healing. They reject as a false dichotomy the choice between getting better oneself and making the world better. These goals, in fact, work in synergistic concert with one another.

"As we work to heal the Earth, the Earth heals us" (Macy, 1991, p. xii). Ecotherapists encourage their clients not only to allow themselves to be nurtured by nature but also to give something back to nature in return, thus establishing a model of reciprocity, mutuality, and balance that carries over to human relationships. The earth gives us everything we need to live; Gaia nurtures our physical bodies completely. When we turn to her to nurture our psyches spiritually, to heal our emotional wounds and traumas, it is fitting that we nurture her in return. Unless we do so, we are only replicating the unbalanced, exploitive, or abusive relationships that have caused us to seek therapy to begin with.

Ecotherapy Approaches

Certain elements of established therapies can be incorporated quite effectively into an ecotherapy approach. "Each of the major clusters of contemporary pschyotherapies offers valuable insights and methods that can be useful in ecotherapy" (Clinebell, 1996, p. 127). A new generation of depth psychologists such as Stephen Aizenstat (1995) are extending the movement initiated by Carl Jung (1976), who presaged that it is not natural disasters nor diseases that threaten the human species but man himself who poses the greatest danger to humankind. Depth psychology is widening the potential union of psyche and world beyond the *human* collective unconscious to the *world* unconscious, the dimension of the psyche that embraces "the relatedness of the inner subjective natures of *all* life" (Yunt, 2001, p. 102). In this vast unconscious realm lies an enormous amount of "wisdom from which the modern mind has become estranged and with which it needs, once again, to regain contact" (Yunt, 2001, p. 101). Depth psychology, therefore, seeks to restore emotional well-being by reconnecting human consciousness to its deepest roots, the matrix of a universal consciousness, and thus recast therapy within a truly ecopsychological frame of reference.

Gestalt Therapy

Gestalt therapy, also, has much to contribute to ecotherapy because it is "inherently ecological in its personality theory, worldview, and methodology. The person is seen as fully embedded in the world, and the world is seen as more like a living organism than like a nonliving mechanism of separate interacting parts" (Cahalan, 1995, p. 216). In Gestalt theory, authentic contact with the world is at the core of emotional health and full human functioning. In an attempt to compensate for the dislocation felt in urban-industrial society, people develop the false identity of "self-as-owner." Defining oneself as owner (of things, land, resources, even qualities) displaces the sense of oneself as a process relating to the world and leads to a lack of groundedness, the empty self, alienation, and disconnectedness. Ecotherapists with a Gestalt orientation use the concept "ecological groundedness" to help their clients regain contact with the world.

William Cahalan (1995), for example, integrates Gestalt theory and methods into his ecotherapy approach by (1) making his office environment accessible to the outdoors and furnishing it with living plants, recycling containers, and so on to ground clients in the natural world and begin to develop ecological consciousness; (2) informing clients that they will explore ways in which they relate to themselves, other people, and other parts of nature; (3) pointing out that breathing itself connects them to the biosphere; (4) asking clients to share memories of nonhuman aspects of their world, especially in their childhoods, to become more aware of how nature can nourish them; (5) walking or sitting outside and engaging with a natural element to show the parallels between interpersonal relating and relating to nature; (6) introducing the image of Gaia as a "living, abiding, self-regulating body within

which we . . . are in constant, often unconscious communion . . . participating in her self-regulation and development" (Cahalan, 1995, pp. 220–221).

Methods used in Gestalt and other therapies that emphasize bodywork help people to experience a renewed physical aliveness dulled by years of submitting to the demands of a technocratic consumer culture. Bodywork should be a fundamental part of ecotherapy "because our bodies are the most obvious, ever-present and inescapable part of the natural world in our lives" (Clinebell, 1996, p. 138). Harmony in our bodily systems is impacted by the harmony or disharmony in the ecosystem; alienation from our own physical bodies produces alienation from the biosphere. Somatic therapies such as yoga, aikido, t'ai chi ch'uan, ideokinesis, autogenic training, the Alexander technique, the Rubenfeld synergy method, Pesso system/psychomotor therapy, Feldenkrais, dance/movement therapy, Hakomi method, and structured integration (also called Rolfing), are just a few of the many therapies that recognize the inextricable interdependence of body and mind. Many of them also have a strong spiritual component as well as being effective stress-reduction techniques.

Bioenergetic Therapy

One of the most influential body-based psychotherapies is Bioenergetics, developed by Alexander Lowen, a student of Wilhelm Reich, the Freudian analyst who believed that muscular holding patterns embodied psychic conflicts. Bioenergetic therapy uses verbal analysis and physical exercises such as breathing and grounding to break through defenses so that emotional-physical-spiritual energies can flow freely. Lowen must have had at least a glimpse of the ecological self when he observed, "As long as the ego dominates the individual, he cannot have the oceanic or transcendental experiences that make life meaningful" (Lowen, 1967, p. 259). When people reconnect with their own bodies, they are able to feel more deeply their spiritual connection to nature.

Gestalt therapy. A therapy that assumes that authentic contact with the world is at the core of emotional health and full human functioning.

Ecofeminist Therapy

Ecofeminist therapy assumes and attends to the parallel between alienation from nature and alienation in other dimensions of a person's life. Because of the patriarchal-technological bias built into society, men receive messages that mitigate against warm, intimate relationships. Patriarchies perpetuate imbalances in men's personalities by overemphasizing masculine traits and derogating female qualities. Often little boys who are taught to suppress feelings of sadness, gentleness, or other "soft" emotions grow up to become either exaggerated versions of men (macho) or hyper-rational and emotionally blocked.

This pattern is evident in the case of a successful aerospace engineer who sought counseling "to get my wife off my back about what she claims is my lack of feelings" (Clinebell, 1996, p. 63). His wife was extremely frustrated because the only feeling her husband seemed to be able to express was anger. Furthermore, he spent most of his time at home in front of the computer. She complained that he did not consult her about decisions that concerned them both and said she was tired of living with a dominating robot. This client had learned the lessons of patriarchy and technopoly well: that the company of machines is preferable to that of other living beings; that feelings are frightening, shameful things to be avoided, if at all possible. By choosing a highly technical profession, the client had placed himself in a corporate climate where these beliefs would most likely be reinforced rather than challenged. In therapy, the parallels between the man's mental problems and his ecological attitudes became apparent when the counselor helped him explore his alienation from the natural world, from his body (the natural world in him), and from most of his intense emotions. As he

> did a deep breathing exercise in one session, long-suppressed tears began to trickle down his cheeks. His bottled-up feelings of painful alienation from his body flowed. These feelings were intertwined dynamically with his feelings that the natural world is something to be named, civilized, or bulldozed into its "place." It became particularly evident that his feelings about "mother earth" were paralleled by

his feelings that women are threatening and need be be controlled or kept at an emotional distance. The latter feelings impacted his behavior with his wife and other women in his life in negative ways—ways that began to change as his earth feelings changed. As he worked through these painful feelings in therapy, his inner emotional channels gradually became more open. What flowed was grief and anger from his lonely cut-offness from himself, people, and the living world, followed by the quiet joy of feeling more alive. Not surprisingly, his sense of positive connection with his wife increased, enhancing both their spiritual and sexual intimacy. (Clinebell, 1996, p. 64)

Methods: Consciousness Raising

Many times people are unaware or only partially aware of how their personal pain can arise from their immersion in the consumer technopoly and their alienation from the biosphere. An ecofeminist approach to therapy often uses **consciousness-raising** techniques to help clients understand the interaction between their presenting problems and the patriarchal values that denigrate women and bring harm to the earth. Sarah Conn describes this technique as "tacking back and forth" between the individual and the larger cultural/ecological level. She works with sexually abused clients by enlarging the scope of their personal experience to include abuse in its various manifestations.

Another ecofeminist counselor helped a client whose life was in disarray economically and personally because of compulsive shopping and mounting debt. In this case, the counselor tried to foster a sense of the client's ecological self by first providing a nonjudgmental context in which her feelings of guilt, shame, frustration, and depression could be expressed. She also pointed out how corporate advertising damages not only a personal sense of adequacy and worth but also depletes the

Consciousness raising. Techniques that help people understand the interaction between their presenting problem and the larger cultural, social, ecological level.

earth's resources in order to sell more and more unneeded products. The client began to regard shopping as a poor substitute for her creative impulses, her ability to identify other enjoyable activities, and her engagement in other forms of satisfaction, pleasure, and creative expression. With her therapist's encouragement, she started to spend some time each day in a natural setting that nurtured her spirit and she began to contribute her talent to an environmental education program for children in her local school system. The focus of therapy had been to expand the client's sense of self beyond "I shop; therefore, I am" and to raise awareness of socially accepted norms that injured her psychological well-being and hurt the environment (Pierce, 1997, p. 44).

Ecoliterature

In addition to suggesting that personal matters are played out against the backdrop of social and ecological contexts, ecotherapists can encourage their clients to expand consciousness in other ways. **Ecoliterature** is replete with beautiful and touching stories of nature experience that evoke strong emotional responses in readers. Many nature writers combine scientific knowledge of nature with a deep spiritual sense of its sacredness. Continuing in the tradition of John Muir and Henry David Thoreau are 20th-century authors such as Aldo Leopold, Loren Eiseley, Barry Lopez, Brian Swimme, Gary Snyder, Annie Dillard, Terry Tempest Williams, Wendell Berry, and many others. Reading such inspirational literature can be an important part of the healing process for the clients of ecotherapists.

Ecofeminist fiction is a new genre of literature that women clients find especially empowering because it features strong women allied with the fragile territory they call home and the nonhuman residents with whom they share the land. Notable among ecofeminist authors is Barbara

---

Ecoliterature. Literature or nature writing that combines scientific knowledge of nature with a deep spiritual sense of its sacredness.

Kingsolver whose novels articulate some major messages of ecopsychology: that conquering the land is tantamount to madness and that "species arrogance" (Mack, 1995) is a force to be resisted with all the considerable resources with which human females are endowed. Women readers, especially, find sustenance and comfort in the stories told in *Prodigal Summer* (Kingsolver, 2000) and *Animal Dreams* (Kingsolver, 1990) about courageous women determined to protect the land and animals they hold dear.

Ecotapes

For clients who respond better to visual media than to bibliotherapy, ecocounselors might consider building an ecotape library from which to lend videos about nature or ecoheroes such as Rachel Carson (Goodwin, 1992), the mother of modern environmentalism, and Julia "Butterfly" Hill (Ficklin, 1998) whose tree-sit to save a stand of redwoods in California gained worldwide attention. A number of popular films available on videotape present characters acting in concert with nature, or opposing antienvironmental forces. The protagonists in *A Civil Action* (Zaillian, 1999) and *Erin Brockovich* (Soderbergh, 2000) both gain personal integrity in the process of battling corporate polluters responsible for poisoning people with toxic chemicals. In these films, empathy for the earth whose water and soil has been contaminated converges with empathy for human beings whose lives and health have been sacrificed on the altar of greed and callousness.

The Native Americans' reverential feeling toward nature pervades *The Education of Little Tree* (Friedenberg, 1998), a touching tale about a Cherokee child learning the traditional ways and insights of his ancestral heritage. *All the Little Animals* (Thomas, 1999), has a Jungian undercurrent in its depiction of a sensitive young man's relationship to the natural world and his mentor's compassionate actions toward the earth's vulnerable creatures. Clients' reactions to these and other ecofilms provide rich material for exploration in therapy.

Griefwork

Many people experience a profound sense of loss when a wooded area in their community is razed in order to build another shopping mall or when they witness another act of violence against the earth. For these clients, feelings of grief similar to those experienced at the death of a loved one are not uncommon. Ecotherapists help their clients work through their feelings of anger, guilt, frustration, sadness, and dread about the deteriorating environment. Group work can be a particularly powerful method for mourning these losses and reaching a point where members' energies can be released into earth-saving activities.

From her extensive experience in despair counseling, JoAnna Macy has discovered several important principles to guide **griefwork.** First, far from being a sign of dysfunction, anguish about the ecocrisis is "a measure of our humanity [and] cannot be reduced to private pathology; it is [only] when we disown our pain for the world that it becomes dysfunctional [by turning] inward in depression and self-destruction, through drug abuse and suicide" (Macy, 1995b, pp. 251–252). People must process information about the environment on an emotional level in order to take responsibility for self-healing and earth-healing. Repressed feeling must be unblocked in order to reconnect with the web of life beyond our separate selves. The safety of an ecotherapy group is an effective format for sharing intense feelings of grief, then planning and taking effective action.

Horticultural Therapy

One of the earliest recorded attempts to heal the psyche through contact with nature occurred in ancient Egypt when court physicians advised royalty to take long walks in the palace gardens to

Griefwork. In ecotherapy, helping clients work through feeling of grief, anger, guilt, frustration, and dread about the deteriorating environment.

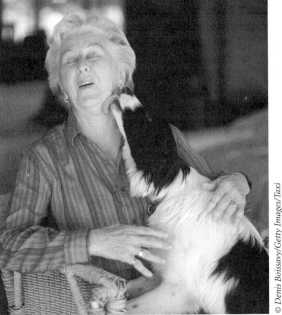

Contact with pets can provide beneficial therapy for human beings.

© Denis Boissavy/Getty Images/Taxi

cure their mental disturbances. Even then, health practitioners recognized the quieting effect of a peaceful natural setting. In the late 18th century, American patriot Dr. Benjamin Rush, sometimes considered the country's first psychiatrist, had his patients engage in farming and gardening. His use of agricultural activities as a treatment modality set the stage for development of an even more comprehensive program at Philadelphia Friends Hospital in the 1800s. Since then, horticultural therapy has become a highly respected specialized profession that is used successfully with many client populations: the disabled, military veterans, prison inmates, troubled youth, the aged, addicts, and others.

Tending to plants, or merely being with plants, heals in various ways. The gardening process teaches "how one's environment affects all living things and how stress and even dying are a natural part of life's cycle" (Davis, 1997, p. 23). Gardening brings people closer to the earth and makes them partners in bringing forth life from the soil. The physical tasks of gardening—weeding, pruning, and planting—reduce stress by dispelling tension, anger, and aggression through bodily activity. The joy and satisfaction that comes from being an active participant in the process of nature generates a sense of protectiveness toward the environment as well as a feeling of trust in nature's life force.

Animal Therapy

It comes as no surprise to those who have loved and cared for a pet at some time in their lives that bonding with a nonhuman creature has salubrious psychological and physiological effects. The growing consensus in the health-care community that contact with animals plays a significant role in reducing stress has led to a proliferation of pet-therapy programs (Ashby, 1992; Clinebell,1996; Colangelo, 1995; Mancuso, 1993; Marino, 1995; Moore, 2001; Niego, 1992). Counselors who make animals part of therapeutic interventions report that the very action of petting an animal has a tremendously calming and soothing effect. Many therapists have seen dramatic breakthroughs when their clients bond with an animal. Residents of nursing homes have responded to pet-therapy dogs or cats after years of shunning human contact. Children too, learn important lessons when given the opportunity to relate to animals. One counseling center in New Jersey brings together "abused and unwanted animals and children from troubled families, to their mutual benefit" (Moore, 2001, p. 132). The unconditional love of these animals is an experience most of the children never had. From their nonhuman friends they learn acceptance, empathy, and what it means to care for another living being.

Like horticultural therapy, animal-assisted or pet therapy has been used successfully in a variety of settings with diverse client populations. "Animal-facilitated therapy has been used in prisons across the country," with inmates caring for retired thoroughbred racehorses (at Walkill in New York), wild mustangs and cattle (at Colorado State Prison), and a variety of other animals. A maximum-security mental hospital in Lima, Ohio,

reported a 50 percent decrease in violence, suicide attempts, and medication levels among patients involved with pet therapy compared to those who were not. "Within the past 30 to 40 years, the healing arts professions have awakened to the inestimable value of pet-assisted therapy programs" (Ashby, 1992, p. 42).

In 1945, Ann Gritt Ashby helped to launch one such program at the Brentwood Neuropsychiatric Hospital in Los Angeles where she worked with returning veterans of World War II. Among her many touching stories is the case of a Hopi Indian who became suicidal after his combat experiences in the Marine Corps. Totally uncommunicative with the medical staff, Ricardo refused to participate in any kind of therapeutic activity until a therapy dog named Rusty befriended him. For weeks, Ricardo would sit on the floor with his arms around Rusty, speaking to him in his native Hopi tongue until the day he told his therapist he was ready to go home to his reservation with Rusty. At this turning point, Ricardo told his therapist that he felt closer to Mother Earth sitting on the floor with Rusty, the only one who understood his problems. One month later, Ricardo was well enough to go home, and although he could not take Rusty with him, he made a ceramic bowl for him as a goodbye gift. A few months later, he wrote his therapist to say that he and his new puppy, Rusty (named after his canine "therapist"), were both doing fine.

Wilderness Therapy

Wilderness therapy is, in a certain sense, the most "radical" of ecotherapy methods because it literally abandons ordinary limits of time and space—the 50-minute session in an indoor office—for several hours, days, or even months in unspoiled terrain. Steven Harper (1995) rejects the use of the word *therapy*, however, because it implies a medical model. "Wilderness practice," as Harper prefers to call his group excursions into the wild, is meant to enliven the senses and restore deadened perceptual powers because at the core of the ecocrisis is "a crisis in perception; we are not truly seeing, hearing, tasting, or consequently, feeling where we are" (Sewall, 1998, p. 165). Whether we refer to this condition as autism (Berry, 1988), anesthesia (Hillman, 1975), or myopia (Abram, 1988), "our blindness has tremendous implications for the quality of relationship between ourselves and the 'more than human world' " (Sewall, 1998, p. 165).

Wilderness experiences produce dramatic shifts in perception characterized by a "nonegoic awareness" (Greenway, 1995, p. 132) in which ego boundaries become permeable enough to feel the oneness of self and nature—the ecological self. Through wilderness therapy, even androcentric, patriarchal perceptions melt away. Men who have been "socialized to dominate nature rather than experience it . . . get beyond their heads, not only in touch with their hearts, but with their bodies" (Voss, as quoted in Clinebell, 1996, p. 224). Participants report that the attentiveness and mindfulness fostered in wilderness therapy brings about a heightened state of awareness, a "peak or transcendent experience" (Maslow, 1964) of sacred connection to the earth.

Robert Greenway (1995), however, cautions against turning wilderness into just another commodity for human use:

> Perhaps the clearest evidence of our recovery will be that we do not demand that wilderness heal us. . . . For a wilderness that must heal us is surely a commodity just as when we can only look at wilderness as a source of endless wealth. . . . If we do use wilderness, let us use it in ways that further its rehabilitation as well as our own. (Greenway, 1995, p. 134–145)

Restoration Therapy

There are many ways in which ecotherapists can help their clients engage in actions that foster a reciprocal, caring relationship with the earth. The "ecological healing circle" (Clinebell, 1996) requires respectful, protective, and nurturent behavior toward nature. Even ostensibly minor actions can promote personal healing as well as earth-healing benefits. A client in an abusive marriage,

for example, regained a sense of control by starting a recycling and composting project. That seemingly simple step began a process of empowerment that led her to a support group where she learned to see the violence she suffered as part of a larger patriarchal system of domination that also harms the earth. From these insights grew a stronger sense of herself as a person within the web of life, sustained by the earth through all her tribulation. Eventually, this woman was able to extricate herself from her destructive marriage and enter into healthier relationships. Thus, small changes in everyday life that may seem insignificant initially can be important points of intervention from which an ecological self begins to emerge.

Another way to demonstrate caring and appreciation for nature is to restore areas that have suffered from human exploitation. Whether it be pruning and weeding, cleaning up contamination, planting trees, or replenishing rivers with fish, **restoration** projects teach people "through their hands and their hearts, to identify with the pain and the healing of the ecosystems that sustain them" (Shapiro, 1995, p. 225). Moreover, the process of restoring nature suggests certain metaphors that "resonate deeply with participants' self-healing work" (Shapiro, 1995, p. 233). The degradation observed while doing restoration work reminds us of the assaults on our personal health and well-being, such as overcrowding, traffic congestion, noise pollution, brutality, and abuse. Restoring balance and health to the environment mirrors the healing process in our own lives.

Summary

The environmental crisis is as much a matter of psychological and emotional health as it is a threat to physical health and survival. Until very recently, health education and health counseling have paid

> **Restoration.** A healing method used by ecotherapists; having clients restore some part of nature that aids in their own healing process.

scant attention to the relationship between human beings and nature. The advent of *ecopsychology* in the late 20th century, however, brought a revisioning of psychological thought and approaches to therapy based upon an ecological conception of the human psyche.

Ecopsychologists believe that the roots of modern psychological distress lie in our estrangement from nature and an inadequate definition of sanity and health. Mainstream psychology has defined the self much too narrowly, ignoring its embeddedness within the ecosystem. A new focus on the *ecological self* "requires fundamental changes in our understanding of human psychology to include the human relationship with the natural world" (Kuhn, 2001, p. 10).

Finding it "strange that we supposed experts and healers of human relations give but passing notice to our extraordinarily unhealthy relationship to the planet as a whole" (O'Connor, 1995, p. 155), ecotherapists are infusing key insights from *deep ecology* and *ecofeminism* into their practice. Those influenced by *deep-ecology* theory urge the disavowal of anthropocentric "attitudes that place human needs solely above the rest of nature" (Kuhn, 2001, p. 11). Ecofeminists reject the androcentric-patriarchal systems of domination and control that lead to various forms of abuse and violence against women and the earth. Both worldviews have contributed to the alienation from nature that poisons both our relationships with one another and the very habitat we depend upon to sustain life.

Because we have learned to see ourselves as separate and *apart* from nature rather than as an integral *part* of nature, we experience feelings of disconnectedness, emptiness, and loneliness that feed the psychopathology of *technoconsumer culture.* Attempts to alleviate these feelings have produced a highly technological, highly commercialized consumer culture characterized by classic symptoms of addiction, depression, anxiety, and muted despair, anguish, and grief about the devastation of our planetary home.

Ecotherapy assumes a connection between healing the wounded human psyche and healing the wounds inflicted on the earth; restoring the health of the individual and restoring the health of the environment are part of the same enterprise. "If professionals do nothing more than encourage people to increase time spent relating intimately with nature, they probably will contribute to their total well-being" (Clinebell, 1996, p. 194). When ecotherapists "prescribe nature," they encourage clients not only to allow themselves to be soothed, nurtured, and rejuvenated by the nonhuman world, but also to care for nature in return. By engaging in animal therapy, horticultural therapy, or restoration activities, clients experience a caring, reciprocal relationship that serves as a model for other interactions in their lives.

Ecotherapy approaches draw on methods from established therapies such as *Gestalt,* various somatic therapies, and *ecofeminist therapy: consciousness-raising,* griefwork, bibliotherapy, videotherapy, bodywork, and wilderness therapy. Any activity that strengthens the human connection with the natural world is potentially healing for both.

Key Terms

androcentrism, 224

anthropocentrism, 224

biophilia, 224

consciousness
   raising, 231

deep ecology, 220

depth psychology, 220

ecofeminism, 220

ecoliterature, 232

ecological self, 224

ecopsychology, 220

ecotherapy, 221

Gestalt therapy, 230

griefwork, 233

restoration, 235

technoconsumer
   culture, 225

Questions for Discussion

1. How does the "egocentric" self differ from the "ecocentric" self?

2. In the view of ecopsychology, what is wrong with patriarchal, androcentric, and anthropocentric worldviews?

3. Describe the reciprocal relationship between the human psyche and the natural world. How

does this relationship affect the notion of what constitutes a healthy person?

4. How might health counselors incorporate ecotherapy strategies and principles?

5. Discuss "sanity" and "insanity" in the framework of the reciprocal relationship between the human psyche and the natural world. Why does ecopsychology seek to redefine these concepts?

Related Web Sites

http://www.ecopsychology.athabascau.ca
Variety of essays, research, and resources for ecopsychology from the Ecopsychology Institute at California State University, Hayward.

http://www.deep-ecology.org
Comprehensive explanation of the ecocentric philosophy of Arne Naess. Gives affiliations and activities of the Institute for Deep Ecology (IDE).

http://www.ecointernet.net
Site dedicated to the study of ecopsychology, cultural ecology, and environmental psychology.

http://www.spiritmoving.com
Explores movement as a way to unblock paths of communication to achieve deeper connections to the world.

http://www.rmetzner-greenearth.org
Publications, activities, and information about the Green Earth Foundation, an educational/research organization founded by ecopsychologist Ralph Metzner.

Health Counseling in the 21st Century

JOSEPH DONNELLY, PH.D.

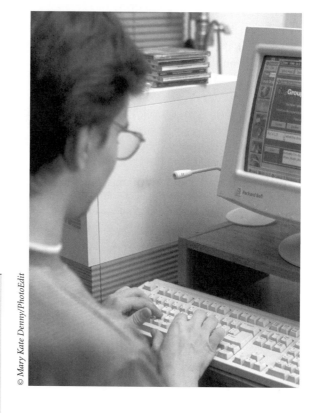

© Mary Kate Denny/PhotoEdit

OBJECTIVES

By the end of this chapter, the reader should be able to:

- Describe how the Internet is being used by the public for health information and counseling

- Understand the benefits and challenges of the new technologies for counselors and clients

- Cite the ethical and legal requirements for online counseling

- Discuss some directions health counselors might take in response to technological and cultural trends

Every professional field must be viewed in the context of the particular cultural and historical period in which it exists. To understand the future of health counseling, one must examine current and future issues affecting both health care and the counseling profession. Changing cultural values and technological developments will no doubt influence health counseling in the 21st century.

The development and widespread use of the Internet has already begun to transform many aspects of American society, such as education, communications, business, and recreation. The Internet has made possible unprecedented access to information, allowing millions of people to find information, advice, and entertainment easily, without leaving their own homes. The Nua Internet Survey of 1998 estimated that there were over 60 million Americans and Canadians online (Izenberg & Lieberman, 1998). The study also found that 82 percent of those who use Web use it to research or find information.

It is estimated that there are currently 15,000 to 20,000 health-related Web sites. According to a survey by Louis Harris & Associates, an Internet research company, 68 percent of adults with Internet access used it to seek medical information, making it the most popular subject on the Web (*Fortune*, Summer 2000 Technology Guide). Health-related services on the Web include health "channels" which contain clusters of related information, chat rooms, and lists of recommended Web sites. Consumers can also utilize questions-and-answer pages, view current health news, search bibliographic databases, find health-care providers, or join discussion and support groups (Izenberg & Lieberman, 1998).

The Internet has made access to information and peer support much easier for both patients and doctors. Yet because much of the material found in health-related Web sites is not regulated, it poses risks for consumers, who may be making health-care decisions based on inaccurate or incomplete information. Individuals are also turning to the Internet for help with personal problems and mental-health concerns. It is estimated that there are thousands of online counseling Web sites, offering a variety of fee-based services to those who would otherwise seek in-person counseling. Sampson, Kolodinsky, and Greeno (1997) attempted to determine how many counseling Web sites there were. A computerized search was done in April 1996, which found 3,764 home pages containing the word "counseling." Although many of the Web sites found did not deal specifically with online counseling, a nonrandom analysis of 401 of these sites led the authors to conclude that there is a substantial amount of online counseling being done on the Web. A month later, the same search yielded 3,983 counseling home pages, a 6 percent increase. At this rate of growth, the annual increase in counseling Web sites would be 55 percent.

There are obvious benefits to online counseling, such as increased access and convenience, but there are also serious risks involved, especially regarding client confidentiality and the maintenance of professional standards and ethics. The Internet has the potential to transform the way people get medical information and health care, and how they seek counseling and support in difficult times. It is clear that the Internet poses a challenge to traditional, accepted methods in both the health care and counseling professions. How these professions adapt to new technologies and the cultural values produced by them may be the most important factor in determining the future of health counseling.

Health Counseling and the Internet

With technological advancements occurring at such a rapid pace, how the Internet is used for health and counseling purposes is likely to change dramatically. We have seen in only a few years the need for legislative and professional response to the increasing amount of counseling activity being conducted on the Internet. Individuals and associations are rushing to enumerate the uses and challenges of new technologies as fast as they arise. It is likely that future generations of health counselors will require a level of techno savvy that counselors never traditionally concerned themselves with or required. The mental-health profession and the medical profession are being affected similarly in terms of greater consumer access to information, but there are important differences too. We will briefly discuss how the public is using the Internet for counseling, and how they are using it for health advice and services. Rather than attempt an exhaustive list in this ever-developing area, we will focus on a few applications and their benefits and pitfalls.

The basic features of the Internet include the use of bulletin boards (BBSs), list servers, discussion groups, email, exchange of text files, data, audio, video, chat—which can be simultaneous, conferencing, and home pages which provide information and may link to other kinds of audio, video, or text (Sampson, Kolodinsky, and Greeno, 1997). Many growing beneficial uses of the Internet have been cited over the past 10 years. Email has been seen as a great resource for the public's health concerns (Hannon, 1996); bulletin-board discussion groups allow counselors to seek assistance dealing with specific types of client issues (Marino, 1996); list servers and information resource collections (such as the ERIC system) can help counselors quickly access information related to a wide variety of counseling issues (Walz, 1996). As far back as 1982, Barnett described a counselor who referred a suicidal individual to counseling on the basis of their online conversations over a chat system on a campus computer network (Barnett, 1982). In 1997 Sampson, Kolodinsky, and Greeno found that the three major types of counseling pages found were: (1) online home pages offering services to potential clients for a fee via email or chat, (2) home pages advertising services, products, and publications, and (3) home pages offering free mental-health or education-related information for the general public. These types likely have not changed dramatically although the number of existing sites assumedly has multiplied annually.

Distance counseling is one of the newer, much-discussed developments we have seen in the counseling professions. There is the simple fact of an increasingly knowledgeable and information-thirsty clientele. Physicians have some ambivalence about the trend of patients surfing the Web for medical information. In a recent survey 37.5 percent of physicians thought the Internet has made patients more knowledgeable about their conditions; 31.6 percent said patients came in to them misinformed. A study in the journal *Cancer* reported that as much as 40 percent of the medical information obtained on the Internet is inaccurate and misleading. The majority of patients bringing information to their doctors bring information on general disease, followed by information about alternative or complementary therapies, drugs, and treatment protocols (Tschida, 1999). This can be seen as a positive trend in that it shows individuals are taking proactive steps to understand their

bodies and their health. This trend is of special pertinence to health counselors who have a vested interest in prevention and promoting health-enhancing behaviors and lifestyles.

There are many ways that patients/clients can access health information on the Internet. They can use health Web-site search engines to search for information and visit general consumer sites and Q&A sites. They can read online health news, and search through bibliographic databases such as Medline. They can visit health sites for professionals. They can find a health provider, join a health discussion or support group, visit a nonprofit, governmental, or educational site for information, or they visit sites devoted to a specific medical or health concern (Izenberg & Lieberman, 1998). Many of these possibilities also apply to mental-health issues and can be utilized similarly by the public. Otherwise underserved populations, such as the homebound, the elderly, those in rural areas, and in some cases minors, have access to an ever-expanding world of information, networking, and services that are in many cases inexpensive or free. Hoagwood and Koretz (1996) estimate that 60–80 percent of children in need of mental-health treatment do not receive it. There are no doubt many factors that contribute to this, but the unfortunate fact remains that 44 million adults lack health insurance according to the U.S. Department of Health and Human Services (2000). We can therefore assume that the low cost of advice and information on the Internet is one of its most powerful attractions. Whether information is accurate or not, the public is seeking it out and it is impacting individual health choices and behaviors.

Let us consider some of the ramifications of just one Internet feature on a population served by health counselors. For people suffering from a specific disease or condition entire Web sites have been created as a sort of clearinghouse for information on symptoms, treatment, and prevention. Often the site works with a physician specialist or team of "experts" who are available for email questions and provide the latest news and articles on the condition. The accuracy of what is posted on these sites may be debatable, but the obvious benefit lay in the networking and sharing of individual experience via billboard, chat, or guest book. Not only can individuals connect with others around the world and hear their reports on symptoms, treatment options, and efficacy, but the format affords an anonymity that many find desirable. In the past in order to get such feedback and support one had to attend a formal support group, which for some stigmatized diseases was very prohibitive—that is, if a group existed at all.

Sites such as these, although potentially a source of misinformation, fill a crucial gap in connecting people across national and state borders who share the same condition. This benefit is less pronounced with conditions that carry no particular stigma but is quite dramatic for those suffering from a sexually transmitted disease—or from an addiction or unwanted pregnancy. The anonymous nature of surfing the Web makes it one of the easiest ways of getting information, particularly for minors. In fact, realistically, it may be the only way minors can get feedback and much-needed information for a condition they have or think they might have. Many minors, especially under 16, lack transportation and the money for clinic visits—they may fear exposure and may not have access for a variety of reasons. They may simply not know where to go to get the help they need. If they have questions about birth control, sexuality, sexual symptoms they are having, pregnancy, and so on, they are likely to look on the Internet for answers first. This is exactly why health counselors need to be aware of the attractions and limitations of the new technology. Surfing the Web may not change a minor's need for counseling, examination, or medical care, but such resources can provide clues as to what kinds of help are not reaching young people most in need.

Health counselors must remember that, while supporting an agenda promoting healthy behaviors and prevention of pregnancy, disease, addiction, abuse, and violence, many young people are undergoing or have already undergone these things. When speaking to young people in a group, obviously the counselor will stress prevention of negative outcomes from the start. But there is as profound a need for ongoing support for individuals who may have been treated or dealt with medically for such problems, but never received the mental-health counseling and support they needed afterward. For instance, a minor (or anyone for that matter) treated for a sexually transmitted disease, or a minor who has had an abortion, may be medically treated and dealt with. But will they receive help with the difficult task of psychological healing and re-integration of their former self-image with a possibly changed self-image? This point is of vital importance, especially when a traumatic episode has been kept secret from parents and peers, which is too often the case. For adolescents dealing with some shame-inducing secret or problem, the Internet may literally be their only perceived source for help and healing that is safe.

Since health counselors work to prevent disease and dangerous behaviors and lifestyles, many of the areas that the profession deals with are controversial and bear considerable social stigma. The U.S. Department of Health and Human Services (2000) recently published Healthy People 2010, a 10-year plan to improve health and prevent disability, disease, and premature death in the United States. The targeted health indicators that were distinguished to improve the overall health and well-being of citizens included mental health, injury and violence, physical activity, overweightness and obesity, tobacco use, substance abuse and responsible sexual behavior. It is important to establish healthy behaviors early since a large proportion of chronic disease and premature death in adulthood arises from behaviors initiated during adolescence (U.S. Department of Health and Human Serivces, 2000). Tackling stigmatizing behaviors in adolescence is particularly difficult since the common avenues of reaching adolescents—through school, parents, and community programs—do not offer them the safety, confidentiality, and accessibility that adults who seek assistance are afforded. The offerings of Internet-based distance counseling in this regard are considerable. The anonymity factor will be an important one for reaching the many different populations of underserved people seeking counseling and assistance for stigmatizing conditions.

Distance Counseling

The ethics of distance counseling have recently received much attention and continue to be defined as the scope of Internet counseling expands (Guterman & Kirk, 1999; Maheu & Gordon, 2000; Oravec, 2000; American Counseling Association, 1999; Reimer-Reiss, 2000). The American Counseling Association (1999) as well as the National Board for Certified Counselors (1999) have published ethical standards for online counseling in response to the proliferation of counseling Web sites. Ethical issues are only one of the challenges associated with this method of service delivery. But there are inherent advantages as well. For mental-health counselors in particular, this method enables them to serve individuals who have illnesses, domestic obligations, and/or live in geographic areas that do not allow for frequent trips to mental-health agencies. In particular, individuals with mental illnesses may not be able to access traditional treatment due to the nature of their disorders (Reimer-Reiss, 2000).

Email systems provide effective techniques for consumer–counselor relations because of their speed, convenience, and efficiency. Although many Americans still do not have email access, the number of those who do is steadily rising. Email is an easy, inexpensive mode for consumers to communicate with their counselors or to engage in group counseling sessions (Reimer-Reiss, 2000). Critics have asserted that conducting groups via distance technologies is an impersonal approach and that the human element is needed in group counseling. However, many individuals find the format more conducive to open and honest expression and less threatening than traditional formats (Ancis, 1998). Also, the anonymity of distance group counseling may allow for less assertive individuals to be more involved than they normally would (Rosenfield, 1997).

Videoconferencing is another technology that is useful in distance counseling. Using this technology, counselors and clients can see and hear each other over vast distances. Software that allows sound and moving pictures to be transmitted can be downloaded over the Internet. Most new computers include a sound card, and digital cameras can be bought for under $250 (Ruskin et al., 1998). These advances enable the public to send and receive real-time audio and video over a computer. In videoconferencing counselors and consumers can read body language and facial expressions, thus closely approximating counseling in person. However it is unlikely that videoconferencing will ever replace face-to-face conferencing. It can be used as an effective supplement, especially for otherwise hard-to-reach clients.

Distance counseling does not come without its challenges for consumers and counselors. The most obvious challenge is the possibility for technical difficulties and failures, in which case counselors should have an alternate plan for service delivery. This might be as easy as using the telephone as a backup. Counselors may have to deal with consumer apprehension about nontraditional counseling sessions. Alimandi, Andrich, and Porqueddu (1995) found that consumers were capable of interacting with distance counselors in a relaxed and natural manner after participating in computer training. Counseling professionals also must have a positive and relaxed attitude toward technology and distance activities if they want them to be effective. Where counselors express frustration or discomfort with technology, a barrier is created to distance counseling. Approximately 50–60 percent of the mental-health professionals surveyed expressed reluctance toward learning about technology (Rosen & Waft, 1995). Many counselors have contended that authentic counseling cannot take place over a distance (Sanders & Rosenfield, 1998). However, general consensus in the field points to the evidence that distance learning can be as effective as traditional approaches.

Distance counseling is meaningless if clients do not have access to the technology. Therefore one of the socioeconomic challenges to distance counseling involves inequitable access to computers and the Internet. The early research into Internet demographics were skewed toward well-educated, affluent, middle-aged males (Who's in line, 1997). However recent research suggests that the demographics are changing and the Internet is being embraced by every age and ethnic group. This trend correlates with low-cost Internet use, mass-marketed online services, employer-provided email accounts, and increased public access to the Internet (Tait, 1999). We have yet to see whether the diversity of users of online counseling services will be in keeping with the growing diversity of Internet users.

The ethics of online counseling cover such areas as confidentiality, establishing the online counseling relationship, and legal considerations. The American Counseling Association has outlined the major ethical standards for Internet online counseling, to be used in conjunction with the latest *ACA Code of Ethics and Standards of Practice (2000)*. Health counselors should be aware of these standards since the profession will likely follow the general trend toward distance and online counseling methods.

The most important ethical point is for counselors to prevent potential breaches of confidentiality. They should provide one-on-one counseling only through "secure" Web sites or email applications that use encryption technology. Encryption protects the transmission of confidential information from access by unauthorized third parties. Counselors therefore should include on their Web site: information about privacy and the limits of confidentiality in the counselor/client relationship; informational notices regarding the security of the counselor's site, the counselor's professional identification, and client information (this last item includes identifying and verifying the identity of clients, and obtaining emergency contact information); and a client waiver and information regarding records of electronic communications and the electronic transfer of client information. In addition the professional counselor should develop an appropriate take-in procedure for potential clients to determine whether online counseling is appropriate for the needs of the client. Counselors must ensure that clients are intellectually, emotionally, and physically capable of using the online counseling services, and of understanding the potential risk and/or limitations of such services.

The second area of main ethical importance is the establishment of the online counseling relationship. After deciding that online counseling is appropriate, counselors should develop a counseling plan that takes into account both the client's individual circumstances and the limitations of online counseling. Counselors should provide clients with a schedule of times during which the online counseling services will be available, including anticipated response times and alternate means of contacting the counselor in the event of an emergency. It is important that professional counselors provide online counseling services only in practice areas within their expertise, and that they do not provide counseling services to clients located in states in which professional counselors are not licensed. In the case of minor or incompetent clients, counselors must obtain the written consent of the legal guardian or other authorized legal representative of the client prior to beginning counseling services.

Finally, in term of legal considerations in online counseling, professional counselors need to confirm that their liability insurance provides coverage for online counseling services. They should confirm that such services are not prohibited by any state or local statutes, regulations or ordinances, codes of professional membership organizations and certifying boards, and/or codes of state licensing boards.

Assessing the Value of Distance/Cybercounseling

Due to the rapidly changing and evolving nature of new technology applications, society at large is presently wrestling with the implications of technology on every aspect of our lives. For therapists and counselors, for whom the one-on-one client contact has always been central, this questioning is even more urgent and necessary at this time. Many therapists are questioning the value of cybercounseling in its various forms. Most counselors and therapists agree that cybercounseling is not and should not be a replacement for in-person therapy. Since most therapists rely to some extent on nonverbal cues when working with a client, this crucial element is eliminated in the online session, in chat rooms, and so on. In addition, a therapist needs to to discriminate which presenting problems might be appropriate to work through in a distance, cybercounseling context. For some problems, Internet-based interaction could be counterproductive to the goals of therapy. For instance, a lack of personal contact could reinforce the very interpersonal behaviors or fears that are limiting the client's functioning. The use of "point and click" technology exclusively could impede the progress of clients who need to learn verbal and nonverbal communication skills.

In Chapter 12, the author highlights a serious concern for the increasingly technological direction of society and how this may be impacting individual psychology and well-being. If we view "cybertherapy" through the lens of ecopsychology, it would seem that the distance, online counselor–client relationship is yet another step toward isolation and dehumanization in a field that has traditionally been centered on the human one-on-one relationship. Yet therapists and counsellors are exploring therapeutic uses of new technology and finding important advantages and assets in it. Time will tell whether the positive benefits of cybercounseling outweigh its dangers and potential negative consequences for clients. At this point in the developing field, each counselor/therapist must decide for him or herself whether his or her values and principles can accommodate the implications of cybertherapy in its varying forms.

Getting Started on the Web

The following information will give the counselor a basic sense of how to get involved with some current "cyber" applications. Possibly the best way to get started is to familiarize yourself with what is out there and how it is being done, namely, by visiting existing Web sites (that is, surfing the Web).

Chat rooms

There are two methods of communication in chat rooms depending on the chat-room software program: synchronous (in real time) and asynchronous (delayed time of a few seconds). A chat room is a designated space in cyberspace where individuals gather around a specific topic, not unlike a room full of people anywhere. Some chat rooms are limited to members of a specific group and some are open chats available to anyone. As of this writing, some free chat rooms currently available are:

> Behavior Online Chat Events at
> *http://behavior.net/chatevents/index.html*

> The Counseling Zone at
> *http://www.couselingzone.com*

You can also create your own chat room for free and invite colleagues and clients by going to: Beeseen at *http://www.beseen.com* and downloading the chat software.

Online Consulting

Online consulting and online coaching is a simple procedure in that the client or client organization communicates with the consultant either through email or in a chat room. Documents can easily be emailed, edited, and revised in common word-processing software. Online consulting also has the advantage of producing an easily printable record of dialogue. There is also the option of creating a Web-based virtual office (intranet) for this purpose. A Web site that currently provides free service of this feature *is http://www.intranets.com.*

Marketing

The Internet offers the counselor considerable opportunities to market their services to a wide audience globally. In order to do this, you must establish a "presence" on the Web. For most people, this means the creation of a Web site. Web-sites can be fairly simple (primarily informational) or complex (involving interactive features). Web site development software, such as Front Page Express, is available for sale at any computer store whereby you can create your own Web site yourself. However, many people opt for hiring a Web-site builder, which can be less time consuming. In addition, the Web-site builder can maintain the site for you and submit it to search engines, which is the next step in terms of making your Web site visible. Once your site is "on the Web" you can add features to create a more interactive environment, such as attaching a chat room. You can also create an online newsletter and attach it to your site. These are indirect ways to market your services through your Web site. More direct ways of marketing include buying advertising space on search engines and other Web pages and purchasing a listing/link on pages designed to advertise your specific type of service. The easiest way to market your site is to be sure it gets listed on as many search engines as possible. A few popular search engines currently are Yahoo at *http://www.yahoo.com,* and Google at *http://www.google.com,* among many others. Most search engines provide information on their site's home page about the process of getting a listing (submitting a Web page). You can also pay for a service that will do this for you. Often Web design, maintenance, and marketing are combined into one package available for a fee. Whether you choose to build your own Web site or have it built, being familiar with your design options and the range of features available is desirable and can be accomplished through simply "surfing the Web" with a critical eye.

Health Promotion in the 21st Century

In this age of information we have seen the consumer's growing access to a variety of information and health tools that were never before available. For the health-counseling profession this may be a positive sign of an increasingly pro-active health-conscious public. We have yet to see whether the public will use the information they find to change unhealthy behaviors and make health-enhancing lifestyle choices as a result. Early on in this chapter statistics showed that a majority of consumers who bring health information to their doctors bring information on alternative treatments. In the last 10 years there has been a steady rise in the popularity of alternative medicine among the general public. There is a demand as never before for organic food and for acceptance of the mind–body connection in creating health. Although still not as mainstream as in Europe, many people are curious and excited by the possibility that there may be complementary low-cost additions to Western medicine. The rising cost of prescription drugs and medical treatment in this country, and the widespread lack of health insurance, make the interest in alternatives understandable. Will this trend affect the direction that health counselors will take toward prevention?

The popularity of ancient mind–body systems such as yoga and tai chi shows that the mainstream is looking for preventative, stress-reducing, life-enhancing modalities. Since these are very much in line with the health counselor's mission, it may be wise to become educated about the benefits and uses of alternative modalities in health counseling. The rise of the information highway and the rise of interest in more holistic modalities reflect a healthy democratization of previously controlled, inaccessible areas. The public has more empowerment to make choices, to understand their choices, and to connect with a global community than ever before. Any empowerment necessarily involves risks and dangers, due to the need for responsibility. A health counselor can assist a client in using information responsibly and translating ideas into concrete reality that protect health and well-being. There are indications that for counselor and client, access to technology can enhance the client–counselor relationship, be cost effective, and be mutually beneficial.

As cultural values change, health counseling will have to change along with them. Some changes we can expect to see in the coming years will be consistent with changes currently happening in marriage and divorce trends, sexual activity/abstinence trends, disease trends (such as AIDS and cancer), and addiction. On a global scale there is increasing awareness of the fragility and exhaustibility of our natural resources, indeed of our basic environment itself. The cancer epidemic in the United States has the general public asking the basic question: What has gone wrong here? There has been a greater focus on environmental causes of disease and even of psychosocial aberrance. Health counselors might begin to address the problem of how to stay healthy in an unhealthy environment, since many consumers have already begun looking for these answers. In general, health counselors should acquaint themselves with the new possibilities in technology and prepare to use them to their full capacity. The profession of health counseling will need to respond appropriately to the changes and demands of a technology-driven society and the culture that it engenders.

Summary

The health-care and counseling fields have been greatly affected by new technological developments such as the Internet and the information highway. It was recently found that medical information is the most popular "subject" on the Web. How the Internet is used for health and/or counseling purposes is likely to change dramatically as advancements occur. There are many ways the public is using the Internet for counseling and health information. These include the use of bulletin boards, discussion groups, email, Web sites dedicated to a specific condition, exchange of text files, individual and organization home pages, and distance counseling. With the advantages of increased convenience and greater accessibility to information come the dangers of misinformation, as well as the practical and ethical challenges for counselors. Future health counselors will need to be aware of the implications of information accessibility on the general public, and specifically on populations often served by health counselors.

Distance counseling is one application likely to affect future counselors who will need a level of techno savvy to adapt to the requirements of an increasingly "online" public. Counselors who practice distance or online counseling need to follow professional standards of legal and ethical practice, the most important being to secure the privacy and security of the counselor-client relationship. Online counseling has the advantages of reaching clients who are underserved, and of being cost effective.

With the increased access to information and health tools, consumers have shown interest in alternative medicine and mind–body systems, and are bringing this information to their doctors. Health counselors should heed this trend and be open to incorporating some of these alternative modalities in their prevention strategies. In general, health counselors will need to understand and be able to utilize the technologies of the 21st century if they are to be successful.

Questions for Discussion

1. What are some of the ethical issues facing counselors who want to practice on the Internet?

2. What are the advantages and disadvantages of online counseling/therapy?

3. How might the counselor–client relationship be affected by not taking place in person, not seeing nonverbal cues, body language, and so on?

4. Do you think that technology will become more and more prominent in the 21st century, or begin to decline eventually? Why?

5. What other cultural or health trends may affect the public well-being in coming years, becoming pertinent to health counselors?

Related Web Sites

http://www.metanoia.org/imhs/index.html.
Site explores e-therapy. When traditional systems fail them, many people are turning to the Internet.

http://www.counselingzone.com/Internet/
Mental Health Counseling and the Internet. A brief history and description of the Internet are presented. Current and po-tential uses of the Internet among mental-health counselors, and ways in which the Internet can be understood from a postmodern perspective, are discussed.

http://www.virtualcs.com/mhi.html
Guide to the Mental Health Internet. Organized by types of resources rather than reviews of whole sites.

http://www.cybertherapy.com/.
Conscious Choices: Online Mental Health Counseling.

Joseph Donnelly, Ph.D.

Dr. Donnelly is a committed advocate of health-education programs, particularly in the area of adolescent health. Since 1997 he has been funded approximately $1.5 million through federal and state agencies to reduce teen pregnancy and the negative outcomes associated with early sexual behavior. Since 1998 he has collaborated with the National Council on Alcoholism and Drug Dependence in helping to reduce drug use within adolescent and pre-adolescent populations. The prevention-intervention programs he has helped to develop have been grounded in the use of communication skills, effective decision making, resistance/refusal skills, self-esteem, and stress management. His expertise has been sought by community organizations and federal and state agencies in the areas of evaluation and program design in alcohol, tobacco, and other drugs, abstinence education, and a multitude of community outreach programs.

Dr. Donnelly is currently an associate professor at Montclair State University in the Program of Health Professions, where he instructs courses in the areas of drug education, health counseling, mental health, and the teaching of health education.

Dr. Donnelly's presentations at the international, national, and state levels have been numerous. He has been a keynote speaker at the New York Counseling Association, New Jersey Dietetic Association, Office of Adolescent Pregnancy Programs, International Council of Self-Esteem, and many other conferences. In addition, he has made over 100 presentations for public schools and local parent organizations. His work in the field of health education and counseling has included over 40 articles published in peer-reviewed publications and trade journals. He acts as a reviewer for several professional health journals, including *Self-Esteem Today*, where he serves as a board member as well.

Dr. Donnelly received his B.S., M.S., and Ph.D. within the specialization of community health education from Southern Illinois University, at Carbondale. He served as a faculty member at Hofstra University for three years, after which he pursued specialization within counseling and psychology at Governor's State University. This specialization culminated in his authorship of the textbook *Mental Health: Dimensions of Self-Esteem and Emotional Well-Being*, published in 2001. Dr. Donnelly has worked in the capacity of author and editor on several textbooks, including *Health Counseling: Application and Theory*. These experiences have helped to solidify his commitment to and passion for health education and counseling, to which he tirelessly devotes his energy.

Joan D. Atwood, Ph.D.

Dr. Atwood is the Director of the Graduate Program in Marriage and Family Therapy at Hofstra University. She is also the Director of the Marriage and Family Therapy Clinic at Hofstra University. She is the past President of the New York State Association for Marriage and Family Therapists and was awarded the Long Island Family Therapist of the Year award for outstanding contributions to the field. Dr. Atwood has published seven books, all relating to the field of marriage and family therapy. In addition, she has published over 100 journal articles on social construction theory and therapy, families in transition, human sexuality issues, and family health issues. She is a Clinical Member and Approved Supervisor of AAMFT; she serves on the editorial board of many journals in the field; she holds diplomate status and is a clinical supervisor on the American Board of Sexology; she has been elected to the National Academy of Social Workers; is a certified Imago therapist; and has served on the President's Commission for Domestic Policy. Among her many projects,

Dr. Atwood is the co-developer of the P.E.A.C.E. Program (Parent Education and Custody Effectiveness), a court-based educational program for parents obtaining a divorce. Dr. Atwood has made numerous TV appearances and radio and newspaper interviews. She is in private practice in individual marriage, and family therapy. Dr. Atwood received her Ph.D. from SUNY Stoneybrook in Social Psychology. She received her M.S.W. From Adelphi University.

Isabel Burk, M.S., C.P.P., C.H.E.S.

Ms. Burk, Director of the Health Network, is a nationally known, award-winning expert on health, prevention, and education issues. She earned her B.S. and M.S. from Lehman College, City University of New York. Ms. Burk is a credentialed prevention professional and a nationally certified health-education specialist, and is a sought-after speaker, trainer, and program developer who has made presentations to more than 45,000 people in 36 states.

Her professional achievements have been honored by the U.S. Department of Health and Human Services, Northeast Center for Safe and Drug-Free Schools, and the New York State Department of Health. Ms. Burk has authored two books and more than 100 feature articles. She has contributed to the Project ALERT curriculum and was a national reviewer for the revised 2002 D.A.R.E. national curriculum. She is an authorized instructor for the New York State Division of Criminal Justice Services, and recently served as Chair of the American School Health Association's Council on Alcohol, Tobacco, and Other Drugs.

Ms. Burk has been a guest on *20/20, CBS This Morning, The View, Phil Donahue,* and *Fox News,* among other TV programs, and writes a monthly online column for The Guidance Channel.

Jon Carlson, Psy.D., Ed.D.

Dr. Carlson is Distinguished Professor in the Division of Psychology and Counseling at Governors State University at University Park, Illinois and Director of the Wellness Clinic in Lake Geneva, Wisconsin. He has authored 30 books and over 120 professional articles. He is the former Editor of the *Journal of Individual Psychology* and Founding Editor of *The Family Journal.* Dr. Carlson has been active as a film producer and developed over 100 professional and trade videos in the areas of psychology, family therapy, brief therapy, parenting, and child therapy. He has completed a 12-video series on behavioral health and health counseling that is available from the American Psychological Association. This series shows how psychologists can work with problems such as pain, sleep, chronic illness, addiction, cancer, and weight management.

Michele M. Fisher, D.P.E.

Dr. Fisher is currently an Associate Professor and Coordinator of the Graduate Program in Physical Education at Montclair State University. She completed her D.P.E. with a concentration in Exercise Physiology at Springfield College in 1995, and joined the faculty of Montclair State University the same year. She also holds a M.S. degree in Cardiac Rehabilitation and Exercise Science from East Stroudsburg University, and a B.S. degree in Biology from Elizabethtown College. Her research interests are in cardiovascular exercise physiology and physical fitness, yielding several peer-reviewed abstracts, presentations, and publications. She also serves as a reviewer for the *Measurement in Physical Education and Exercise Science Journal,* has chaired the research committee for the Eastern District Association (EDA) of the American Alliance for Health, Physical Education, Recreation and Dance (AAHPERD), and is on the Executive Board of the New Jersey Association for Health, Physical Education, Recreation, and Dance (NJAHPERD). Dr. Fisher has been recognized as the College Teacher of the Year by NJAHPERD in 2002 and is the 2000 recipient of the Mabel Lee Award by AAHPERD. She is also certified as an exercise specialist by the American College of Sports Medicine.

Eva S. Goldfarb, Ph.D.

Dr. Goldfarb has been a sexuality educator and author since 1987. She is coauthor of *Our Whole Lives: Sexuality Education for Grades 10–12* and *Our Whole Lives: Sexuality Education for Grades 4–6*, two sexuality-education curricula that are part of the groundbreaking *Our Whole Lives* life-long curriculum series. Coauthor of *Filling the Gaps*, a book on hard-to-teach topics in human sexuality, Dr. Goldfarb has spent her career preparing future sexuality educators, teaching courses, leading workshops, consulting on media projects, conducting seminars, and developing curricula in the areas of human sexuality and sexual health. She is also the author of numerous articles in the area of sexuality education.

Dr. Goldfarb is currently an Associate Professor in the Program of Health Professions at Montclair State University, specializing in Human Sexuality Education. She also sits on the Board of Directors of SIECUS (The Sexuality Information and Education Council of the United States).

Dr. Goldfarb was awarded an honorary doctorate of humane letters in 2001 for her work on the *Our Whole Lives* curricula. Previously, she earned her B.A. degree from Trinity College in Hartford, Connecticut, her M.A. from the Annenberg School of Communications at the University of Pennsylvania; and her Ph.D. in educational leadership in human sexuality from the Graduate School of Education, also at the University of Pennsylvania.

Jerrold S. Greenberg, Ph.D.

Dr. Greenberg is a Professor in the Department of Public and Community Health at the University of Maryland. Dr. Greenberg earned his B.A. and M.A. degrees from The City College of New York, and continued his education at Syracuse University where he earned his Ph.D. Dr. Greenberg has taught at Syracuse University, Boston University, and the State University of New York at Buffalo before accepting his current position at the University of Maryland in 1979. Dr. Greenberg has written over 40 books on such topics as elder care, health, stress management, physical fitness, wellness, health-education ethics, methods of health education, and service-learning. In addition, he has published approximately 80 articles in professional journals and lay magazines, and has made hundreds of presentations at professional conferences, work-site seminars, and before other groups.

Among Dr. Greenberg's honors are the American School Health Association's Distinguished Service Award; selection as Alliance Scholar by the American Alliance for Health, Physical Education, Recreation, and Dance; the Presidential Citation, the Certificate of Appreciation, and the Scholar Award of the American Association for Health Education; selection as a finalist for the Thomas Ehrlich Faculty Award for Service-Learning of Campus Compact; and inclusion in *Who's Who in America*, *Outstanding Young Men of America*, and *Who's Who in World Jewry*. Dr. Greenberg has also served on the editorial boards of the professional journals *Health Education* and *The Journal of School Health*; and as a reviewer for other professional journals such as the *Michigan Journal of Community Service Learning*.

Dr. Greenberg is a national leader in service-learning in health education and founder of the Service-Learning in Health Education Interest Group listserv comprised of health educators from across the United States. He also authored and edited a new book published by the American Association for Health Education (AAHE) entitled *Service-Learning in Health Education* and conducted Train-the-Trainer workshops based on that book for health educators at the AAHE convention.

Arden Greenspan-Goldberg, M.S.W., A.C.S.W., B.C.D.

Ms. Goldberg is a nationally known speaker and clinician in private practice for over 25 years, specializing in eating disorders, and women's, teen, and family issues. She earned her M.S.W. from Hunter College School of social work, City University of New York. Her Post Masters training was at The National Institute for the Psychotherapies in New York where she earned two certificates in psychotherapy and psychoanalysis.

As a former adjunct professor of psychology at St. Thomas Aquinas College she taught the introduction and treatment of eating disorders and psychology of women. Ms. Greenspan-Goldberg is a former columnist for Gannett's *Rockland Journal News*. Her advice column "ask arden" was geared toward teen and family issues. Her clinical cases and advice have appeared in numerous articles in *The Ladies Home Journal*, "Can This Marriage Be Saved," *Women's Own, Family Circle* magazine, and in newspapers.

Ms. Greenspan-Goldberg was President and Fellow of the Rockland Chapter of the New York State Society for Clinical Social Workers. She is a board-certified diplomate in clinical social work with the American Board of Examiners and with the National Association of Social Workers, and a member of both the National Eating Disorder Organization, and the American Federation of Television and Radio Actors (AFTRA).

Ms. Greenspan-Goldberg has been a guest expert on *The View*, *Sally Jesse Rafael*, *Maury Povich*, MSNBC cable, and has appeared on a regular basis on *Good Day New York*.

Luis Montesinos, Ph.D.

Dr. Montesinos is currently an Associate Professor at the Psychology Department of Montclair State University. He also serves as the Director for the New Faculty program, a campus-wide initiative that introduces new faculty to the culture and procedures of the University. He obtained his M.A. from the Behavior Analysis and Therapy, and his Ph.D. at the Rehabilitation Institute of Southern Illinois University at Carbondale. A native of Chile, Dr. Montesinos also holds a degree of Psychologist from the Universidad Catolica in that country.

With more than 25 years of experience in academia Dr. Montesinos has taught as visiting professor in universities in Spain, Chile, and Colombia. He has published numerous articles in the United States and Latin America and is fre-

quently invited as guest speaker at international conferences.

Gloria Pierce, Ph.D.

Dr. Pierce is professor of Counseling, Human Development, and Educational Leadership at Montclair State University where she also directed an innovative mentoring program for new faculty at MSU for 6 years. She holds a Ph.D. and M.A. from Columbia University, a M.A. in human development from Fairleigh Dickinson University, and a B.A. from Douglass College, Rutgers University. She has lectured and published work in several areas of expertise, including stress and burnout, management and organization development, mentoring, feminist counseling, ecopsychology, and ecofeminism.

Elizabeth Schroeder, M.S.W.

Ms. Schroeder is a professional trainer and consultant in the areas of sexuality, counseling, and non-profit administration and supervision. She has provided trainings throughout the United States to youth-serving professionals and teens; presented at national conferences; written about sexuality issues and training for national newsletters, magazines, and monographs; and is a sexuality expert for the award-winning Web site, Sex, Etc. She is the author of the 5th edition of *Taking Sides: Controversial Issues in Family and Interpersonal Relationships*, (Fall 2002), and of a chapter on Nepal for the upcoming edition of the *International Encyclopedia of Sexuality*. The former Associate Vice President of Education and Training at Planned Parenthood of New York City, Ms. Schroeder established the agency's first professional training institute for social service and school professionals. As the Manager of Education and Special Projects at Planned Parenthood Federation of America, she coordinated the production of their multiple-award-winning video kit for families with adolescent children, "Talking About Sex: A Guide for Families." She is a recipient of the national Apple Blossom Award, which recognizes a

Planned Parenthood Education or Training Director who has "risen quickly to the forefront with new ideas, energy, and commitment."

An adjunct instructor of Human Sexuality and Health Counseling at Montclair State University, Ms. Schroeder earned a M.S.W. from New York University, and is pursuing a doctorate in Human Sexuality Education at Widener University.

Len Sperry, M.D., Ph.D.

Dr. Sperry is currently Clinical Professor of Psychiatry and Preventive Medicine at the Medical College of Wisconsin in Milwaukee, Wisconsin, and Professor and Director of the Doctoral Program in Counseling at Barry University in Miami Shores, Florida. He is a licensed psychologist and physician who has practiced health counseling and psychotherapy for over 30 years. Dr. Sperry is a Fellow of the American Psychological Association and a Diplomate in Clinical Psychology of the American Board of Professional Psychology, Inc. In addition, he is board certified by the American Board of Psychiatry and Neurology and by the American Board of Preventive Medicine. He is on the editorial board of nine journals and has published nearly 300 articles and book chapters and more than 38 professional books. The second edition of *Health Promotion and Health Counseling* is in press. The recipient of the Harry Levinson Award from the American Psychological Association, his work on health counseling is featured in the "Chronic Illness" video of the APA video series "Behavioral Health Issues."

Shahla Wunderlich, Ph.D., R.D.

Dr. Wunderlich is currently a Professor of Food and Nutrition at Montclair State University, Upper Montclair, New Jersey. She received a B.S. degree in Food Technology and Nutrition from Pahlavi University, Shiraz, Iran, and an M.S. degree in Nutrition from the American University of Beirut, Beirut, Lebanon. She earned her Ph.D. from the Massachusetts Institute of Technology, Cambridge, MA, in Nutritional Biochemistry and Metabolism. Dr. Wunderlich's research findings in the areas of nutrition assessment, maternal and child nutrition, HIV, and diabetes have been published in the *Journal of the American Dietetic Association, Topics in Clinical Nutrition, Nutrition Today,* and the *Journal of the American Association of Diabetes Educators* among others. Dr. Wunderlich has also served as a reviewer for many nutrition textbooks.

Dr. Wunderlich is the recipient of many awards, including the American Dietetic Association Outstanding Dietetic Educator award, the Sandoz Nutrition Dietetic Educator Practice Award, and the United Nations International Children's Fund (UNICEF) Award. Dr. Wunderlich is a registered dietitian, a certified nutrition specialist, and a Fellow of the American College of Nutrition. She is an active member of the American Dietetic Association, the American Society for Nutritional Sciences, the Federation of American Societies for Experimental Biology, and the New Jersey Dietetic Association.

GLOSSARY

Abstinence To refrain completely from a substance or activity.

Addiction When one feels dependent, controlled, or negatively influenced by a behavior or substance.

Affect How a person expresses their emotional state, usually reflecting the circumstances of a person's life.

Androcentrism Male-centered, or patriarchal, belief system that overvalues masculine qualities and denigrates the feminine.

Anorgasmia Lack of orgasm in females which usually has psychological causes.

Anthropocentrism A human-centered worldview which ordains all living things to be inferior to human beings, justifying exploitation and abuse of the nonhuman world.

Assessment An initial estimation of the patient's understanding of the need for treatment, the treatment regimen, and the degree of mastery of any requisite skills necessary for compliance.

Attitude of gratitude Learning to be grateful for what one has, while not denying or ignoring reality.

Autonomy The ethical principle that people should be free to decide their own course of action as long as they do no harm to others.

Behavioral analysis and therapy A counseling approach that assumes that behavior is lawful and obeys certain principles that can be discerned through careful analysis; the application of learning principles to deviant (abnormal) behavior.

Behavioral assessment Initial gathering of client's behavioral information that may be done through interviews, direct observation, self-monitoring, analogue assessment, study of antecedents and consequences, and so on.

Behavioral contract A written document usually signed by the individual and one or more persons by which both parties commit to a particular behavioral program.

Beneficence The ethical principle to do good—not doing harm is not good enough. Includes benefits and balancing benefits and harms.

Biophilia The profound innate love of nature evidenced in children.

Biopsychosocial A term that describes the roles biological, psychological, and social factors play in a person's general health.

Body composition The relative percentage of fat and fat-free tissues (muscles, bone, and water) in the body.

Boundaries Physical or psychological parameters within which a counselor works with a client.

Cessation The stopping or "quitting" of a particular behavior.

Client Any individual with whom the counselor interacts.

Client-centered Helping a client make a well-informed decision, rather than doing what a counselor thinks is in the best interest of the client.

Codes of ethics Standards, principles, responsibilities, and rules expressing the duties of professionals to whom the codes apply.

Coercion Encouraging, motivating, and influencing clients to behave in certain ways that health counselors believe to be in the client's best interests.

Cognitive behavior therapy A grouping of techniques which are based on the assumption that behavior change can be achieved by altering cognitive processes, since maladaptive cognitive processes are the main factors responsible for maladaptive behaviors.

Cognitive restructuring   A type of cognitive behavioral therapy that attempts to restructure faulty thinking and negative self-statements into more positive ideas.

Coming out   The process of acknowledging one's gay, lesbian, or bisexual attractions and identity to oneself and disclosing them to others.

Communication skills   Methods of effective communication, practiced as sender and receiver, using verbalization and nonverbal messages.

Compensation   One of the two basic principles of aging—If there are any losses in function or capacity of organs or body systems there will be a tendency to compensate for it somehow.

Consciousness raising   Techniques that help people understand the interaction between their presenting problem and the larger cultural, social, ecological level.

Counseling relationship   The context in which the process of therapy is experienced and enacted.

Counseling termination   Weaning a client from the counseling relationship if he or she is exhibiting pseudodependency, or if it is in the client or counselor's best interest.

Counselor   Any educational or health professional who is in a position to provide information or services to a client.

Death and dying   Death is a process of transition that starts with dying and ends with being dead. Also refers to the point at which a person is declared physically dead. Dying is the irreversible and progressive period in which the organism loses its viability.

Deep ecology   The philosophical idea that there needs to be a widening and deepening of the self to include all other forms of life.

Defense mechanisms   Strategies, usually subconscious, that a person uses to protect or defend her or himself against anxiety and perceived psychological threats.

Defenses   Ways in which a person attempts to protect her or himself against anxiety. These can include denial, rationalization, regression, and so on.

Denial   A defense in which a person acts as if something is not real, or ignores a situation or circumstance.

Dependence   Compulsive and uncontrollable use of a substance or practice of a behavior.

Depth psychology   A branch of psychology that seeks to restore emotional well-being by reconnecting human consciousness to its deepest roots, the matrix of a universal consciousness within an ecological frame of reference.

Determinism   The belief that prior experience, not free will, directs the course of our lives.

Developmental tasks   The maturational skills necessary for a healthy relationship including (1) positive self-image, (2) individuation, (3) expression of love without feeling depleted, (4) willingness to assume responsibility and care-taking and (5) a balance of emotions and reasoning.

Disease prevention   Any efforts, activities or information whose purpose is to prevent diseases and promote good health.

Eating disorder   When a person uses food as a coping mechanism to punish, deprive, or self-soothe in order to deal with feelings of pain, depression, and so on. These include anorexia nervosa, bulimia, and binge eating.

Ecofeminism   A form of feminism/ecology that rejects the male-centered system of domination and control that leads to violence against women and the earth.

Ecoliterature   Literature or nature writing that combines scientific knowledge of nature with a deep spiritual sense of its sacredness.

Ecological self   A shift in perception, often through a wilderness experience, characterized by an awareness in which one feels the oneness of self and nature.

Ecopsychology　Psychology that embraces an ecological conception of the human psyche, wherein the roots of modern psychological distress lie in the estrangement from nature and inadequate definitions of sanity.

Ecotherapy　A form of therapy that assumes a connection between healing the wounded human psyche and healing the wounds inflicted on the earth.

Effective communication　Communication characterized by listening, receptivity, specificity, honesty, respect, and nonjudgment.

Energy balance　When a person's energy consumed (calories) per day closely matches his or her energy expenditure.

Endorphins　The natural chemical responsible for good feelings; a natural opiate released in the body.

Epidemiological transition　The change in health habits by which developing countries not only adopt the economic development model of the industrialized countries, but also inherit its high incidence of chronic conditions and unhealthful behavioral patterns.

Erectile dysfunction (impotence)　The persistent or recurrent inability of a man to attain or maintain an erection in order to engage in satisfying sexual activities requiring this response.

Ethical dilemmas　Instances when two or more ethical principles compete with each other, leading to different determinations of morality.

Ethical principles　Guidelines used to determine whether a situation or decision is moral or immoral; for example, nonmaleficence, beneficence, autonomy, and so on.

Ethics　A system by which one determines whether an action is moral or immoral.

Exercise　Planned physical activity designed to improve physical fitness.

Family planning　The conscious decision one makes about having a family, including when to have children, how many, and how far apart.

Female Arousal Disorder　Persistent or recurrent inability to attain or maintain sufficient vaginal lubrication and swelling to engage in satisfying sexual activities; can also be a persistent lack of arousal, excitement, or pleasure.

Female Orgasmic Disorder (inhibited female orgasm)　Persistent or recurrent delay in or absence of orgasm following sexual arousal and excitement, when orgasm is desired.

Free Association　A technique originally developed by Freud, where the client is instructed to say anything that comes to mind, in hopes of extricating unconscious information.

Functional analysis　The process of testing hypotheses regarding the functional relations among antecedents, target behaviors and consequences; used in the behavioral approach.

Gestalt therapy　A therapy that assumes that authentic contact with the world is at the core of emotional health and full human functioning.

Griefwork　In ecotherapy, helping clients work through feeling of grief, anger, guilt, frustration, and dread about the deteriorating environment.

Hassles　Minor stressing events encountered on a daily basis that can take a toll on one's health.

Health　A state of complete physical, mental, and social well-being and not merely the absence of disease or infirmity.

Health counseling　A form of health education that describes various approaches and methods for assisting individuals to reduce or prevent the progression of disease as well as to improve health status and functioning.

Health expectancy　The number of years that a person can expect to live in a positive state of self-sufficiency.

Health-focused psychotherapy　Psychotherapeutic interventions for health issues that tend to focus more on core personality dynamics and psychotherapeutic assessment.

Health promotion: Actions directed to achieve and maintain health through the empowerment of individuals and communities.

Health-promotion counseling   Provided by a health-promotion specialist to improve lifestyle and health behaviors. Uses assessment and educational methods aimed toward skill-building and often uses interventions designed to increase clients' perceptions of control and self-efficacy.

Healthy People 2010   Developed by the U.S. Department of Health and Human Services, a 10-year plan of health objectives for the nation based on two goals—to increase the quality and years of healthy life and to eliminate health disparities.

Healthy relationships   Relationships in which positivity, growth, effective communication, and mature giving and receiving of love are standard.

HIV (human immunodeficiency virus)   The virus that can lead to AIDS, that is transmitted through the body fluids blood, semen, vaginal discharge, and breast milk.

Hypoactive Sexual Desire Disorder or **Inhibited Sexual Desire (ISD)**   A lack of interest in sexual activity, in males and females.

Intervention   When a health counselor makes suggestions, observations, assessment or referral to aid another person.

Justice   The ethical principle that each person should be treated fairly and similarly given the circumstances, not treated the same.

Life event   Changes in one's life routine that can be stressful.

Life expectancy   The number of years that on average we can expect to live.

Locus of control   A person's perceptions of the degree of control they have over events that affect their lives (external vs. internal).

Logo therapy   A kind of existential therapy developed by Victor Frankl, that focuses on individual power and freedom to create our lives.

Maximum range of life   The number of years a species can be expected to live; generally, six times the time elapsed between birth and maturity.

Medical-care counseling   A kind of health counseling that takes place in the medical setting, whose goal is to improve health status by implementing the health prescription or recommendation.

Morality   A judgment about whether an action is "good" or "right," "bad" or "wrong." Refers to specific situations or events.

Nonmaleficence   The ethical principle that describes the position "whatever else is done, do no harm."

Noticing   When a counselor shares with the client something the counselor has observed.

Nutrition   A well-balanced meal plan that includes nutrient-dense foods, fruits, vegetables, grains, lean meats or meat alternatives, and low-fat dairy foods which supply no more than 30 percent of calories as fat.

Obesity   Excessive fat deposits in adipose tissue, having a Body Mass Index (BMI) of 30 or more.

Occupational stress   Stress on the job that may be comprised of sources of stress at work, stressors from outside of work and/or individual characteristics that contribute to an unwanted stress response.

Paraphrasing   When a counselor takes a client's statement or concept and puts it into simpler, more concise, yet still nonjudgmental terms.

Patient education   Also called "psychoeducation." Is provided by physician extenders such as nurses, social workers, health educators, and so on, in a clinical setting. It is often directed at a specific health concern that the physician deems problematic. The goal is to improve patient understanding, skill, and compliance with health prescription.

Physical activity   Any body movement that is brought about through contraction of skeletal muscles and results in an increase in energy expenditure.

Placebo A substance that contains no catalystic effects, that is used in medicinal experiments; literally mean "I will please" in Latin.

PLISSIT A model for sexual counseling, meaning Permission, Limited Information, Specific Suggestions, and Intensive Therapy.

Premature ejaculation When a male has a persistent or recurrent experience of ejaculation with minimal sexual stimulation before he and his partner wish it.

Preorgasmia A term of for females who have never experienced an orgasm.

Primary aging Aging that occurs as a consequence of the passage of time and is unavoidable.

Primary prevention The first level of prevention characterized by education and the provision of appropriate information.

Psychoneuroimmunology (PNI) The scientific investigation of how the brain affects the body's immune cells and how the immune system can be affected by behavior.

Rapport A process by which the counselor creates a comfortable, warm trusting relationship with a client.

Reductionist thinking An overly simplistic way of looking at something or thinking, reducing its complexity or subtlety.

Referral When a counselor who is not qualified to work with a client's presenting issue refers the client to another counselor.

Reinforcement A behavioral technique that uses consequences to increase the likelihood of future occurrence of a behavior; can be positive or negative.

Relapse A temporary setback, a lapse, a return to unhealthy coping that can occur in the recovery process.

Relapse prevention Measures taken to ensure that behavorial changes made will be maintained in everyday life; Preparing a client for a lapse by teaching the client coping skills that can be directly used in high risk situations.

Relaxation techniques Techniques that result in decreased heart rate, blood pressure, respiration and muscle tension, such as meditation, mindfulness, and diaphragmatic breathing.

Restoration A healing method used by ecotherapists; having clients restore some part of nature that aids in their own healing process.

Secondary aging Aging that occurs because of environmental events and the adoption of certain behavioral patterns, and which could be avoided.

Secondary prevention The stage of prevention when a problem has been isolated and a specific focus identified. The client's need for assistance is more apparent and important.

Self-disclosure When a person shares personal information about him or her self with another person.

Self-management An aim of health counseling which requires health-oriented skills, a belief in one's ability to address life challenges, and an environment that encourages positive development.

Sexual assault/ sexual violence Any unwanted sexual attention, touching, or coercive action or behaviors, including rape; incest; sexual, verbal, or physical harassment; child molestation; marital rape; indecent exposure; and voyeurism.

Sexual dysfunction Disorders that can be physical or psychological, based on values and beliefs, stress, fatigue, anxiety, or a combination of factors that inhibit sexual expression.

Sexual orientation One of the four components of a person's sexual identity, which describes a person's attraction to and behavior with their own or opposite gender.

Sexual pain disorder—dyspareunia A recurrent or persistent pain in the genital area during sexual stimulation or intercourse.

Sexually transmitted infections (STI) Infections that are transmitted from person to person through sexual contact.

Social health   Refers to communities, friends, and families and the way an individual experiences him or herself as part of a social system.

Social support   The assistance received by the others in one's life, which may be emotional, financial, spiritual, practical or informational in nature.

Stages of counseling process   Four stages or phases that evolve throughout the course of counseling and/or therapy. These are the (1) engagement, (2) assessment, (3) intervention, and (4) maintenance stages.

Stress   The combination of a stressor and stress reactivity.

Stress management   The practice of obtaining an optimal level of stress in one's life, or helping a client to do so.

Stress psychophysiology   The physical chain reaction to a stressor, which involves the secretion of hormones, and the increase of heart rate and oxygen consumption.

Stress reactivity   Changes in the body in response to a stressor that include increased heart rate, blood pressure, and respiratory rate.

Stressors   The small everyday pressures and hassles of life that can accumulate and lead to stress.

Successful aging   Maintaining a low risk of disease and disability, good cognitive and physical functioning and an active participation in society throughout all stages of life.

Technoconsumer culture   In ecotherapy, the highly technological, commercialized consumer culture that is characterized by addiction, anxiety, despair, and anguish about the devastation of the planet.

Tertiary prevention   The third level of prevention, when intense counseling is necessary.

Theoretical (perfect use) failure rate   An estimate of the percentage of times a method of contraception would be expected to fail to prevent an unintended pregnancy under the best possible conditions if used perfectly.

Theories of aging   The rationale for how and why we age; usually either assuming the existence of a set "program" for aging or assuming that "mistakes" or "accidents" cause aging to occur.

Transactional Analysis   A form of cognitive behavioral therapy developed by Eric Berne; it focuses on the interactions between individuals through different ego states.

Traps and pitfalls of relationships   Many mechanisms, conscious and subconscious, that can undermine and negatively impact a relationship. These can include defenses such as denial, projection, devaluation, and so on.

Type A behavior pattern   A behavior pattern comprised of a sense of time urgency, excessive competitive drive, aggressiveness, impatience, and free-floating hostility.

Typical use (actual use) failure rate   An estimate of the failure rate of a contraceptive method including factors of human error, carelessness, and technical failure.

Vaginismus   The persistent or recurrent involuntary contraction of the perineal muscles surrounding the outer third of the vagina, making it difficult or impossible for penetration to take place.

Value   Estimation of worth developed over many years through numerous experiences and encounters that determine the weighting of ethical principles.

Variability   One of the two basic principles of aging—that aging varies dramatically between people and this variation increases with age.

Withdrawal   A psychological and/or physical syndrome experienced when one addicted to a substance for a prolonged period does not ingest the substance.

REFERENCES

Chapter 1

Beitman, B. (1987). *The Structure of Individual Psychotherapy.* New York: Guilford.

Browers, R. T. (2001). Counseling in mental health and private practice. In D. Cappuzzi & D. R. Gross (eds.) *Introduction to the Counseling Profession, 3rd Ed,* pp. 316–337. Needham Heights, MA: Allyn & Bacon.

Donnelly, J., Eburne, N., & Kittleson, M. (2001). *Mental Health: Dimensions of Self-Esteem & Emotional Well-Being.* Boston, MA: Allyn & Bacon.

Duncan, B., Solovey, A., & Rusk G. (1992). *Changing the Rules: A Client-Directed Approach to Therapy.* New York: Guilford.

Engel, G. (1977). The need for a new medical model: A challenge to biomedical science. *Science, 196,* 129–136.

Gelso, C. J., & Fretz, B. R. (2001). *Counseling Psychology.* Fort Worth, TX: Harcourt College Publishers.

Glanz, K., Lewis F., & Rimer, B. (1997). *Health Behavior and Health Education: Theory, Research, and Practice, 2nd Edition.* San Francisco: Jossey-Bass.

Hershenson, D. B., & Berger, G. P. (2001). The state of community counseling: A survey of directors of CACREP-accredited programs. *Journal of Counseling & Development, 79,* 188–193.

Janis, I. (1983). *Short-term Counseling: Guidelines Based on Recent Research.* New Haven: Yale University Press.

Jordan-Marsh, M., Gilbert, J., Ford, J., & Kleeman, C. (1984). Lifestyle intervention: A conceptual framework. *Patient Education and Counseling, 6,* 29–38.

Lambert, M. (1992). Implication of psychotherapy outcome research for eclectic psychotherapy. In J. Norcross, (ed.) *Handbook of Eclectic Psychotherapy,* pp. 436–462. New York: Brunner/Mazel.

Levant, R. (1986). *Psychoeducational Approaches to Family Therapy and Family Counseling.* New York: Springer.

Marlatt, G. A., & Gordon, J. (1985). *Relapse Prevention: Maintenance Strategies in the Treatment of Addictive Behaviors.* New York: Guilford.

Miller, S., Duncan, B., & Hubble, M. (1997). *Escape From Babel: Toward a Unifying Language Or Psychotherapy Practice.* New York: Norton.

Miller, W.R. & Rollnick, S. (1991). *Motivational Interviewing: Preparing People for Change.* New York: Guilford.

National Commission for Health Education, Inc. (2000). *Competencies Update Project: Promoting Quality Assurance in Health Education.* Allentown, PA: National Commission for Health Education, Inc. Available at http://www.nchec.org/CUPpress_release.htm

O'Donnell, M. (1989). Definition of health promotion: Part III: Stressing the impact of culture. *American Journal of Health Promotion, 3(3),* 1–8.

Orlinsky, D., Grawe, K. & Parks, B. (1994). Process and outcome in psychotherapy. In Bergin, A. Bergin, & S. Garfield, (eds.) *Handbook of Psychotherapy and Behavior Change, 4th Edition,* pp. 270–576. New York: Wiley.

Pistole, M. Carole, & Roberts, Amber (2002). Mental health counseling: Toward resolving identity confusions. *Journal of Mental Health Counseling, 24(1),* 1–19.

Redman, B. (2001). *The Practice of Patient Education, 9th Ed.* St. Louis: Mosby.

Rogers, C. (1951). *Client-Centered Therapy.* Boston: Houghton Mifflin.

Sperry, L. (1986). The ingredients of effective health counseling: Health beliefs, compliance and relapse prevention. *Individual Psychology, 42,* 279–287.

Sperry, L. (1999). *Cognitive Behavior Therapy of the DSM-IV Personality Disorders.* New York: Brunner/Mazel.

Sperry, L., Brill, P., Howard, K., & Grissom, G. (1996). *Treatment Outcomes in Psychotherapy and Psychiatric Interventions.* New York: Brunner/Mazel.

Sperry L. (1988). Biopsychosocial therapy: An integrative approach for tailoring treatment. *Individual Psychology, 44(2),* 225–235.

Sperry, L., Lewis, J., Carlson, J., & Englar-Carlson, M. (2002). *Health Promotion and Health Counseling.* Boston: Allyn & Bacon.

Strupp, H. (1995). The psychotherapist's skills revisited. *Clinical Psychology, 2,* 70–74.

Tappe, Marlene K., & Galer-Unti, Regina A. (2001). Health educator's roles in promoting health literacy & advocacy for the 21st century. *Journal of School Health, 71(10),* 477–483.

U.S. Department of Health and Human Services (2000). *Healthy People 2010: Understanding and Improving Health.* Washington, DC: Government Printing Office.

World Health Organization (1948). *The First Ten Years of the World Health Organization.* Geneva: World Health Organization.

CHAPTER 2

Engel, G. L. (1980). The clinical application of the biopsychosocial model. *American Journal of Psychiatry, 137*, 535–544.

Fouad, N. A., & Brown, M. J. (2000). Role of race and social class in development: Implications for counseling psychology. In Steven D. Brown and Robert W. Lent (eds.) *Handbook of Counseling Psychology, 3rd Edition*, pp. 379–408. New York: Wiley.

Gladding, S. J. (2001). *The Counseling Dictionary*. Upper Saddle River, NJ: Prentice Hall.

Hedgepeth, E. & Helmich, J. (1996). *Teaching about Sexuality and HIV: Principles and Methods for Effective Education*. New York: New York University Press.

Hoffman, M. A., & Driscoll, J. M. (2000). Health promotion and disease prevention: A concentric biopsychosocial model of health status. In Steven D. Brown and Robert W. Lent, (eds.) *Handbook of Counseling Psychology, Third Edition*, pp. 532–567. New York: Wiley.

Klages, M. (1997). Psychoanalysis and Sigmund Freud. *University of Colorado at Boulder*. Available at http://www. colorado.edu/English/ENGL2012Klages/freud.html

Martin, C. (2001) "Melanie Klein." *PsycheMatters*. Available at http://www.psychematters.com/bibliographies/klein.htm

Ormont, L. R. (1992). *The Group Therapy Experience*. New York: St. Martin's Press.

Rossides, D. W. (1997) *Social Stratification: The Interplay of Class, Race, and Gender, 2nd Edition*. Upper Saddle River, NJ: Prentice Hall.

Savvides, P. (2001) "Jean Piaget." Available at http://www.psychlinks.cjb.net; http://www.brittanica.com.

Shane, E. M. (1989) Mahler, Kohut, and infant research: Some comparisons. In *Self Psychology: Comparisons and Contrasts*, D. W. Detrick and S. P. Detrick, (eds.) Hillsdale, NJ: The Analytic Press.

Sharkey, W. (1995). "Erik Erikson." *Department of Psychology, Muskingum College*. Available at http://muskingum. edu/~psychology/psycweb/history/erikson.htm.

Sobel, D. S. (1995) Rethinking medicine: Improving health outcomes with cost-effective psychosocial interventions. *Psychosomatic Medicine, 57*, 234–244.

Uchino, B. N., Cacioppo, J. T., & Kiecolt-Glaser, J. K. (1996) The relationship between social support and physiological processes: A review with emphasis on underlying mechanisms and implications for health. *Psychological Bulletin, 119*, 488–531.

Wilson, P. M. (1991). *When Sex is the Subject: Attitudes and Answers for Young Children*. Santa Cruz, CA: ETR Associates.

CHAPTER 3

Bayles, M. (1981). *Professional Ethics*. Belmont, CA: Wadsworth.

Beauchamp, T. L., and Childress, J.F. (1989). *Principles of Biomedical Ethics*. New York: Oxford University Press.

Brammer, L. M. and MacDonald, G. (1996). *The Helping Relationship: Process and Skills, 6th Edition*. Boston: Allyn & Bacon.

Buchanan, D. R. (2000). *An Ethic of Health Promotion: Rethinking the Sources of Human Well-Being*. New York: Oxford University Press.

Butler, J. T. (2001) *Principles of Health Education and Health Promotion*. Belmont, CA: Wadsworth.

Capwell, E. M., Smith, B. J., Shirreffs, J., & Olsen, L. K. (2000). Development of a unified code of ethics for the health education profession: A report of the national task force on ethics in health education. *Journal of Health Education, 31*, 212–214.

Coalition of National Health Education Organizations. (2000). Code of ethics for the health education profession. *Journal of Health Education, 31*, 216–217.

Diaz, R. M., Ayala, G., Bein, E., Henne, J., & Marin, B. V. (2001). The impact of homophobia, poverty, and racism on the mental health of gay and bisexual Latino men. *American Journal of Public Health, 91*, 927–932.

Gilman, S. E., Cochran, S. D., Mays, V. M., Hughes, M., Ostrow, D., & Kessler, R. C. (2001). Risk of psychiatric disorders among individuals reporting same-sex sexual partners in the national morbidity survey. *American Journal of Public Health, 91*, 933–939.

Greenberg, J. S. (1978). Health education as freeing. *Health Education, 9*, 20–21.

Greenberg, J. S. (1985). Iatrogenic health education disease. *Health Education, 16*, 4–6.

Greenberg, J. S. (2001). *The Code of Ethics for the Health Education Profession: A Case Study Book*. Sudbury, MA: Jones and Bartlett.

Hiller, M. D. (1987). Ethics and health education: Issues in theory and practice. In P. M. Lazes, H. Kaplan, and K. A. Gordon, (eds.) *The Handbook of Health Education*. Rockville, MD: Aspen.

Jecker, N. S. (1997). Introduction to the methods of bioethics. In N. S. Jecker, A. R. Jonsen, & R. A. Pearlman, (eds.) *Bioethics: An Introduction to History, Methods, and Practice*, pp. 113–125. Sudbury, MA: Jones and Bartlett.

Johnson, D. W. (1997). *Reaching Out: Interpersonal Effectiveness and Self-Actualization, 2nd Edition.* Boston: Allyn & Bacon.

Last, J. M. (1998). *Public Health and Human Ecology, 2nd Edition.* Stamford, CT: Appleton and Lange.

Lewis, J. A., Sperry, L., & Carlson, J. (1993). *Health Counseling.* Pacific Grove, CA: Brooks/Cole.

O'Connell, J. K., and Price, J. H. (1983). Ethical theories for promoting health through behavioral change. *Journal of School Health,* 53, 476–479.

Pellegrino, E. D. (1981). Health promotion as public policy: The need for moral groundings. *Preventive Medicine*, 10, 371–378.

Razak, A. and Schoenwald, P. (1989). Case study. *Issues and Insights* 1,1.

Ryan, C. and Futterman, D. (2001). Social and developmental challenges for lesbian, gay, and bisexual youth. *SIECUS Reports*, 29, 5–18.

Thiroux, J. P. (1995). *Ethics: Theory and Practice, 5th Edition.* Englewood Cliffs, NJ: Prentice Hall.

Wolfe, A. (2001). *Moral Freedom: The Search for Virtue in a World of Choice.* New York: Norton.

CHAPTER 4

Allgoewer, A., Wardle, J., & Steptoe, A. (2001). Depressive symptoms, social support, and personal health behaviors in young men and women. *Health Psychology*, 20, 223–227.

Antoni, M. H., Lehman, J. M., Klibourn, K. M., Boyers, A. E., Culver, J. L., Alferi, S. M., et al. (2001). Cognitive-behavioral stress management intervention decreases the prevalence of depression and enhances benefit finding among women under treatment for early-stage breast cancer. *Health Psychology,* 20, 20–32.

Baer, D., Wolf, M. M., & Risley, T. R. (1968). Some current dimensions of Applied behavior analysis. *Journal of Applied Behavior Analysis*, 1, 91–97.

Baer, D., Wolf, M. M., & Risley, T. R. (1987). Some still-current dimensions of applied behavior analysis. *Journal of Applied Behavior Analysis*, 20, 313–328.

Carver, C. S., & Scheier, M. F. (1990). Origins and functions of positive and negative affect: A control-process view. *Psychological Review*, 97, 19–35.

Ellis, A. (1997). Using rational emotive behavior therapy techniques to cope with disability. *Professional Psychology: Research & Practice*, 28, 17–22.

Ellis, A. & Abrams, M. (1994). *How to Cope with a Fatal Illness.* New York: Barricade Books.

Epstein, L. H., Saelens, B. E., Myers, M. D., & Vito, D. (1997). Effects of decreasing sedentary behaviors on activity choice in obese children. *Health Psychology*, 16, 107–113.

Hains, A. A., & Szyjakowski, M. (1990). A cognitive stress-reduction intervention program for adolescents. *Journal of Counseling Psychology*, 37, 79–84.

Jason, L. A., & Burrows, B. (1983). Transition training for high school seniors. *Cognitive Therapy and Research*, 7, 79–92.

Kazdin, A. E. (2001). *Behavior Modification in Applied Settings, 6th Edition.* CT: Wadsworth.

Kiselica, M. S., Baker, S. B., Thomas, R. N., & Reedy, S. (1994). Effects of stress inoculation training on anxiety, stress, and academic performance among adolescents. *Journal of Counseling Psychology*, 41, 335–342.

Kramer, F. M., Jeffery, R. W., Snell, M. K., & Forster, J. L. (1986). Maintenance of successful weight loss over 1 year: Effects of financial contracts for weight maintenance or participation in skills training. *Behavior Therapy*, 17, 295–301.

Krasner, L., & Ullmann, L. P. (1973). *Behavior Influence and Personality.* New York: Holt, Rinehart & Winston.

Lombard, D. N., Lombard, T., & Winett, R. A. (1995). Walking to meet health guidelines: The effect of prompting frequency and prompt structure. (1994). *Health Psychology*, 14, 164–170

Marlatt, G. A., & Gordon, J. R. (eds.) (1985). *Relapse Prevention: Maintenance Strategies in the Treatment of Addictive Behaviors.* New York: Guilford.

Meichenbaum, D. H. (1977). *Cognitive-Behavior Modification: An Integrative Approach.* New York: Plenum.

Meichenbaum, D. H. (1985). *Stress Inoculation Training.* Elmsford, NY: Pergamon Press.

Mermelstein, R., Lichtenstein, E., & McIntyre, K. (1983). Partner support and relapse in smoking-cessation programs. *Journal of Consulting and Clinical Psychology*, 51, 465–466.

Miller, D. L., & Kelley, M. L. (1994). The use of goal setting and contingency contracting for improving children's homework. *Journal of Applied Behavior Analysis*, 27, 73–84.

Miltenberg, R. G. (2001). *Behavior Modification: Principles and Procedures, 2nd Edition.* Connecticut: Wadsworth.

Pellios, L., Morren, J., Tesch, D., & Axelrod, S. (1999). The impact of functional analysis methodology on treatment choice for self-injurious and aggressive behavior. *Journal of Applied Behavior Analysis*, 32, 185–195.

Premack, D. (1959). Toward empirical behavior laws I: Positive reinforcement. *Psychological Review*, 66, 219–233.

Preston, K. L., Umbricht, A., Wong, C. J., Epstein, D. H. (2001). Shaping cocaine abstinence by successive approximation. Journal of Counseling of Psychology, 69(4), 643–654.

Prochaska, J. O., & DiClemente, C. C. (1984). *The Transtheoretical Approach: Crossing Traditional Boundaries of Therapy.* Homewood, IL: Dow Jones-Irvin.

Simkin, L. R., & Gross, A. M. (1994). Assessment of coping with high-risk situations for exercise relapse among healthy women. *Health Psychology, 13,* 274–277.

Sullum, J., & Clark, M. M. (2000). Predictors of exercise relapse in a college population. *Journal of the American College Health,* 48, 175–179.

Wysocki, T., Hall, G., Iwata, B., & Riordan, M. (1979). Behavioral management of exercise: Contracting for aerobic points. *Journal of Applied Behavior Analysis,* 12, 55–64.

Chapter 5

Ainsworth, B. E., Haskell, W. L., Leon, A. S., Jacobs, Jr., D. R., Montoye, H. J., Sallis, J. F., & Paffenbarger, Jr., R. S. (1993). Compendium of physical activities: Classification of energy costs of human physical activities. *Medicine and Science in Sports and Exercise,* 1, 71–80.

American College of Sports Medicine (2000). *ACSM's Guidelines for Exercise Testing and Prescription,* 6th Ed. Philadelphia, PA: Lippincott Williams & Wilkins.

American Dietetic Association (1997). Position of the American Dietetic Association: weight management. *Journal of the American Dietetic Association,* 97, 71–74.

Balady, G. J., Chaitman, B., Driscoll, D., Foster, C., Froelicher, E., Gordon, N., Pate, R., Rippe, J., & Bazzarre, T. (1998). American College of Sports Medicine and American Heart Association Joint Position Statement: Recommendations for cardiovascular screening, staffing, and emergency policies at health/fitness facilities. *Medicine and Science in Sports and Exercise,* 30, 1009–1018.

Blair, S. N., Kampert, J. B., Kohl, H. W. III, Barlow, C. E., Macera, C. A., Paffenbarger, R. S., & Gibbons, L. W. (1996). Influences of cardiorespiratory fitness and other precursors on cardiovascular disease and all-cause mortality in men and women. *Journal of the American Medical Association,* 276, 205–210.

Blair, S. N., Kohl, H. W. III, Barlow, C. E., Paffenbarger, R. S., Gibbons, L. W., & Macera, C. A. (1995). Changes in physical fitness and all-cause mortality: A prospective study of healthy and unhealthy men. *Journal of the American Medical Association,* 273, 1093–1098.

Canadian Society for Exercise Physiology. (1994). *PAR-Q and You.* Glouchester, Ontario: Canadian Society for Exercise Physiology.

Chapelot, D., Aubert, R., Marmonier, C., Chabert, M., & Louis-Sylvestre, J. (2000). An endocrine and metabolic definition of the internal interval in humans: Evidence for a role of leptin on the prandial pattern through fatty acid disposal. *American Journal of Clinical Nutrition,* 72, 421–431.

Gross, W. C., & Daynard, M. D. (eds.) (1997). *Commercial weight loss products and programs. What consumers stand to gain and lose?* Washington, D.C.: Report of Presiding Panel Federal Trade Commission.

Jakicic, J. M., Clark, K., Coleman, E., Donnelly, J. E., Foreyt, J., Melanson, E., Volek, J., & Volpe, S. L. (2001). American College of Sports Medicine Position Statement: Appropriate intervention strategies for weight loss and prevention of Weightregain for adults. *Medicine and Science in Sports and Exercise,* 33, 2145–2156.

Kern, P. A. (1997). Potential role of TNFa and lipoprotein lipase as candidate gene for obesity. *Journal of Nutrition,* 1917S–1922S.

King, A. C., & Martin, J. E. (2001). Physical activity promotion: Adoption and maintenance. *In ACSM's Resource Manual for Guidelines for Exercise Testing and Prescription, 4th Ed.* Philadelphia: Lippincott Williams & Wilkins.

Koplan, J. P., & Dietz, W. H. (1999). Caloric imbalance and public health policy. *Journal of the Medical Association,* 282, 1579–1585.

Kushi, L. H., Fee, R. M., Folsom, A. R., Mink, P. J., Anderson, K. E., & Sellers, T. A. (1997). Physical activity and mortality in postmenopausal women. *Journal of the American Medical Association,* 277, 1287–1292.

Levine, A. S., & Billington, C. J. (1997). Why do we eat? A neural system approach. *Annual Review of Nutrition,* 17, 596–619.

Mahan, K. L., & Escott-Stump, S. (2000). *Krause's Food, Nutrition, and Diet Therapy, 10th Ed.* Philadelphia, W. B. Saunders Company.

Miller, M. A. (1985). A calculated method for determination of ideal body weight. *Nutrition Support Services,* vol. 31–33.

National Institute of Health (2000). *Practical Guide for Identification, Evaluation, and Treatment of obesity and Overweight in the US uses 703 rather than 705 for calculating BMI.* Washington, D.C.: US Department of Health and Human Services.

National Institute of Health. Obesity Evaluation Initiative (1998). *Clinical Guidelines on the Identification, Evalu-*

ation, and Treatment of Overweight and Obesity in Adults. Washington, D.C.: US Department of Health and Human Services.

National Institute of Health (1992). *Overweight and Obesity in Adults.* Washington, DC: US Department of Health and Human Services.

Oldways Preservation and Exchange Trust. (2000). *The Mediterranean Diet Pyramid.* Boston, MA.

Paffenbarge, R. S., Kampert, J. B., Lee, I., Hyde, R. T., Leung, R. W., & Wing, A. L. (1994). Changes in physical activity and other lifeway patterns influencing longevity. *Medicine and Science in Sports and Exercise,* 26, 857–865.

Pate, R. R., Pratt, M., Blair, S. N., Haskell, W. L., Macera, C. A., Bouchard, C., et al. (1995). Physical activity and public health: A recommendation from the Centers for DiseaseControl and Prevention and the American College of Sports Medicine. *Journal of the American Medical Association,* 273, 402–407.

Pollock, M. L., Gaesser, G. A., & Butcher, J. D. (1998). The recommended quantity and quality of exercise for developing and maintaining cardiorespiratory and muscular fitness, and flexibility in healthy adults. *Medicine and Science in Sports and Exercise,* 30, 975–991.

Russell R., Rasmussen H., & Lichtenstein A. H. (1999). Modified Food Guide Pyramid for people over seventy years. *Journal of Nutrition,* 129, 751–53.

Shape of America! (1998). *Guidelines for Treatment of Adult Obesity, 2nd Ed.* Bethesda, MD: The American Obesity Association.

Sigman-Grant, M. (1996). Stages of change: A framework for nutrition interventions. *Nutrition Today,* 31, 162–167.

United States Department of Agriculture. (1999) USDA Center for Nutrition and Policy Promotion. Washington, DC. Program AID 1649.

United States Department of Health and Human Services (1998–1999). *Healthy People 2000 Review.* USDHHS, CDC, National Center for Health Statistics.

United States Department of Health and Human Services (2000). *Healthy People 2010: Understanding and Improving Health, 2nd Ed.* Washington, D.C.: U.S. Government Printing Office.

United States Department of Health and Human Services (1996). *Physical Activity and Health: A Report of the Surgeon General.* Atlanta, GA: U.S. Dpartment of Health and Human Services, Centers for Disease Control and Prevention, National Center for Chronic Disease Prevention and Health Promotion.

United States Department of Health and Human Services, Public Health Service, Centers for Disease Control and Prevention, National Center for Chronic Disease Prevention. http://www.cdc.gov/nccdphp/

Whitney, E. N., & Rolfes, S. R. (2002). *Understanding Nutrition, 9th Ed.* Belmont, CA: Wadsworth Group/Thomson Learning.

CHAPTER 6

10th Special Report to U.S. Congress on Alcohol and Health, U.S. Department of Health and Human Services, Public Health Service, National Institutes of Health & National Institute on Alcohol Abuse and Alcoholism. June, 2000. NIH#00-1583.

Alcoholics Anonymous Twelve Steps and Twelve Traditions, 1986. New York: AA World Services.

Alcoholism treatment assessment instruments (1998). [Online] [NIAAA Treatment Handbook Series 4: Assessing Alcohol Problems]. Bethesda, MD: NIAAA (10/19/00) http://silk.nih.gov/silk/niaaa1/publication/assinstr.htm

Allen, J. P.; Columbus, M.; and Fertig, J. Assessment in Alcoholism Treatment: An Overview. In: NIAAA Treatment Handbook Series 4, *Assessing Alcohol Problems: A Guide for Clinicians and Researchers.* NIH publication no. 95-3745, 1995.

American Psychiatric Association (2000). Diagnostic and Statistical Manual of Mental Disorders, Fourth Edition. Washington, D.C.: American Psychiatric Publishers.

Anderson, K. (2001). Internet use among college students: An exploratory study. *American Journal of College Health,* 50(1), 21–26.

Approaches to Drug Abuse Counseling. National Institute on Drug Abuse (NIDA), US Department of Health and Human Services, National Institutes of Health. Rockville, MD, 2000.

Boren, J. J., Onken, L. S., Carrol, K. M., (Eds.) (2000) *Approaches to Drug Abuse Counseling.* National Institute on Drug Abuse/National Institutes of Health, Bethesda MD.

Brick, J., & Erickson, C. K. (1998). *Drugs, the Brain and Behavior: The Pharmacology of abuse and dependence.* New York: The Haworth Medical Press.

Brownell, K., & Foreyt, J. (1986). The Eating Disorders: Summary and Integration. In *Handbook of Eating Disorders: Physiology, Psychology and Treatment of Obesity, Anorexia, and Bulimia.* USA: Basic Books. pp. 503–513.

Bulik, C., & Johnson, C. (2001 Spring). Brave New World: The Role of Genetics in the Prevention and Treatment of Eating Disorders. *Outlook,* 14(1), 1–4.

Council on Compulsive Gambling of New Jersey 2002. Found online at http://www.800gambler.org, accessed January 28, 2002.

Carbonari, J. P. & DiClemente, C. C. (2000). Using transtheoretical model profiles to differentiate levels of alcohol abstinence success. *Journal of Consulting & Clinical Psychology*, (68): 810–818.

Carney, M. M. & Kivlahan, D. R. (1995). Motivational subtypes among veterans seeking substance abuse treatment: Profiles based on stages of change. *Psychology of Addictive Behaviors.* 9(2):135–142.

Cohall, A. (Ed.). (1997). Keeping Adolescents Healthy. *Patient Care*, pp. 56–65, 70, 77–83. *Coexisting Conditions Assessment and Treatment of Patients with Coexisting Mental Illness and Alcohol and other Drug Abuse Treatment.* (1995.) United States Department of Health and Human Services, Public Health Service. Substance Abuse and Mental Health Service Administration. Improvement Protocol (TIP) Series 9.

Davis, W. (2001). A word from the editor. *Perspective: Professional Journal of the Renfrew Center Foundation,* 7(1), 1–2.

DiClemente, C. C. & Bellino, L. E. (1999) Motivation for Change and Alchoholism Treatment. *Alcohol Research & Health 23*: 86–93.

DiClemente, C. C. & Prochaska, J. O. (1998). Toward a comprehensive, transtheoretical model of change: Stages of change and addictive behaviors. In Miller, W. R. and Heather, N., (Eds.), *Treating Addictive Behaviors. 2nd edition.* New York: Plenum.

DiClemente, C. C. & Scott, C. W. (1997). Stages of Change: Interactions with treatment compliance and involvement. In: Onken, L. S., Baline, J. D., & Boren, J. J., (Eds.) *Beyond the Therapeutic Alliance: Keeping the Drug-Dependent Individual in Treatment.* Rockville, MD: National Institute on Drug Abuse.

DiClemente, C. C. & Hughes, S. O. (1990.) Stages of change profiles in outpatient alcoholism treatment. *Journal of Substance Abuse,* (2), 217–235.

Eating Disorders Awareness and Prevention, Inc. website: http://www.edap.org, accessed April, 2002.

Effectiveness of Substance Abuse Treatment White Paper, United States Department of Health and Human Services, Public Health Service (1995). Rockville, Maryland.

Fairburn, C. (1993). A clinical perspective: Why all the fuss? NEDO Web site. Fallon, P., Katzman, M., & Wooley, S. (eds.) (1994). *Feminist Perspectives on Eating Disorders.* New York: Guilford.

Fallon, P., Katzman, M., & Wooley, S., (Eds.) (1004). *Feminist Perspectives on Eating Disorders.* New York: Guilford.

Farber, S. (1998 Fall), The Body Speaks, the Body Weeps: Eating Disorders, Self Mutilation and Body Modifications. *Perspective: Professional Journal of the Renfrew Center Foundation,* (4)2, 8–9.

Farber S. (2000). *When the body is the target: Self harm, Suffering and Traumatic Attachments.* Jason Aronson, Inc.

Favazza, A., DeRosear, L., & Conterio, K. (1989). Self mutilation and eating disorders. *Suicide and Life Threatening Behavior,* 19(4), 352–361.

Fuller, R., & Hiller-Sturmhofel, S. (1999). Alcoholism Treatment in the United States. *Alcohol Research & Health,* 23(2), 69–77.

Gaesser, G. (2001a). How is obesity best defined? *Perspective: Professional Journal of the Renfrew Foundation,* 7, 3.

Gaesser, G. (2001b) Big Fat Lies: The Truth About Your Weight and Your Health. In *Perspective,* 7(1), 6.

Garner, D, & Garfinkel (1979). The Eating Attitudes Test: An index of the symptoms of anorexia nervosa. *Psychological Medicine,* 9, 273–279.

Garner, D, Olmsted, M. P., & Polivy, J. (1983). Development and validation of a multidimensional eating disorder inventory for anorexia and bulimia. *International Journal of Eating Disorders,* 2, 15–34.

Gerstein, D. R., Foote, M. L., Ghadialy, R., U. S. Substance Abuse and Mental Health Services Administration, Office of Applied Studies (1999). *The Prevalence and Correlates of Treatment for Drug Problems.* DHHS #0497-D-01. Rockville, MD: SAMHSA, OAS.

Gidwani, G. P., & Rome, E. S. (1997). Eating disorders. *Clinical Obstetrics and Gynecology,* 40(3), 601–615.

Grant, B. F., & Dawson, D. A. (1997). Age at Onset of Alcohol Use and Its Association with DSM-IV Alcohol Abuse and Dependence, *Journal of Substance Abuse,* 9, 103–110.

Greenspan-Goldberg, A. (April 1991). "Eating Disorders in the Athlete." National Institute for the Psychotherapies professional newsletter.

Grilo C. M. (1998) The assessment and treatment of binge eating disorder. *Journal of Practical Psychiatry and Behavioral Health* (4), 191–201.

Hsu, G. I. K. (1996). *Epidemiology of the Eating Disorders.* Psychiatric Clinics of North America, 19(4), 681–697.

Isenberg, Marc & Rhoads, Rick. (2001) The Student Athlete Survival Guide. McGraw-Hill, Inc.

Johnson, C. (1985). The initial consultation for patients with bulimia and anorexia nervosa. In D. M. Garner, & P. E. Garfinkel (eds.) *Handbook of Psychotherapy for Anorexia Nervosa and Bulimia*, pp. 19–51. New York: Guilford Press.

Johnson, C. & Pure, D. (1986) Assessment of Bulimia. In Brownell, K. & Forety, J., (eds.), *Handbook of Eating Disorders.* USA: Basic Books.

Leshner, A. (1999). Science-based view of drug addiction and its treatment. *Journal of the American Medical Association, 282*(14), 1314–1316.

Levenkron, S. (1999). *Cutting: Understanding and Overcoming Self-Mutilation.* New York: Norton.

Levine, M. A short list of salient warnings signs for eating disorders. Presented at the 13th National NEDO Conference, Columbus Ohio.

Matlin, M. (1993). *The Psychology of Women.* Fort Worth, TX: Harcourt Brace College Publishers.

National Institute on Drug Abuse, DHHS, National Institutes of Health (1998). *Nicotine Addiction* (publication #0467-A30). Washington, D.C.: U. S. Government Printing Office.

National Institute on Drug Abuse, National Institutes of Health (1999). *Principles of Drug Addiction Treatment: A Research-Based Guide.* United States Department of Health and Human Services, Public Health Services.

National Institute of Health, National Institute of Diabetes & Digestive & Kidney Diseases (1993). *Binge Eating Disorder.* Publication #94–3589.

Partnership for a Drug-Free America. *1999 Partnership Attitude Tracking Study: Parents.* Conducted by Audits & Surveys Worldwide. Released April, 1999. (www. drugfreeamerica.org)

Pipher, M. (1994). *Reviving Ophelia. Saving the Selves of Adolescent Girls.* New York: Putnam.

Pokovny, A. D.; Miller, B. A.; & Kaplan, H. B. (1972). The Brief Mast: A Shortened Version of the Michigan Alcohol Screening Test. *American Journal of Psychiatry,* 129, 342–345.

Prochaska, J. O. (1994). Strong and weak principles for progressing from precontemplation to action on the basis of twelve problem behaviors. *Health Psychology,* 13(1), 47–51.

Prochaska, J. O., DiClemente, C. C., & Norcross, J. C. (1992). In search of how people change: Applications to addictive behaviors. *American Psychology* 47(9). 1102–1114.

Prochaska, J. O., Norcross, J. C., & DiClemente, C. C. (1994). *Changing for Good.* New York: Avon Books.

Prochaska, J. O., Velicer, F. V., Rossi, J. S., Goldstein, M. G., Marcus, B. H., Rakowski, W., Fiore, C. Harlow L., Redding, C. A., Rosenbloom, & D., Rossi, S. R. (1994). Stages of change and decisional balance for 12 problem behaviors. *Health Psychology,* 13(1), 39–46.

Resnick, M. D., Bearman, P. S., Blum, R. W., Bauman, K. E., Harris, K. M., Jones, Tabor, J.; Beuhring T., Sieving-R. E., Shew, M. Ireland, M., Bearinger, L. H. Udry, J. R., (1997). Protecting adolescents from harm: Findings from the National Longitudinal Study on Adolescent Health. *Journal of the American Medical Association,* 9(10), 832–843.

Rhoads, Rick, (2001) *The Money Sucker Machine: The Truth About Gambling and How It Destroys Lives.* A Game Publishing.

Schneider Institute for Health Policy (2001). Substance Abuse: the Nation's Number One Health Problem—Key Indicators for Policy Update Brandeis University.

Smoking-Attributable Mortality and Years of Potential Life Lost Editorial Note—1997. *Morbidity and Mortality Weekly Report,* 46(20): 444–451.

Stukard, A., Sorensen, & Schulsinger, F. (1980). Use of the Danish Adoption Register for the Study of Obesity and Thinness. In S. Kety (ed.) *The Genetics of Neurology and Psychiatric Disorders.* New York: Raven Press.

Substance Abuse: the Nation's Number One Health Problem. Key Indicators for Policy Update. Schneider Institute for Health Policy, Brandeis University, 2001.

Summary of Findings from the 1999 National Household Survey on Drug Abuse, U.S. Department of Health and Human Services, Substance Abuse and Mental Health Services Administration, Office of Applied Studies, SMA 00-3466, 2000.

Tobacco Facts. (2001). The University of Wisconsin Center for Tobacco Research and Intervention, http://www. ctri.wisc.edu/sub_dept/quick_facts/qtftobaccofacts. html

Treating Tobacco Use and Dependence. Quick Reference Guide for Clinicians, (2000 October.) U.S. Public Health Service. http://www.surgeongeneral.gov/-tobacco/tobaqrg.htm

SAMHSA Office of Applied Studies DHHS, OAS (1999*). Substance Use and Mental Health Characteristics by Employment Status,* DHHS #SMA99-3311, Rockville, MD: SAMHSA, OAS.

U.S. Department of Health and Human Services, Substance Abuse and Mental Health Services Administration, Office of Applied Studies (1999). *Summary of Findings from the 1999 National Household Survey on Drug Abuse.* SMA 00-3466, 2000.

U.S. Department of Health and Human Services, Public Health Service, National Institutes of Health & National Institute on Alcohol Abuse and Alcoholism (2000*). 10th Special Report to U.S. Congress on Alcohol and Health.* NIH#00-1583.

U.S. Department of Health and Human Services, Public Health Service. (1995). *Coexisting Conditions Assessment and Treatment of Patients with Coexisting Mental Illness and Alcohol and other Drug Abuse Treatment.* Substance Abuse and Mental Health Service Administration. Improvement Protocol (TIP) Series 9.

Weiss, R. D, Griffin, M. L., Najavits, L. M., Kogan, J., Hufford, C., & Thompson, H., Albeck J., Bishop S., Daley D., Mercer, D. Simon-Onken, L., & Siqueland, L. (1996). Self-help activities in cocaine dependent patients entering treatment: Results from the NIDA Collaborative Cocaine Study. *Drug and Alcohol Dependence*, 43, 79–86.

Willioughby, F. W. & Edens, J. F. (1996). Construct validity and predictive utility of the Stages of Change Scale for alcoholics. *Journal of Substance Abuse 8*, (3), 275–291.

Wolf, Naomi (1991*). The Beauty Myth: How Images of Beauty are Used Against Women*. New York: Morrow.

Young, K. S. (1998). A therapist guide to access and treat internet addiction. Published on http://www.net. addiction.com.

Zerbe, K. J. (1995). *The Body Betrayed*. Carlsbad, CA: Gurze Books.

CHAPTER 7

Assertive Conflict Resolution Communication Skills (2001). Found online at http://www.csulb.edu/~tstevens/c14-lisn.htm.

Atwood, J. (1994). The mating game: What we know and what we don't know. *Journal of Couples Therapy*, 4, 1–2.

Atwood, J. (1993). Social constructionist couple therapy. *The Family Journal: Counseling and Therapy for Couples and Families*, 1(2),116–130.

Atwood, J. (1992). Comprehensive Marital Therapy. *Journal of Couples Therapy*, 3, 41–65.

Atwood, J. & Maltin, L. (1992). The tasks and traps of relationships. *Journal of Couples Therapy*, 3(4), 111–134.

Doherty, B. (2000). *Intentional Marriage: Your Rituals Will Set You Free*. A presentation at the Fourth Annual Smart Marriages Conference, Denver, Colorado, July, 2000. Found online at http://www. smartmarriages.com.

Gottman, J. (1994). *Why Marriages Succeed or Fail . . . and How You Can Make Yours Last*. New York: Simon & Schuster.

Gottman, J., and Silver, N. (1999). *The Seven Principles for Making Marriage Work*. New York: Three Rivers Press.

Hendrix, H. (1988). *Getting the Love You Want*. New York: Simon & Schuster.

Hendrix, H. (1992*). Keeping the Love you Find*. New York: Simon & Schuster.

Hendrix, H., & Hunt, H. (1994). *The Couples Companion: Meditations and Exercises for Getting the Love you Want*. New York: Simon & Schuster.

How to Share What's in your Heart with Your Spouse. (2001). Found online at http://www.marriage. about/library/how to/htfeel.htm?once=true.

Mahler, M., Pine, F., Bergman, A. (1975). The Psychological Birth of the infant. New York: Basic Books.

Robinson, J. (1997). *Communication Miracles for Couples*. California: Conari Press.

Scharff, D. & Scharff, J. (1991). Object Relations Couples Therapy. New Jersey: Jason Aronson, Inc.

Signs of Healthy Relationships. (2001). Found online at http://www.the.net/wise/relationships/healthy_relationships.htm.

Sollee, D. (1996). Divorce Predictor. Found online at http://www.smartmarriages.com

Sollee, D. (1997). A conference that asks: Are you smart enough to have a smart marriage? Found online at http://www.smartmarriages.com.

The U.S. Census Bureau (2001). Divorce and Marriage Statistics. Found online at http://www.aamft.org.

Weiner-Davis, M. (2000). Healing from Infidelity. *The Divorce Busting Newsletter*, April 20, 2001. Found online at http://www.weiner-davis.com.

CHAPTER 8

American Psychological Association (2001). Answers to Your Questions About Sexual Orientation and Homosexuality. Available at www.apa.org/pubinfo/orient.html.

Annon, J. (1976). *The Behavioral Treatment of Sexual Problems, Vol 1. Brief therapy*. New York: Harper & Row Publishers Inc.

Bell, A., Weinberg, N., & Hammersmith, S. (1981). *Sexual preference: Its Development in Men and Women*. Bloomington, IN: Indiana University Press.

Blonna, R., & Levitan, J. (2000). *Healthy Sexuality*, Englewood, CO: Morton.

Cates, W. (1999). Estimates of the Incidence and Prevalence of Sexually Transmitted Diseases in the United States. *Sexually Transmitted Diseases*, 26(4) (April 1999), s2–s7.

CDC—Centers for Disease Control and Prevention (2000). Tracking the Hidden Epidemic: Trends in STDs in the United States 2000 Found online at http://www.cdc.gov/nchstp/dstd/Stats_Trends/Trends2000.pdf.

Eng, T. R. & Butler, W. T. (eds) (1997). *Summary, The Hidden Epidemic: Confronting* STDs Washington, DC: Academy Press, Institute of Medicine.

Fischl, M., Dickinson, D., Scott, G., Klimas, N., Fletcher, M., & Parks, W. (1987). Evaluation of heterosexual partners, children, and household contacts of adults with AIDS. *Journal of the American Medical Association*, 257, 640–644.

Florida Department of Health (2001). HIV Testing Options Found online at http://www9.myflorida.com

Garofalo. R., Wolf, R. C., Kessel, S., Palfrey, J., & Du Rant, R. H. (1998). The association between health risk behaviors and sexual orientation among a school-based sample of adolescents. *Pediatrics*, 101(5), 895–902.

Gary Kelly, *Sexuality Today*, 7th ed. pp. 316–319.

Green, B. (1994). Sexual Disorders. Found online at http://www.priory.com/sex.htm.

Kaiser Family Foundation (1998). The Kaiser Family Foundation/Glamour 1998 Survey of Men and Women on Sexually Transmitted Diseases: Press Release. Found online at http://www.kff.org/archive/repro/survey/glamour1998/glamour_rel.html

Kinsey, A., Pomeroy, W. and Martin, C., (1948). Sexual Behavior in the Male. Philadelphia: Saunders.

Kinsey, A., Pomeroy, W. Martin, C., and Gebhard, P. (1953). Sexual Behavior in the Human Female. Philadelphia: Saunders.

Koch, P. (1995). *Exploring Our Sexuality*, Dubuque, IA: Kendall/Hunt.

Laumann, E. O., Gagnon J. H., Michael R. T., & Michaels S. (1994). *The Social Organization of Sexuality: Sexual Practices in the Unites States*. Chicago: University of Chicago Press.

Lifson, A. (1988). Do alternate modes for transmission of human immunodeficiency virus exist? *Journal of the American Medical Association*, 152, 1353–1357.

Michael, R., Gagnon, J., Laumann, E., & Kolata, G. (1994). *Sex in America: A Definitive Survey*. Boston: Little, Brown.

Nichols, M. (1989). Sex therapy with lesbians, gay men, and bisexuals. In R. R. Leiblum & R. C. Rosen (eds.) *Principles and Practice of Sex Therapy*, 2nd Ed. New York: Guilford.

Pregnancy Options (2001) Planned Parenthood of Connecticut, Inc. Available online at http://www.ppct.org/medical/services/preg-options/options.html

Remafedi, G., Resnick, M., Blum, R., & Harris, L. (1992). Demography of sexual orientation in adolescents. *Pediatrics*, 89(4), 714–721.

Rodecker, M. M., Bullard, D. G. (1981). Basic issues in sexual counseling of persons with physical disabilities. In D. G. Bullard, and S. E. Knight, (eds) *Sexuality & Physical Disability: Personal Perspectives*. St. Louis: Mosby.

Saewyc, E. M., Bearinger, L. H., Blum, R. W., & Resnick, M. D. (1999). Sexual intercourse, abuse and pregnancy among adolescent women: Does sexual orientation make a difference? *Family Planning Perspectives*, 31(3) (May/June), 127–131.

Sexual Assault Victim Advocate, Larimer Center For Mental Health (2001). Found online at http://www.fortnet.org/sava/

Sexually Transmitted Diseases (2001). Planned Parenthood of New York City. Found online at http://www.ppnyc.org/facts/faq/stds.html

Strong, B., & De Vault, C. (1994). *Human Sexuality*. Mountain View, CA: Mayfield.

The Hidden Epidemic: Confronting Sexually Transmitted Diseases (1996). Washington DC: National Academy Press.

Weerakoon, P. (2001). Human Sexuality Course, University of Sydney. Found online at http://www.cchs.usyd.edu.au/bio/sex2000/

World Health Organization (1975). Education and treatment in human sexuality: The training of health professionals. *Technical Report, Series 572*, Section 2.1.

Zilbergeld, B. (1992) The New Male Sexuality. New York: Bantam.

CHAPTER 9

Albert, M. S., Servage, C. R., Jones, K., Seeman, T., Blazer, D. & Rowe, J. W. (1995). Predictors of cognitive change in older persons: MacArthur studies of successful aging. *Psychology and Aging*, 10(4), 578–589.

Adams, R. G., Blieszner, R. (1995). Aging well with friends and family. *American Behavioral Scientist*, 39(2), 209–224.

Berkman, L. F., & Breslow, L. (1983). Health and Ways of Living: Findings from the Almeda County Study. New York: Oxford University Press.

Bishop, C. E. (1999). Where are the missing elders? The decline in nursing home use, 1985 and 1995. *Health Affairs*, 18, 146–155.

Burack, O. R. (1996). The effects of list making on recall in young and old adults. *Journal of Gerontology*, Series B: Psychological and Social Sciences, 51B (4), 226.

Cohen, G. (2000). Loneliness in later life. *American Journal of Geriatric Psychiatry*, 8, 273–275.

Corr, C. and Corr, D. (1992). Adult hospice day care. Death Studies, 16(2), 155–172.

Flowers, N. (2000). In-home assessment and counseling of the elderly, in Nancy Newton & Kadi Sprengle (eds.) *Psychosocial Interventions in the Home: Housecalls*. New York: Springer Publishing.

Giordano, J. A. (2000). Effective communication and counseling with older adults. *International Journal of Aging & Human Development*, 51, 315–324.

Goldstein, M., Pinto, B., Marcus, B., Lynn, H., Jette, A., McDermott, S., et al.(1999). Physician-based physical activity counseling for middle-aged and older adults: A randomized trial. *Annals of Behavioral Medicine*, 21, 40–47.

Gordon, T. J. (1987). Medical breakthroughs: Cutting the toll of killer diseases. *The Futurist*, January–February, 21, 15–17.

Greider, K. Making our minds last a lifetime. *Psychology Today*, November–December, 29(6), 42 (1996).

Hermanson, B. (1988). Beneficial six year outcome of smoking cessation in older men and women with coronary disease. *New England Journal of Medicine*, 319, 13–65.

Hickey, T., Wolf, F. M., Robins, L. S., Wagner, M. B., & Harik, W. (1995). Physical activity training for functional mobility. *The Journal of Applied Gerontology*, 14(4) 357–371.

Kastenabum. R. (2000). Counseling the elderly dying patient, in Victor Molinari (ed.) Professional Psychology in Long-Term Care: A Comprehensive Guide. New York: Hatherleigh Press.

Kelner, M. (1995). Activists and delegators: Elderly patients preferences about control at the end of life. *Social Sciences and Medicine*, 41(4), 537–545.

King, A. C. (1991). Mini Series: Exercise and aging. *Annals of Behavioral Medicine*, 13(3), 87–90.

Langer, N. (2001). The role of gerontology in retirement counseling. *Gerontology & Geriatrics Education*, 21, 81–87.

Lewis, M. M. (2001). Spirituality counseling and the elderly: An introduction to spiritual life review. *Journal of Adult Development*, 8(4), 231–240.

Lovett, S. B. (1989). Processes of aging: enhancement of the later years. In R. A. Winett, A.C. King, & D. G. Altman (eds.) *Health Psychology and Public Health.* New York: Pergamon General Psychology Series.

Morgan, J. N. (1986). Unpaid productive activity over the life course. In Institute of Medicine/ National Research Council (eds.) *America's Aging: Productive Roles in an Older Society.* Washington, DC: National Academy Press.

Perlmulter, M., & Hall. E. (1985). *Adult Development and Aging, 2nd Edition.* New York: John Wiley and Sons.

Rowe, J. W. (1999) Geriatrics prevention and the remodeling of Medicare. *New England Journal of Medicine*, 340, 720–721.

Rowe, J. W., & Kahn, R. L. (1998). *Succesful Aging.* New York: Pantheon Books.

Sabin, E. P. (1993). Social relationships and mortality among the elderly. The *Journal of Applied Gerontology*, 12(1), 44–60.

Schaie, K. W. (1994). The course of adult intellectual development. *American Psychologist*, 49, 304–313.

Schaie, K. W. (1996). Intellectual development in adulthood: The Seattle Longitudinal Study. New York: Cambridge University Press.

Schaie, K. W., & Willis, S. L. (1986). Can decline in intellectual functioning be reversed? *Developmental Psychology*, 22(2), 223.

Segraves, R. T., & Segraves, K. R. (1995). Human sexuality and aging. *Journal of Sex Education and Therapy*, 21(2), 88.

Shock, N., Greulich, R., & Andres, R. (1984). Normal human aging: the Baltimore longitudinal study of aging (BLSA). The Gerontology Research Center, NIA, NIH. Washington, D.C.: U.S. Government Printing Office.

Snowdon, D. A. (1997). Aging and Alzheimer's disease: lessons from the Nun study. *The Gerontologist*, 37(2), 150.

Spillman, B. C., & Lubitz, J. (2000). The effect of longevity on spending for acute and long-term care. *New England Journal of Medicine*, 11, 1409–1424.

Uhlmann, R. F., Pearlman, R. A., & Cain, K. C. (1988). Physicians' and spouses' predictions of elderly patients' resuscitation preferences. *Journal of Gerontology Medical Sciences*, 43, M115–121.

Unger, J. B., Anderson, Johnson, C., & Marks, G. (1997). Functional decline in the elderly evidence for direct and stress buffering protective effects of social interactions and physical activity. *Annals of Behavioral Medicine*, 13(3), 87–90.

Verbrugge, L. M. (1984). Longer life but worsening health? Trends and health in mortality of middle-aged and older persons. *Milbank Quarterly*, 62, 475.

Whittemore, R., Rankin, S. H., Callahan, C. D., Leder, M. C., & Carroll, D. L. (2000). The peer advisory experience providing social support. *Qualitative Health Research*, 10, 260–277.

World Health Organization (1997). *The World Health Report 1997: Conquering Suffering, Enriching Humanity.* The World Report Series.

World Health Organization (1998). *The World Health Report 1998: Life in the 21st Century: A Vision for All.* The World Report Series.

The World Health Report 2000. Health Systems: Improving Performance.

CHAPTER 10

American Psychiatric Association (1994). *Diagnostic and Statistical Manual of Mental Disorders, 4th edition.* Washington DC: APHA.

Berne, E. (1972). *What Do You Say After You Say Hello?* New York: Grove Press.

Brooks, D. K., & Weikel, W. J. (1986). Mental health counseling in an historical perspective. In W. J. Weikel & A. J. Palmo (eds.), *Foundations of Mental Health Counseling,* pp. 5–28. Springfield, IL: Charles C Thomas.

Carson, R. C., Butcher, J. N., & Mineka, S. (1996). *Abnormal Psychology and Normal Life, 10th ed.* New York: Harper Collins.

Carter, Rosalynn (1996). "A Positive Link of Mind and Body," *Los Angeles Times* editorial, May 7.

Clark, A.J. (1995). Projective techniques in the counseling process. *Journal of Counseling & Development,* 73, 311–315.

Current Health 2 (1995). December, 22(4), 26–28.

Dinkmeyer, D. C., Pew, W. L., & Dinkmeyer, D. C. Jr. (1979). *Adlerian Counseling and Psychotherapy.* Monterey: Brookes/Cole.

Donnelly, J., Eburne, N., & Kittelson, M. (2001*). Mental Health—Dimensions of Self-Esteem, & Emotional Well-Being.* Boston: Allyn & Bacon.

Eisenberg, Leon (1997). Psychiatry and health in low-income populations. *Comprehensive Psychiatry,* 38, March/April.

Frankl, V. (1979). The will to meaning. In *Foundations and Application of Logotherapy.* New York: Simon & Schuster.

Freud, S. (1935). A General Introduction to Psychoanalysis. New York: Liveright.

Goleman, Daniel (1995). *Emotional Intelligence.* New York: Bantam Books.

Harris, Rothenberg International (1999). Value to Companies: What research Says. Found online at http://info@harrisrothenberg.com

Hollenbeck, W., Donnelly, J., & Eburne, N. (2001). *Mental Health—Dimensions of Self-Esteem, & Emotional Well-Being, Teacher's Manual.* Boston: Allyn & Bacon.

Levinthal, C. (1988). *Messengers of Paradise: Opiates and the Brain.* New York: Doubleday. Library of Congress Web site http://www.loc.gov/exhibits/treasures. 2001.

Library of Congress website (2001). http://www.governmentguide.com

McCassey, J. H (1898). How to limit the over-production of defectives and criminals. *The Journal of the American Medical Association.* Found online at http://www.jama.ama-assn.org

National Institutes of Mental Health (2000). Mental health: A report of the Surgeon General. Chapter One. Available Online: http://www.nimh.nih.gov/ mhsgrpt/chapter1/sec1.html#mind_body

National Mental Health Association Web site: http://www.nmha.org. 2002

National Institute of Health (1997). Disease Specific Estimates of Direct and Indirect Costs of Illness and NIH Update. Washington: US Department of Health and Human Services.

Robbins, J. (2000). Wired for Sadness. *Discover,* 21(4), 76–82.

SAMSHA report (1998). Available at http://www. samsha. gov

Siegel, Bernie S. (1986). *Love, Medicine & Miracles.* New York: Harper and Row.

SGRMH (1999). Available at http://www.psi-solutions. org/cf/dec/mentalhealth.html

Smith, H. B. & Robinson, G. P. (1995). Mental health counseling: Past, present and future. Journal of Counseling and Development, 74, 158–162.

Szasz, T. (1987) *Insanity, The Idea and Its Consequences.* New York: Wiley.

Turner, Clair E. (1951). *Community Health Educator's Compendium of Knowledge.* Englewood Cliffs NJ: Prentice-Hall.

Viney, W., & Zorich, S. (1982). Contributions to the history of psychology XXIX: Dorothea Dix. *Psychological Reports,* 50, 211–218.

Waiswol, N. (1995). Projective techniques as psychotherapy. *American Journal of Psychotherapy,* 73(3), 311–316.

Wallace, W. A. (1986). *Theories of Counseling and Psychotherapy: A Basic Issues Approach.* Boston: Allyn & Bacon.

Wartik, Nancy (1997). Missed diagnosis: Why depression goes untreated in women. *American Health,* June.

Washburn, Lindy (2000). "Did She Have to Die?" *The Bergen Record,* 25 June.

CHAPTER 11

Anderson, G. E. (1972). College Schedule of Recent Experience. Master's thesis, North Dakota State University.

Ballinger, J. C., Davidson, J. R., Lecrubier, Y., Nutt, D. J., Foa, E. B., Kessler, R. C., McFarlane, A. C., & Shalev, A. Y. (2000). Consensus statement on posttraumatic stress disorder from the international consensus group on depression and anxiety. *Journal of Clinical Psychiatry,* 61, 60–66.

Barling, J., Bluen, S. D., & Moss, V. (1990). Dimensions of Type A behavior and marital dissatisfaction. *Journal of Psychology,* 124, 311–319.

Bauer, M. E., Vedhara, K., Perks, P., Wilcock, G. K., Lightman, S. L., Shanks, N. (2000). Chronic stress in caregivers of dementia patients associated with reduced lymphocyte sensitivity to glucocorticoids. *Journal of Neuroimmunology,* 103, 84–92.

Bensin, H. & Zipper, M. Z. (2000). *The Relaxation Response.* New York: Morrow.

Bernhard, J.D., Kristeller, J., & Kabat-Zinn, J. (1988). Effectiveness of relaxation and visualization techniques as an adjunct to phototherapy and photo chemotherapy of psoriasis. *Journal of the American Academy of Dermatology, 19,* 573–574.

Bluen, S. D., Barling, J., & Burns, W. (1990). Predicting sales performance, job satisfaction, and depression by using the achievement strivings and impatience-irritability dimensions of Type A behavior. *Journal of Applied Psychology, 75,* 212–216.

Cooper, C. L. and Marshall, J. (1978). Occupational sources of stress: A review of the literature relating to coronary heart disease and mental ill health. *NIOSH Proceedings of Occupational Stress Conference.* Cincinnati, OH: National Institute of Occupational Safety and Health, p. 9.

Cruess, D. G., Leserman, J., Petitto, J. M., Golden, R. N., Szuba, M. P., Morrison, M. F., & Evans, D. L. (2001). Psychosocial-immune relationships in HIV disease. *Seminal Clinical Neuropsychiatry, 6,* 241–251.

DeLongis, A., Coyne, J. C., Dakof, G., Folkman, S., & Lazarus, R. (1982). Relationship of daily hassles, uplifts, and major life events to health status. *Health Psychology, 1,* 119–136.

Feiner, R. D., Farber, S. S., & Primavera, J. (1983). Transition in stressful life events: A model of primary prevention. In R. D. Feiner, L. A. Jason, J. N. Moritsugu, & SS. Farber *Preventive Psychology: Theory, Research and Practice.* New York: Plenum.

Forman, J. W. & Myers, D. (1987). *The Personal Stress Reduction Book.* Englewood Cliffs, NJ: Prentice Hall.

Friedman, M. & Rosenman, R. H. (1974). *Type A Behavior and Your Heart.* Greenwich, CT: Fawcett.

Girdano, D. A., Everly, G. S, & Dusek, D. E. (1993). *Controlling Stress and Tension, 4th Edition.* Englewood Cliffs, NJ: Prentice Hall.

Greenberg, J. S. (2002). *Comprehensive Stress Management, 7th Edition.* New York: McGraw-Hill.

Hennessy, M. B., Deak, T., & Schiml-Webb, P. A. (2001). Stress-induced sickness behavior: An alternative hypothesis for responses during maternal separation. *Developmental Psychobiology, 39,* 76–83.

Holahan, C. K., Holahan, C. J., & Belk, S. S. (1984). Adjustment in aging: The role of life stress, hassles, and self-efficacy. *Health Psychology, 3,* 315–328.

Holmes, T. H., & Rahe, R. H. (1967). The social readjustment rating scale. *Journal of Psychosomatic Research, 11,* 213–218.

Kabat-Zinn, J. et al. (1992). Effectiveness of a meditation-based stress reduction program in the treatment of anxiety disorders (1987). *American Journal of Psychiatry, 149,* 936–943.

Kabat-Zinn, J. et al. (1987). Four-year follow-up of a meditation-based program for the self-regulation of chronic pain: Treatment outcomes and compliance. *The Clinical Journal of Pain, 2,* 159–173.

Kanner, A. D. et al. (1981). Comparison of two modes of stress management: Daily hassles and uplifts versus major life events. *Journal of Behavioral Medicine, 4,* 1–39.

Kiecolt-Glaser, J. K., McGuire, L., Robles, T. F., & Glaser, R. (2002a). Emotions, morbidity, and mortality: New perspectives from psychoneuroimmunology. *Annual Review of Psychology, 53,* 83–107.

Kiecolt-Glaser, J. K., McGuire, L., Robles, T. F., & Glaser, R. (2002b). Psychoneuroimmunology and psychosomatic medicine: Back to the future. *Psychosomatic Medicine, 64,* 15–28.

Koskenvuo, M., Kaprio, J., Rose, R. J., Kesaniemi, A., & Sarna, S. (1988). Hostility as a risk factor for mortality and ischemic heart disease in men. *Psychosomatic Medicine, 50,* 330–340.

Krucoff, C., & Krucoff, M. (2000). *Healing Moves: How to Cure, Relieve, and Prevent Common Ailments with Exercise.* New York: Harmony Books.

Manuck, S. B. et al. (1992). Does cardiovascular reactivity to mental stress have prognostic value in post-infarction patients? A pilot study. *Psychosomatic Medicine, 54,* 102–108.

Matich J. and Sims, L. (1992). A comparison of social support variables between women who intend to breast or bottle feed. *Social Science Medicine, 34,* 919–927.

Meichenbaum, D. (1977). *Cognitive-Behavior Modification.* New York: Plenum.

Moynihan, J. A., Karp, J. D., Cohen, N., & Ader, R. (2000). Immune deviation following stress odor exposure: Role of endogenous opoids. *Journal of Neuroimmunology, 102,* 145–153.

Pelletier, K. R. (1977). *Mind as Healer, Mind as Slayer.* New York: Dell Publishing Company.

Pred, R. S., Spence, J. T., & Helmreich, R. L. (1986). The development of a new scale for the Jenkins Activity Survey measure of the Type A construct. *Social and Behavioral Science Documents, 16,* No. 2679.

Princeton Study (1989). Student stress lowers immunity. *Brain Mind Bulletin, 14*(1), 7.

Rein, G., Atkinson, M., & McCraty, R. (1995). The physiological and psychological effects of compassion and anger: Part 1 of 2. *Journal of Advancement in Medicine, 8,* 87–105.

Rosenhan, D. L. and Seligman, M. E. P. (1995). *Abnormal Psychology.* New York: Norton.

Shekelle, R. B. et al. (1983). Hostility, risk of coronary heart disease and mortality. *Psychosomatic Medicine,* 45,109–114.

Solomon, Z., Mikulincer, M., and Hobfill, S.E. (1987). Objective versus subjective measurement of stress and social support: Combat related reactions. *Journal of Consulting and Clinical Psychology,* 55, 557–583.

Spiegel, D., & Sephton, S. E. (2001). Psychoneuroimmune and endocrine pathways in cancer: Effects of stress and support. *Seminal Clinical Neuropsychiatry,* 6, 252–265.

Stang, P., Von Korff, M., & Galer, B. S. (1998). Reduced labor force participation among primary care patients with headache. *Journal of General Internal Medicine,* 13, 296–302.

Steptoe, A. (1997). The link between stress and illness. *Journal of Psychosomatic Research,* 35, 633–644.

Stoney, C. M., & Engebretson, T. O. (2000). Plasma homocysteine concentrations are positively associated with hostility and anger. *Life Sciences,* 66, 2267–2275.

"Stress." *Newsweek,* June 14, 1999, p. 61.

Waning, E., & Castleman, M. (1984). Healing your aching back. *Medical Self-Care,* 26–29.

Weiman, C.G. (1977). A study of occupational stressors and the incidence of disease/risk. *Journal of Occupational Medicine,* 19, 119–122.

Wolpe, J. (1973). *The Practice of Behavior Therapy.* New York: Pergamon Press.

Yang, E. V., & Glaser, R. (2002). Stress-induced immunomodulation and the implications for health. *International Immunopharmacology,* 2, 315–324.

Zarski, J. J. (1984). Hassles and health: A replication. *Health Psychology,* 3, 243–251.

CHAPTER 12

Abram, D. (1988). Merleau-Ponty and the voice of the earth. *Environmental Ethics,* 10 , 101–120.

Aizenstat, S. (1995). Jungian psychology and the world unconscious. In T. Roszak, M. E. Gomes, & A. D. Kanner, (eds.) *Ecopsychology: Restoring the earth, healing the mind,* pp. 92–100. San Francisco: Sierra Club Books.

Armstrong, J. (1995). Keepers of the earth. In T. Roszak, M. E. Gomes, & A. D. Kanner, (eds.) *Ecopsychology: Restoring the Earth, Healing the Mind,* pp. 316–324. San Francisco: Sierra Club Books.

Ashby, A. G. (1992, July) Healing war's wounds. *Dogworld,* 40–43.

Bateson, G. (1972). *Steps to an Ecology of Mind.* New York: Chandler Publishing Co.

Bear, S., Mulligan, C., Nufer, P., & Wabun (1989). *Walk in Balance: The Path to Healthy, Happy, Harmonious living.* New York: Simon & Schuster.

Berry, T. (1988). *The Dream of the Earth.* San Francisco: Sierra Club Books.

Berry, T. (1999). *The Great Work.* New York: Bell Tower.

Bly, R. (1996). *The Sibling Society.* New York: Vintage Books.

Buber, N. (1958). *I and Thou.* New York: Scribner.

Cahalan, W. (1995). Ecological groundedness in Gestalt therapy. In T. Roszak, M. E. Gomes, & A. D. Kanner, (eds.) *Ecopsychology: Restoring the Earth, Healing the Mind,* pp. 216–223. San Francisco: Sierra Club Books.

Churchill, W. (1994). *Indians Are Us? Culture and Genocide in Native North America.* Monroe, ME: Common Courage Press.

Clinebell, H. (1996). *Ecotherapy: Healing Ourselves, Healing the Earth.* New York: Haworth Press.

Cohen, M. J. (1997). *Reconnecting with Nature.* Corvallis, OR: Ecopress.

Colangelo, L. L. (1995). A calming presence. Asbury Park Press, AA1, AA5.

Conn, S. A. (1995). When the earth hurts, who responds? In T. Roszak, M. E. Gomes, & A. D. Kanner, (eds.) *Ecopsychology: Restoring the Earth, Healing the Mind,* pp. 156–171. San Francisco: Sierra Club Books.

Conn, S. A. (1998). Living in the earth: Ecopsychology, health and psychotherapy. *The Humanistic Psychologist,* 26 (1, 2, 3), 179–198.

Cushman, P. (1990). Why the self is empty: Toward a historically situated Psychology. *American Psychologist,* 45, 599–611.

Davis, S. (1997, September). Using horticulture as an effective vehicle in counseling various populations. *Counseling Today,* 20–30.

Devall, B., & Sessions, G. (1985). *Deep Ecology: Living As if Nature Mattered.* Layton, Utah: Gibbs Smith.

Devereux, P., Steele, J., & Kubrin, D. (1989). *Earthmind.* New York: Harper and Row.

Dodson Gray, E. (1982). *Patriarchy As a Conceptual Trap.* Wellesley, MA: Roundtable Press.

Eaton, E. (1982). *The Shaman and the Medicine Wheel.* Wheaton, IL: Theosophical Publishing House.

Ficklin, J. (producer) (1998). *Luna: The Stafford Giant Tree Sit.* [Videotape]. Headwaters Action, P.O. Box 2198, Redway, CA 95560.

Friedenberg, R. (director) (1996). The Education of Little Tree. [Videotape]. Paramount.

Garrett, M. (1998). Walking On the Wind. Santa Fe, NM: Bear & Company Publishing.

Glendinning, C. (1994). My Name is Chellis & I'm in Recovery from Western Civilization. Boston: Shambhala.

Glendinning, C. (1995). Technology, trauma, and the wild. In T. Roszak, M. E. Gomes, & A. D. Kanner, (eds.) *Ecopsychology: Restoring the Earth, Healing the Mind,* pp. 41–54. San Francisco: Sierra Club Books.

Goodwin, N. (producer). (1992). *Rachel Carson's Silent Spring.* [Videotape]. PBS Video.

Gore, A. (1992). *Earth in the Balance.* New York: Plume.

Greenway, R. (1995). The wilderness effect and ecopsychology. In Roszak, T., Gomes, M., & Kanna, A. D. (eds) Ecophychology: Restoring the Earth, Healing the Mind. Hawyard, CA: California State University, Ecopsychology Institute.

Harper, S. (1995). The way of wilderness. In T. Roszak, M. E. Gomes, & A. D. Kanner, (eds.) *Ecopsychology: Restoring the Earth, Healing the Mind,* pp. 183–200. San Francisco: Sierra Club Books.

Heart, B. (1998). *The Wind Is My Mother.* New York: Berkeley Books.

Hillman, J. (1975). *Re-visioning Psychology.* New York: Harper Row.

Hillman, J. (1992, May/June). Is therapy turning us into children? *New Age Journal,* 60–65, 136–140.

Hillman, J. & Ventura, M. (1992). *We've Had a Hundred Years of Psychotherapy and the World's Getting Worse.* New York: HarperCollins.

Hoffman, C. (1998). The hoop and the tree: An ecological model of health. *The Humanistic Psychologist* 26 (1, 2, 3), 154.

Ivey, A. E., Ivey, M. B., & Simek-Morgan, L. (1993). *Counseling and Psychotherapy: A Multicultural Perspective,* 3rd Ed. Boston: Allyn & Bacon.

Jeffers, R. (1977). *The Double Axe.* New York: Liveright.

Jung, C. G. (1976). The symbolic life. In RFC Hull (trans.), *Collected Works of C. G. Jung,* 18, Princeton, NJ: Princeton University Press.

Kalb, C. (2001, January 22). Seeing a virtual shrink. *Newsweek,* 54–56.

Kanner, A. D., & Gomes, M. E. (1995). The all-consuming self. In T. Roszak, M. E. Gomes, & A. D. Kanner, (eds.) *Ecopsychology: Restoring the Earth, Healing the Mind,* pp. 77–91. San Francisco: Sierra Club Books.

Kanner, A. D. (1998). Mount Rushmore syndrome: When narcissism rules the earth. *The Humanistic Psychologist,* 26(1, 2, 3), 101–121.

Kuhn, J. L. (2001). Toward an ecological humanistic psychology. *Journal of Humanistic Psychology,* 41(2), 9–24.

Kingsolver, B. (1990). *Animal Dreams.* New York: HarperCollins.

Kingsolver, B. (2000). *Prodigal Summer.* New York: Harper Collins.

Lovelock, J. (1979). *Gaia: A New Look at Life on Earth.* Oxford: Oxford University Press.

Lowen, A. (1967). *The Betrayal of the Body.* London: Collier Macmillan, Ltd.

Mack, J. E. (1995). The politics of species arrogance. In T. Roszak, M. E. Gomes, & A. D. Kanner, (eds.) *Ecopsychology: Restoring the Earth, Healing the Mind,* pp. 279–287. San Francisco: Sierra Club Books.

Macy, J. (1991). *World as Lover, World as Self.* Berkeley, CA: Parallax Press.

Macy, J. (1995a). Interview by Karla Arens. *Wild Duck Review,* 1, 1–3.

Macy, J. (1995b). Working through environmental despair. In T. Roszak, M. E. Gomes, & A. D. Kanner, (eds.) *Ecopsychology: Restoring the Earth, Healing the Mind,* pp. 240–259. San Francisco: Sierra Club Books.

Mancuso, D. (1993, September 21). Hounds of love. *Asbury Park Press,* B1, B2.

Mander, J. (1991). *In the Absence of the Sacred.* San Francisco: Sierra Club Books.

Margulis, L. & Lovelock, J. (1975, Summer). The atmosphere as circulatory system of the biosphere—the Gaia hypothesis. *CoEvolution Quarterly,* 30–40.

Marino, T. W. (1995, January). Has mental health gone to the dogs? *Counseling Today,* 10–11, 22.

Maslow, A. H. (1964). *Religions, Values, and Peak-Experiences.* New York: Penguin Books.

Matthiessen, P. (1984). *Indian Country.* New York: Penguin Books.

McGaa, E. (1990). *Mother Earth Spirituality.* San Francisco: Harper.

Metzner, R. (1991). Psychologizing deep ecology: A review essay. *ReVision* 13(3), 147–152.

Metzner, R. (1995). The psychopathology of the human-nature relationship. In T. Roszak, M. E. Gomes, & A. D. Kanner, (eds.) *Ecopsychology: Restoring the Earth, Healing the Mind,* pp. 55–67. San Francisco: Sierra Club Books.

Miles, M. B. (1981). *Learning to Work in Groups: A Practical Guide for Members & Trainers.* New York: Teachers College Press, Columbia University.

Moore, K. (2001, June 26). The best in breed. *Asbury Park Press,* B2.

Naess, A. (1986). Self realization: An ecological approach to being in the world. In G. Session (ed.), *Deep Ecology for the 21st Century,* 225–239.

Naisbitt, J. (1982). *Megatrends: Ten New Directions Transforming Our Lives.* New York: Warner Books, Inc.

Niego, M. (1992, Summer). Rx: Animals, *ASPCA Animal Watch,* 9–13.

O'Connor, T. (1995). Therapy for a dying planet. In T. Roszak, M. E. Gomes, & A. D. Kanner, (eds.) *Ecopsychology: Restoring the Earth, Healing the Mind,* pp. 149–155. San Francisco: Sierra Club Books.

Oskamp, S. (2000). A sustainable future for humanity? *American Psychologist* 55(5), 496–508.

Pearce, J. C. (1977). *Magical Child.* New York: Bantam Books.

Pierce, G. (1997, July). Finding the connection between self and the environment. *Counseling Today,* 44.

Postman, N. (1992). *Technopoly: The Surrender of Culture to Technology.* New York: Alfred A. Knopf.

Roszak, T. (1978). *Person/Planet.* Garden City, NY: Anchor Books.

Roszak, T. (1992). *The Voice of the Earth.* New York: Touchstone.

Roszak, T. (1995). Where psyche meets Gaia. In T. Roszak, M. E. Gomes, & A. D. Kanner, (eds.) *Ecopsychology: Restoring the Earth, Healing the Mind,* pp. 1–17. San Francisco: Sierra Club Books.

Roszak, T., Gomes, M. E., & Kanner, A. D. (eds.), *Ecopsychology: Restoring the Earth, Healing the Mind,* pp. 122–135. San Francisco: Sierra Club Books.

Scarce, R. (1990). *Eco-Warriors: Understanding the Radical Environmental Movement.* Chicago: Noble Press.

Sewall, L. (1998). Looking for a worldview: Perceptual practice in an ecological age. *The Humanistic Psychologist,* 26(1, 2, 3), 163–167.

Shapiro, E. (1995). Restoring habitats, communities, & souls. In T. Roszak, M. E. Gomes, & A. D. Kanner, (eds.) *Ecopsychology: Restoring the earth, Healing the Mind,* pp. 224–239. San Francisco: Sierra Club Books.

Shepard, P. (1982). *Nature and Madness.* San Francisco: Sierra Club Books.

Shepard, P. (1995). *Nature and madness.* In T. Roszak, M. E. Gomes, & A. D. Kanner, (eds.) *Ecopsychology: Restoring the Earth, Healing the Mind,* pp. 21–40. San Francisco: Sierra Club Books.

Soderbergh, S. (director). (2000). *Erin Brockovich.* [Videotape]. Universal.

Thomas, J. (director). (1999). *All the Little Animals.* [Videotape]. Lions Gate.

Wilson, E. O. (1984). *Biophilia.* Cambridge, MA: Harvard University Press.

Winter, D. (2000). Some big ideas for some big problems. *American Psychologist,* 55(5), 516–522.

Worrell, J., & Remer, P. (1992). *Feminist Perspectives in Therapy.* New York: Wiley.

Yunt, J. (2001). Jung's contribution to an ecological psychology. *Journal of Humanistic Psychology,* 41(2), 96–121.

Zaillian, S. (director). (1999). *A Civil Action.* [Videotape]. Touchstone.

EPILOGUE

Alimandi. L, Andrich, R., & Porqueddu, B. (1995). Teleworking in connection with technical aids for disabled persons. *Journal of Telemedecine and Telecare,* 1, 165–172.

American Counseling Association (1999, October). Ethical Standards for Internet On-Line Counseling. Available online at www.counseling.org/gc/cybertx.htm

Ancis, J. R. (1988). Cultural competency training at a distance: Challenges and strategies. *Journal of Counseling and Development,* 76, 134–142.

Barnett, D. C. (1982). A suicide prevention incident involving the use of the computer. *Professional Psychology,* 13, 565–570.

Fortune, Summer 2000 Technology Guide. Doctor's in the house, p 233.

Guterman, J. & Kirk,, M. (1999). Mental health counselors and the Internet. *Journal of Mental Health Counseling,* 21, 309–326.

Hannon, K. (1996, May 13) Upset? Try cybertherapy. *U.S. News and World Report,* 81,83.

Hoagwood, K., & Koretz, D. (1996). Embedding prevention services within systems of care: Strengthening the nexus for children. *Applied and Preventive Psychology,* 5, 225–234.

Izenberg, N,. & Lieberman, D. (1998). The Web, communication trends and children's health part 3: The Web and health consumers. *Clinical Pediatrics,* 37(5), 275–286.

Marino, T. W. (1996, January). Counselors in cyberspace debate whether client discussions are ethical. *Counseling Today,* 8.

National Board for Certified Counselors (1997, December 1). Standards for the ethical practice of web counseling. Available online at www.nbcc.org/ ethics/wcstanard.htm

Oravec, J. (2000). Internet and computer technology hazards: Perspectives for family counseling. *British Journal of Guidance and Counseling,* in press.

Reimer-Reiss, Marti L. (2000). Utilizing Distance Technology for Mental Health Counseling. *Journal of Mental Health Counseling,* 22(3), 189–204.

Rosenfield, M. (1997). *Counseling by Telephone.* London: Sage.

Ruskin, K. J., Palmer, A., Hagenouw, M., Lack, A., & Dunnill, R. (1998). Internet teleconferencing as a clinical tool for anesthesiologists. *Journal of Clinical Monitoring and Computing,* 14, 183–189.

Sampson, J. P., Kolodinsky, R. W., & Greeno, B. P. (1997). Counseling on the information highway: Future possibilities and potential problems. *Journal of Counseling and Development,* 75, 203–212.

Sanders, P., & Rosenfield, M. (1998). Counseling at a distance: Challenges and new initiatives. *British Journal of Guidance and Counseling,* 26, 5–10.

Tait, A. (1999). Face-to-face and at a distance: The mediation of guidance and counseling through the new technologies. *British Journal of Guidance and Counseling,* 27, 113–122.

Tschida, Molly (1999). Log on, plug in, check it out. *Modern Physician,* 3(10), 35–49.

U.S. Department of Health and Human Services (2000). *Healthy People 2010* (Conference ed., Vols. 1 & 2). Washington, D.C.: Author. (Also available online at www.health.gov/healthypeople)

Walz, G. R. (1996). Using the I-Way for career development. In R. Feller & G. Walz (eds) Optimizing life transitions in turbulent times: *Exploring Work, Learning and Careers* (pp. 415–427). Greensboro: University of North Carolina, ERIC Clearinghouse on Counseling and Student Services.

Who's in line to log on. (1997). *Forecast,* 17(10), 1–2.

INDEX